HEALTH AND THE GUT

THE EMERGING ROLE OF INTESTINAL MICROBIOTA IN DISEASE AND THERAPEUTICS

HEALTH AND THE GUT

THE EMERGING ROLE OF INTESTINAL MICROBIOTA IN DISEASE AND THERAPEUTICS

Edited by
William Olds

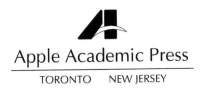

Apple Academic Press

TORONTO   NEW JERSEY

Apple Academic Press Inc.	Apple Academic Press Inc.
3333 Mistwell Crescent	9 Spinnaker Way
Oakville, ON L6L 0A2	Waretown, NJ 08758
Canada	USA

©2015 by Apple Academic Press, Inc.

First issued in paperback 2021

Exclusive worldwide distribution by CRC Press, a member of Taylor & Francis Group
No claim to original U.S. Government works

ISBN 13: 978-1-77463-204-8 (pbk)
ISBN 13: 978-1-77188-072-5 (hbk)

Library of Congress Control Number: 2014941128

Library and Archives Canada Cataloguing in Publication

Health and the gut: the emerging role of intestinal microbiota in disease and therapeutics/ edited by William Olds.

Includes bibliographical references and index.
ISBN 978-1-77188-072-5 (bound)
1. Intestines--Microbiology. 2. Intestines--Diseases. I. Olds, William, editor

QR171.I6H42 2014   612.3'3   C2014-903540-3

Apple Academic Press also publishes its books in a variety of electronic formats. Some content that appears in print may not be available in electronic format. For information about Apple Academic Press products, visit our website at **www.appleacademicpress.com** and the CRC Press website at **www.crcpress.com**

ABOUT THE EDITOR

WILLIAM OLDS, MSc

William Olds has an undergraduate degree from University of Michigan, and is currently working on his PhD at Yale University in the laboratory of Tian Xu. His current research focuses on satiety signals from the gut and how that communication to the brain breaks down in the pathogenesis of obesity.

CONTENTS

ACKNOWLEDGMENT AND HOW TO CITE

The editor and publisher thank each of the authors who contributed to this book, whether by granting their permission individually or by releasing their research as open source articles or under a license that permits free use, provided that attribution is made. The chapters in this book were previously published in various places in various formats. To cite the work contained in this book and to view the individual permissions, please refer to the citation at the beginning of each chapter. Each chapter was read individually and carefully selected by the editor; the result is a book that provides a nuanced study of the gut microbiome and its implications on human health. The chapters included examine the following topics:

- Chapter 1 serves as a good introduction to the gut microbiome field and the concepts that we will explore further in this book.
- Chapter 2 highlights and critically examines exciting developments in our understanding of the link between obesity and the gut microbiota.
- Chapter 3 discusses potential mechanisms by which probiotics can help prevent obesity.
- Chapter 4 shows how obesity can cause the microbiota to "leak" out of the gut and induce inflammation, wreaking havoc on the body.
- Numerous gut microflora studies in humans have suggested a link between the loss of *Bacteriodetes* family members and obesity. However, the roles of *Bacteriodetes* (if any) in obesity have remained elusive. Chapter 5 investigates how one member has the ability to fight obesity.
- Chapter 6 investigates more probiotics that combat obesity.
- Thus far, we have focused on the gut microflora themselves, but the interaction between the gut epithelial cells and microbes is just as important. chapter 7 highlights what keeps the microbiota in their home in the gut and how the intestinal epithelial cells contribute to the composition of microflora community.
- Chapter 8 highlights the necessity of keeping a tight lid on the microbiota for health.
- Chapter 9 discusses how modulating the gut microflora populations through synbiotic food (a special chocolate-covered biscuit!) can help improve health.

- Chapter 10 reviews the extent to which diet contributes to microbial diversity and health.
- Chapter 11 explains how the Western diet and medical advances have negatively impacted our gut microbiomes and presents emerging therapies to increase biodiversity in the gut microbiome.
- As the title indicates, Chapter 12 focuses on the relationship between the health in elderly individuals and the microbiome and the potential of dietary interventions. This will be a field to watch as the "Baby Boomer" generation enters retirement and physicians search for ways to mitigate the strain on healthcare.
- Chapter 13 explores how the microbiome influences drug efficacy, adding another layer of complexity for physicians when treating patients.
- Chapter 14 details the most famous microbiome intervention strategy: fecal transplantations. The method's strengths, weaknesses, and future directions are reviewed here

LIST OF CONTRIBUTORS

Young-Tae Ahn
Korea Yakult Co., Ltd., Yongin, Gyeonggi, Republic of Korea

Eric J. Alm
Broad Institute, Massachusetts Institute of Technology and Harvard University, Cambridge, Massachusetts, United States of America and Civil and Environmental Engineering, Massachusetts Institute of Technology, Cambridge, Massachusetts, United States of America and Biological Engineering, Massachusetts Institute of Technology, Cambridge, Massachusetts, United States of America

Ramy K. Aziz
The Egyptian Bioinformatics and Systems Biology Network (EgyBio.net), Cairo, Egypt, Department of Microbiology and Immunology, Faculty of Pharmacy, Cairo University, Cairo, Egypt, Current address: Systems Biology Research Group, UC San Diego, 9500 Gilman Drive, La Jolla, CA, 92093-0412, USA

Siddheshvar Bhela
Departments of Neurology and Immunobiology, Yale School of Medicine, New Haven, Connecticut, United States of America

Harald Brüssow
BioAnalytical Sciences, Food and Health Microbiology, Nestlé Research Center, Lausanne, Switzerland

Patrizia Brigidi
Department of Pharmaceutical Sciences, University of Bologna, Bologna, Italy

Craig R. Campbell
Discipline of Physiology, Bosch Institute, University of Sydney, Sydney, Australia

Marco Candela
Department of Pharmaceutical Sciences, University of Bologna, Bologna, Italy

Paola Gauffin Cano
Microbial Ecology and Nutrition Research Group, Institute of Agrochemistry and Food Technology (IATA), National Research Council (CSIC), Valencia, Spain

Paola Carnevali
R&D Food Microbiology & Bioprocess Research, Barilla G&R f.lli SpA, Parma, Italy

Ian D. Caterson
Boden Institute of Obesity, Nutrition, Exercise and Eating Disorders, University of Sydney, Sydney, Australia

Eugene B. Chang
Department of Medicine, The University of Chicago, Chicago, Illinois, USA

Antonis Chatzigiagkos
Laboratory of Pathology, Faculty of Veterinary Medicine, Aristotle University of Thessaloniki, Thessaloniki, Greece

Myung-Sook Choi
Center for Food and Nutritional Genomics, Kyungpook National University, Daegu, Republic of Korea and Department of Food Science and Nutrition, Kyungpook National University, Buk-gu, Daegu, Republic of Korea

David I. Cook
Discipline of Physiology, Bosch Institute, University of Sydney, Sydney, Australia

Federica Cruciani
Department of Pharmaceutical Sciences, University of Bologna, Bologna, Italy

Eline Dejonckheere
Department for Molecular Biomedical Research, VIB, Ghent, Belgium and Department of Biomedical Molecular Biology, Ghent University, Ghent, Belgium

Riet De Rycke
Department for Molecular Biomedical Research, VIB, Ghent, Belgium and Department of Biomedical Molecular Biology, Ghent University, Ghent, Belgium

Suzanne Devkota
Joslin Diabetes Center, Harvard Medical School, Boston, Massachusetts

Willem M. de Vos
Laboratory of Microbiology, Wageningen University, Wageningen, the Netherlands, Department of Veterinary Biosciences, Faculty of Veterinary Medicine, University of Helsinki, Helsinki, Finland, and Department of Bacteriology and Immunology, Medical Faculty, University of Helsinki, Helsinki, Finland

Anuwat Dinudom
Discipline of Physiology, Bosch Institute, University of Sydney, Sydney, Australia

Sahar El Aidy
Department of Experimental Oncology, European Institute of Oncology, Milan, Italy

Susan E. Erdman
Division of Comparative Medicine, Massachusetts Institute of Technology, Cambridge, Massachusetts, United States of America

Annelies Geirnaert
Laboratory of Microbial Ecology and Technology (LabMET), Ghent University, Ghent, Belgium

Kris Gevaert
Department of Medical Protein Research, VIB, Ghent, Belgium and Department of Biochemistry, Ghent University, Ghent, Belgium

Maria Elisabetta Guerzoni
Department of Food Science, University of Bologna, Bologna, Italy

Connie W. Y. Ha
School of Molecular Bioscience, University of Sydney, Sydney, Australia

David A. Hafler
Departments of Neurology and Immunobiology, Yale School of Medicine, New Haven, Connecticut, United States of America and Broad Institute, Massachusetts Institute of Technology and Harvard University, Cambridge, Massachusetts, United States of America

Filip Van Hauwermeiren
Department for Molecular Biomedical Research, VIB, Ghent, Belgium and Department of Biomedical Molecular Biology, Ghent University, Ghent, Belgium

Andrew J. Holmes
School of Molecular Bioscience, University of Sydney, Sydney, Australia

M. José Huertas
Instituto de Bioquímica Vegetal y Fotosíntesis, Centro de Investigaciones Isla de la Cartuja, Universidad de Sevilla-CSIC, Av. Américo Vespucio 49, 41092, Seville, Spain.

Chul-Sung Huh
Korea Yakult Co., Ltd., Yongin, Gyeonggi, Republic of Korea

Nicholas H. Hunt
Molecular Immunopathology Unit, Bosch Institute and Sydney Medical School, University of Sydney, Sydney, Australia

Yassin M. Ibrahim
Division of Comparative Medicine, Massachusetts Institute of Technology, Cambridge, Massachusetts, United States of America

Ian B. Jeffery
Department of Microbiology, University College Cork, College Road, Cork, Ireland and Alimentary Pharmabiotic Centre, University College Cork, College Road, Cork, Ireland

Sean M. Kearney
Division of Comparative Medicine, Massachusetts Institute of Technology, Cambridge, Massachusetts, United States of America and Biological Engineering, Massachusetts Institute of Technology, Cambridge, Massachusetts, United States of America

Markus Kleinewietfeld
Departments of Neurology and Immunobiology, Yale School of Medicine, New Haven, Connecticut, United States of America and Broad Institute, Massachusetts Institute of Technology and Harvard University, Cambridge, Massachusetts, United States of America

Jessica R. Lakritz
Division of Comparative Medicine, Massachusetts Institute of Technology, Cambridge, Massachusetts, United States of America

Yan Y. Lam
Boden Institute of Obesity, Nutrition, Exercise and Eating Disorders, University of Sydney, Sydney, Australia

Tatiana Levkovich
Division of Comparative Medicine, Massachusetts Institute of Technology, Cambridge, Massachusetts, United States of America

Claude Libert
Department for Molecular Biomedical Research, VIB, Ghent, Belgium and Department of Biomedical Molecular Biology, Ghent University, Ghent, Belgium

Sofie Lodens
Department for Molecular Biomedical Research, VIB, Ghent, Belgium and Department of Biomedical Molecular Biology, Ghent University, Ghent, Belgium

Carlos López-Otin
Departamento de Bioquimica y Biologia Molecular, Instituto Universitario de Oncologia, Universidad de Oviedo, Oviedo, Spain

Robin A. McGregor
Center for Food and Nutritional Genomics, Kyungpook National University, Daegu, Republic of Korea

Carmen Michán
Campus de Rabanales, Department of Biochemistry and Molecular Biology, Universidad de Córdoba, Edificio Severo Ochoa C-6, 2a Planta, 14071, Córdoba, Spain.

Andrew J. Mitchell
Molecular Immunopathology Unit, Bosch Institute and Sydney Medical School, University of Sydney, Sydney, Australia

Ángela Moya
Microbial Ecology and Nutrition Research Group, Institute of Agrochemistry and Food Technology (IATA), National Research Council (CSIC), Valencia, Spain

Maurice Ndagijimana
Department of Food Science, University of Bologna, Bologna, Italy

Jan Oscarsson
AstraZeneca R&D, Mölndal, Sweden

Maureen J. Ostaff
Dr. Margarete Fischer-Bosch-Institute of Clinical Pharmacology, Stuttgart, Germany and University of Tuebingen, Germany

Paul W. O'Toole
Department of Microbiology, University College Cork, College Road, Cork, Ireland and Alimentary Pharmabiotic Centre, University College Cork, College Road, Cork, Ireland

Do-Young Park
Korea Yakult Co., Ltd., Yongin, Gyeonggi, Republic of Korea

Se-Hoon Park
Korea Yakult Co., Ltd., Yongin, Gyeonggi, Republic of Korea

Alison Perrotta
Civil and Environmental Engineering, Massachusetts Institute of Technology, Cambridge, Massachusetts, United States of America

Theofilos Poutahidis
Division of Comparative Medicine, Massachusetts Institute of Technology, Cambridge, Massachusetts, United States of America and Laboratory of Pathology, Faculty of Veterinary Medicine, Aristotle University of Thessaloniki, Thessaloniki, Greece

Mariam R. Rizkallah
The Egyptian Bioinformatics and Systems Biology Network (EgyBio.net), Cairo, Egypt and The American University in Cairo, New Cairo, Egypt

Rama Saad
The Egyptian Bioinformatics and Systems Biology Network (EgyBio.net), Cairo, Egypt and The
American University in Cairo, New Cairo, Egypt

Arlette Santacruz
Microbial Ecology and Nutrition Research Group, Institute of Agrochemistry and Food Technology
(IATA), National Research Council (CSIC), Valencia, Spain

Yolanda Sanz
Microbial Ecology and Nutrition Research Group, Institute of Agrochemistry and Food Technology
(IATA), National Research Council (CSIC), Valencia, Spain

Christopher Smillie
Civil and Environmental Engineering, Massachusetts Institute of Technology, Cambridge, Massachusetts, United States of America

An Staes
Department of Medical Protein Research, VIB, Ghent, Belgium and Department of Biochemistry,
Ghent University, Ghent, Belgium

Eduard Friedrich Stange
Department of Gastroenterology, Robert Bosch Hospital, Stuttgart, Germany

Len H. Storlien
Boden Institute of Obesity, Nutrition, Exercise and Eating Disorders, University of Sydney, Sydney,
Australia

Mi-Kyung Sung
Center for Food and Nutritional Genomics, Kyungpook National University, Daegu, Republic of
Korea and Department of Food and Nutrition, Sookmyung Women's University, Seoul, Republic of
Korea

Pieter Van den Abbeele
Laboratory of Microbial Ecology and Technology (LabMET), Ghent University, Ghent, Belgium

Roosmarijn E. Vandenbroucke
Department for Molecular Biomedical Research, VIB, Ghent, Belgium and Department of Biomedical
Molecular Biology, Ghent University, Ghent, Belgium

Tom Van de Wiele
Laboratory of Microbial Ecology and Technology (LabMET), Ghent University, Ghent, Belgium

Elien Van Wonterghem
Department for Molecular Biomedical Research, VIB, Ghent, Belgium and Department of Biomedical
Molecular Biology, Ghent University, Ghent, Belgium

Bernard J. Varian
Division of Comparative Medicine, Massachusetts Institute of Technology, Cambridge, Massachusetts, United States of America

Willy Verstraete
Laboratory of Microbial Ecology and Technology (LabMET), Ghent University, Ghent, Belgium

Beatrice Vitali
Department of Pharmaceutical Sciences, University of Bologna, Bologna, Italy

Jan Wehkamp
Dr. Margarete Fischer-Bosch-Institute of Clinical Pharmacology, Stuttgart, Germany and University of Tuebingen, Germany and Department of Gastroenterology, Robert Bosch Hospital, Stuttgart, Germany

Sae-Rom Yoo
Department of Food Science and Nutrition, Kyungpook National University, Buk-gu, Daegu, Republic of Korea

Rina Yu
Center for Food and Nutritional Genomics, Kyungpook National University, Daegu, Republic of Korea and Department of Food Science and Nutrition, University of Ulsan, Ulsan, Republic of Korea

INTRODUCTION

For generations, we have been indoctrinated with the belief that bacteria are illness-causing scourges. The shocking truth is that there are more bacterial cells in your gut than in your entire body. Even more incredible is that more and more research is revealing that these so-called "gut germs" keep us healthy, rather than leading to sickness. There are numerous strains of bacteria living in the human gut at any time and, like a rainforest or a barrier reef, the gut is a complex habitat. This intestinal ecosystem of bacteria is called the gut microbiome. This nascent field is rapidly evolving and has exciting implications for health. In this text, we will:

1. Introduce readers to the gut microbiota field.
2. Highlight the emerging role of the microbiome in obesity.
3. Explore the relationship between the immune system and gut microbes.
4. Look at the implications of this field for therapy.

William Olds

The book begins with an introductory chapter by Devkota and Chang, which aims to present and evaluate the recent findings that contribute to our understanding of the functional impact of diet on the enteric microbiome and outcomes of disease. Nutrients in excess and in deficiency have significant impact on gut microbial communities in both rodents and humans, acting directly on the microbiota or indirectly via altering host physiology. Furthermore, the effects of diet on the microbiome in determining health or disease can differ substantially depending on the age and environment of the individual. Dietary compounds can have profound short-term and long-term effects on the assemblage of the gut microbiome, which in turn affects the host–microbe interactions critically important for intestinal, metabolic, and immune homeostasis. Until recently, the mechanisms underlying these effects were poorly understood. However, new insights have now been gained, made possible through the application of advanced technologies and bioinformatics, novel experimental models, and human research. As a result, our conceptual framework for understanding the impact of diet on the gut microbiome, health, and disease has advanced considerably, bringing the promise of better tools of risk assessment, diagnostics, and therapeutic intervention in an age of personalized medicine.

Chapter 2, a short review by Huertas and Michán, introduces the second section, which focuses on the connection between gut microbiome and obesity. The article highlights some of the recent developments in the field, and how our understanding of the connections between these two topics is connected.

A recent epidemiological study showed that eating fast food items such as potato chips increased likelihood of obesity, whereas eating yogurt prevented age-associated weight gain in humans. It was demonstrated previously in animal models of obesity that the immune system plays a critical role in this process. In Chapter 3, Poutahidis and colleagues examined human subjects and mouse models consuming Westernized "fast food" diet, and found CD4+ T helper (Th)17-biased immunity and changes in microbial communities and abdominal fat with obesity after eating the Western chow. In striking contrast, eating probiotic yogurt together with Western chow inhibited age-associated weight gain. The authors went on to test whether a bacteria found in yogurt may serve to lessen fat pathology by using purified *Lactobacillus reuteri* ATCC 6475 in drinking water. Surprisingly, we discovered that oral *L. reuteri* therapy alone was sufficient to change the pro-inflammatory immune cell profile and prevent abdominal fat pathology and age-associated weight gain in mice regardless of their baseline diet. These beneficial microbe effects were transferable into naïve recipient animals by purified CD4+ T cells alone. Specifically, bacterial effects depended upon active immune tolerance by induction of Foxp3+ regulatory T cells (Treg) and interleukin (Il)-10, without significantly changing the gut microbial ecology or reducing ad libitum caloric intake. The article's finding that microbial targeting restored CD4+ T cell balance and yielded significantly leaner animals regardless of their dietary "fast food" indiscretions suggests population-based approaches for weight management and enhancing public health in industrialized societies.

In Chapter 4, Lam and colleagues investigated the relationship between gut health, visceral fat dysfunction and metabolic disorders in diet-induced obesity. C57BL/6J mice were fed control or high saturated fat diet (HFD). Circulating glucose, insulin and inflammatory markers were measured. Proximal colon barrier function was assessed by measuring transepithelial resistance and mRNA expression of tight-junction proteins. Gut microbiota profile was determined by 16S rDNA pyrosequencing. Tumor necrosis factor (TNF)-α and interleukin (IL)-6 mRNA levels were measured in proximal colon, adipose tissue and liver using RT-qPCR. Adipose macrophage infiltration (F4/80+) was assessed using immuno-histochemical staining. HFD mice had a higher insulin/glucose ratio (P= 0.020) and serum levels of serum amyloid A3 (131%; P = 0.008) but reduced circulating adiponectin (64%; P = 0.011). In proximal colon of HFD mice compared to mice fed the control diet, transepithelial resistance and mRNA expression of zona occludens 1 were reduced by 38% (P<0.001) and 40% (P = 0.025) respectively and TNF-α mRNA level was 6.6-fold higher (P= 0.037). HFD reduced *Lactobacillus* (75%; P<0.001) but increased *Oscillibacter* (279%; P = 0.004) in fecal microbiota. Correlations were found between abundances of *Lactobacillus* (r = 0.52; P = 0.013) and *Oscillibacter* (r = −0.55; P = 0.007) with transepithelial resistance of the proximal colon. HFD increased macrophage infiltration (58%; P = 0.020), TNF-α (2.5-fold,P<0.001) and IL-6 mRNA levels (2.5-fold; P = 0.008) in mesenteric fat. Increased macrophage infiltration in epididymal fat was also observed with HFD feeding (71%; P = 0.006) but neither TNF-α nor IL-6 was altered. Perirenal and subcutaneous adipose tissue showed no signs of inflammation in HFD mice. The current results implicate gut dysfunction, and attendant inflammation of contiguous adipose, as salient features of the metabolic dysregulation of diet-induced obesity.

Associations have been made between obesity and reduced intestinal numbers of members of the phylum *Bacteroidetes*, but there is no direct evidence of the role these bacteria play in obesity. In Chapter 5, Guaffin Cano and colleagues evaluate the effects of *Bacteroides uniformis* CECT 7771 on obesity-related metabolic and immune alterations. Adult (6–8 week) male wild-type C57BL-6 mice were fed a standard diet or a high-fat-diet HFD to induce obesity, supplemented or not with *B. uniformis* CECT 7771 for seven weeks. Animal weight was monitored and histologic, biochemical, immunocompetent cell functions, and features of the faecal microbiota were analysed after intervention. The oral administration of *B. uniformis* CECT 7771 reduced body weight gain, liver steatosis and liver cholesterol and triglyceride concentrations and increased small adipocyte numbers in HFD-fed mice. The strain also reduced serum cholesterol, triglyceride, glucose, insulin and leptin levels, and improved oral tolerance to glucose in HFD fed mice. The bacterial strain also reduced dietary fat absorption, as indicated by the reduced number of fat micelles detected in enterocytes. Moreover, *B. uniformis* CECT 7771 improved immune defence mechanisms, impaired in obesity. HFD-induced obesity led to a decrease in TNF-α production by peritoneal macrophages stimulated with LPS, conversely, the administration of *B. uniformis* CECT 7771 increased TNF-α production and phagocytosis. Administering this strain also increased TNF-α production by dendritic cells (DCs) in response to LPS stimulation, which was significantly reduced by HFD. *B. uniformis* CECT 7771 also restored the capacity of DCs to induce a T-cell proliferation response, which was impaired in obese mice. HFD induced marked changes in gut microbiota composition, which were partially restored by the intervention. Altogether, the findings indicate that administration of B. uniformis CECT 7771 ameliorates HFD-induced metabolic and immune dysfunction associated with intestinal dysbiosis in obese mice.

In Chapter 6, Park and colleagues aim to investigate the functional effects of probiotic treatment on the gut microbiota, as well as liver and adipose gene expression in diet-induced obese mice. Male C57BL/6J mice were fed a high-fat diet (HFD) for 8 weeks to induce obesity, and then randomized to receive HFD+probiotic (*Lactobacillus curvatus* HY7601 and *Lactobacillus plantarum* KY1032, n = 9) or HFD+placebo (n = 9) for another 10 weeks. Normal diet (ND) fed mice (n = 9) served as non-obese controls. Diet-induced obese mice treated with probiotics showed reduced body weight gain and fat accumulation as well as lowered plasma insulin, leptin, total-cholesterol and liver toxicity biomarkers. A total of 151,061 pyrosequencing reads for fecal microbiota were analyzed with a mean of 6,564, 5,274 and 4,464 reads for the ND, HFD+placebo and HFD+probiotic groups, respectively. Gut microbiota species were shared among the experimental groups despite the different diets and treatments. The diversity of the gut microbiota and its composition were significantly altered in the diet-induced obese mice and after probiotic treatment. The authors observed concurrent transcriptional changes in adipose tissue and the liver. In adipose tissue, pro-inflammatory genes (TNFα, IL6, IL1β and MCP1) were down-regulated in mice receiving probiotic treatment. In the liver, fatty acid oxidation-related genes (PGC1α, CPT1, CPT2 and ACOX1) were up-regulated in mice receiving probiotic treatment. The gut microbiota of diet-induced obese mice appears to be modulated in mice receiving probiotic treatment. Probiotic treatment might reduce diet-induced obesity and modulate genes associated with metabolism and inflammation in the liver and adipose tissue.

We survive because we adapted to a world of microorganisms. All our epithelial surfaces participate in keeping up an effective barrier against microbes while not initiating ongoing inflammatory processes and risking collateral damage to the host. Major players in this scenario are antimicrobial peptides (AMPs). Such broad-spectrum innate antibiotics are in part produced by specialized cells but also widely sourced from all epithelia as well as circulating inflammatory cells. AMPs belong to an ancient defense system found in all organisms and participated in a preservative co-evolution with a complex microbiome. Particularly interesting interactions between host barrier and microbiota can be found in the gut. The intestinal cell lining not only has to maintain a tightly regulated homeostasis during its high-throughput regeneration, but also a balanced relationship towards an extreme number of mutualistic or commensal inhabitants. Chapter 7, by Ostaff and colleagues, describes how recent research suggests that advancing our understanding of the circumstances of such balanced and sometimes imbalanced interactions between gut microbiota and host AMPs should have therapeutic implications for different intestinal disorders.

Several pathological processes, such as sepsis and inflammatory bowel disease (IBD), are associated with impairment of intestinal epithelial barrier. In Chapter 8, Vandenbroucke and colleagues investigated the role of matrix metalloproteinase MMP13 in these diseases. The authoras observed that MMP13$^{-/-}$ mice display a strong protection in LPS- and caecal ligation and puncture-induced sepsis. We could attribute this protection to reduced LPS-induced goblet cell depletion, endoplasmic reticulum stress, permeability and tight junction destabilization in the gut of MMP13$^{-/-}$mice compared to MMP13$^{+/+}$ mice. Both in vitro and in vivo, the authors found that MMP13 is able to cleave pro-TNF into bioactive TNF. By LC-MS/MS, they identified three MMP13 cleavage sites, which proves that MMP13 is an alternative TNF sheddase next to the TNF converting enzyme TACE. Similarly, they found that the same mechanism was responsible for the observed protection of the MMP13$^{-/-}$ mice in a mouse model of DSS-induced colitis. The article identified MMP13 as an important mediator in sepsis and IBD via the shedding of TNF. Hence, it proposes MMP13 as a novel drug target for diseases in which damage to the gut is essential.

The human gut harbors a diverse community of microorganisms which serve numerous important functions for the host wellbeing. Functional foods are commonly used to modulate the composition of the gut microbiota contributing to the maintenance of the host health or prevention of disease. In Chapter 9, Vitali and colleagues characterized the impact of one month intake of a synbiotic food, containing fructooligosaccharides and the probiotic strains *Lactobacillus helveticus* Bar13 and *Bifidobacterium longum* Bar33, on the gut microbiota composition and metabolic profiles of 20 healthy subjects. The synbiotic food did not modify the overall structure of the gut microbiome, as indicated by Polymerase Chain Reaction-Denaturing Gradient Gel Electrophoresis (PCR-DGGE). The ability of the probiotic *L. helveticus* and *B. longum* strains to pass through the gastrointestinal tract was hypothesized on the basis of real-time PCR data. In spite of a stable microbiota, the intake of the synbiotic food resulted in a shift of the fecal metabolic profiles, highlighted by the Gas Chromatography Mass Spectrometry Solid Phase Micro-Extraction (GC-MS/SPME) analysis. The extent of short chain fatty acids (SCFA), ketones, carbon disulfide and methyl acetate was significantly affected by the synbiotic food consumption. Furthermore, the Canonical discriminant Analysis of Principal coordinates (CAP) of GC-MS/SPME profiles allowed a separation of the stool samples recovered before and after the consumption of the functional food. In this study the authors investigated the global impact of a dietary intervention on the gut ecology and metabolism in healthy humans. They demonstrated that the intake of a synbiotic food leads to a modulation of the gut metabolic activities with a maintenance of the gut biostructure.

In particular, the significant increase of SCFA, ketones, carbon disulfide and methyl acetate following the feeding period suggests potential health promoting effects of the synbiotic food.

It is well established that diet influences the health of an individual and that a diet rich in plant-based foods has many advantages in relation to the health and well-being of an individual. What has been unclear until recently is the large contribution of the gut microbiota to this effect. As well as providing basic nutritional requirements, the long-term diet of an animal modifies its gut microbiota. In adults, diets that have a high proportion of fruit and vegetables and a low consumption of meat are associated with a highly diverse microbiota and are defined by a greater abundance of *Prevotella* compared to *Bacteroides*, while the reverse is associated with a diet that contains a low proportion of plant-based foods. Furthermore, it is becoming increasingly clear that the effect of the microbial ecology of the gut goes beyond the local gut immune system and is implicated in immune-related disorders, such as IBS, diabetes and inflamm-ageing. In Chapter 10, Jeffery and O'Toole investigate the evidence that a balanced diet leads to a balanced, diverse microbiota with significant consequences for healthy ageing by focusing on conditions of interest.

Accumulating evidence demonstrates the intimate association between human hosts and the gut microbiome. Starting at birth, the sterile gut of the newborn acquires a diverse spectrum of microbes, needed for immunological priming. However, current practices (caesarean sections, use of formula milk) deprive newborns from being exposed to this broad spectrum of microbes. Unnecessary use of antibiotics and excessive hygienic precautions (e.g. natural versus chlorinated drinking water) together with the Western diet further contribute to a decreased microbial diversity in the adult gut. This has been correlated with recurrent *Clostridium difficile* infection, inflammatory bowel diseases and obesity, among others. A healthy gut microbiome is thus characterized by a diverse network of metabolically interacting microbial members. In this context, Chapter 11, by Van den Abbeele and cooleages, reviews several existing and novel approaches to manage the gut microbiome. First, prebiotic compounds should be re-defined in the sense that they should enhance the ecological biodiversity rather than stimulating single species. Recent studies highlight that structurally different polysaccharides require specific primary degraders but also enhance a similar network of secondary degraders that benefit from cross-feeding. A faecal transplantation is a second approach to restore biodiversity when the microbiota is severely dysbiosed, with promising results regarding *C. difficile*-associated disease and obesity-related metabolic syndromes. A final strategy is the introduction of key microbial network units, i.e. pre-organized microbial associations, which strengthen the overall microbial network of the gut microbiome that supports human health.

One hundred years ago, Metchnikoff associated human health, and particularly healthy ageing, with a specific type of gut microbiota. Classical culture methods associated a decrease in bifidobacteria and an increase in enterobacteria with ageing. Chapter 12, by Brüssow, describes how modern molecular methods blurred this simple picture and documented a substantial inter-individual variability for the gut microbiome even when stratifying the elderly subjects according to health status. Nutritional interventions with resistant starch showed consistent gut microbiota changes across studies from different geographical areas and prebiotic supplementation induced a 10-fold increase in gut bifidobacteria. However, in the ELDERMET study, microbiota changes do not precede, but follow the changes in health status of elderly subjects possibly as a consequence of diet changes.

The influence of resident gut microbes on xenobiotic metabolism has been investigated at different levels throughout the past five decades. However, with the advance in sequencing and pyrotagging technologies, addressing the influence of microbes on xenobiotics had to evolve from assessing direct metabolic effects on toxins and botanicals by conventional culture-based techniques to elucidating the role of community composition on drugs metabolic profiles through DNA sequence-based phylogeny and metagenomics. Following the completion of the Human Genome Project, the rapid, substantial growth of the Human Microbiome Project (HMP) opens new horizons for studying how microbiome compositional and functional variations affect drug action, fate, and toxicity (pharmaco-microbiomics), notably in the human gut. The HMP continues to characterize the microbial communities associated with the human gut, determine whether there is a common gut microbiome profile shared among healthy humans, and investigate the effect of its alterations on health. In

Chapter 13, Saad and colleagues offer a glimpse into the known effects of the gut microbiota on xenobiotic metabolism, with emphasis on cases where microbiome variations lead to different therapeutic outcomes. The authors discuss a few examples representing how the microbiome interacts with human metabolic enzymes in the liver and intestine. In addition, they attempt to envisage a roadmap for the future implications of the HMP on therapeutics and personalized medicine.

While practised for over thousand years, there is presently a renaissance in the interest of using of faecal transplantations to modify the intestinal microbiota of patients. This clinical practice consists of delivering large amounts of bowel microbes in various forms into the intestinal tract of the recipient that usually has been cleared previously. The major reason for the popularity of faecal transplantations is their effectiveness in treating a variety of diseases. Hence, there is a need to develop this procedure to the next level. While there are various developments to select, standardize and store the donor microbiota, it is more challenging to understand the intestinal microbial communities and develop ways to deliver these via robust biotechnological processes. The various approaches that have been followed to do so are discussed in Chapter 14, where de Vos also addresses the concept of the minimal microbiome, as well as the production of the synthetic communities that can be instrumental in new therapeutic avenues to modify the intestinal microbiota.

PART I

INTRODUCTION:
THE RAINFOREST IN THE GUT

CHAPTER 1

NUTRITION, MICROBIOMES, AND INTESTINAL INFLAMMATION

SUZANNE DEVKOTA AND EUGENE B. CHANG

1.1 INTRODUCTION

The gastrointestinal tract is both the largest endocrine and immune organ in the entire body—an evolutionary adaptation owing largely to the continual influx of food products we consume and need to digest. With over 50 known gut hormone genes and a multitude of bioactive peptides, and a mucosal surface harboring a dense microbial community, it is no wonder that dysbiosis and imbalances of the gastrointestinal tract have been implicated in an array of diseases throughout the body. In this review, we will discuss the latest research in the area of diet–microbe interactions and offer perspective on the influence of diet in maintaining immune homeostasis in the gut, and provide insight into new therapeutic pathways.

Reprinted with permission from Wolters Kluwer Health. Devkota S and Chang EB. Nutrition, Microbiomes, and Intestinal Inflammation. Current Opinions in Gastroenterology **29** *(2013): 603–607. doi:10.1097/MOG.0b013e328365d38f.*

1.2 DIETARY IMPACT ON REDEFINING SYMBIOSIS

The relationship with our intestinal microbiota has traditionally been viewed as a commensal relationship in which one member benefits (us), whereas the other member remains neither harmed nor helped (bacteria). This thinking stemmed from our understanding of the enteric microbiota's role in aiding in the breakdown of otherwise indigestible dietary components and, in the case of soluble fiber, using these substrates to produce beneficial byproducts for us such as short-chain fatty acids. However, we now realize that this relationship is mutualistic in most cases, in which both members distinctly benefit. More recently, Chow and Mazmanian [1] have introduced the concept of the pathobiont which are bacteria that coexist with the commensal bacteria in a healthy individual, but typically in very low abundance. However, given the opportunity or positive selection criteria that enhances their fitness, these microbes bloom and exhibit pathogenic properties, in many cases causing immune activation and inflammation. What precipitates these changes has only recently become clear. Recent studies, for instance, have demonstrated that dietary components can promote the emergence of pathobionts from the commensal microbiota, either through direct interactions with the microbiota or indirectly by altering the host physiology that initiates downstream effects capable of impacting microbial communities and causing dysbiosis and disease.

1.3 DIRECT AND INDIRECT EFFECTS OF DIETARY COMPONENTS AND STARVATION ON THE GUT MICROBIOME

Koeth et al. [2&] showed us that specific dietary components can have unexpected consequences such as promoting atherosclerosis by directly affecting the gut microbiota. In this study, humans consuming excessive amounts of dietary L-carnitine through food sources such as red meat (an 8-oz sirloin steak challenge in this case) resulted in a bacterial profile characterized by enriched *Prevotella* and decreased *Bacteroidetes*, that is, a profile similar to that of 'free-range' omnivores, in contrast to that of vegetarians or vegans. It was found that when L-carnitine was consumed, elevated serum levels of trimethylamine oxide (TMAO) were observed, as a result of microbial conversion of its precursor trimethylamine (TMA). These investigators had previously reported similar findings in mice, where the increased blood levels of TMAO were shown to rapidly accelerate atherosclerosis. Although a specific pathobiont was not identified, the collective diet-induced shifts of the microbial community appeared to favor more efficient metabolism of L-carnitine, resulting in the production of TMAO [3]. Dietary fats have also been shown to have profound and sustained effects on gut microbial composition of humans [4] and mice when compared to low-fat diets, but these changes are highly dependent on the source or type of the dietary fat. Specifically, it was found that different dietary fats affected the proportion of glycine versus taurine conjugation of hepatic bile acids. More hydrophobic fats, such as those derived from highly saturated and processed dairy sources (e.g. anhydrous milkfat), promoted the growth of a sulfite-reducing pathobiont, *Bilophila wadsworthia*, by creating a substrate-rich environment high in taurocholic acid and low in glycocholic acid. In contrast, fat derived from unsaturated safflower oil or a low-fat diet created a biliary profile roughly equal in its proportion of taurocholic to glycocholic acid. By altering the hepatic metabolism to favor taurocholate production, bioavailable organic sulfur found in taurine was introduced to the colonic bacteria and prompted the growth of *B. wadsworthia*. Under these conditions, *B. wadsworthia* became a pathobiont by promoting a robust antigen-specific T-helper type 1 (Th1) immune response leading to colitis, but only in the IL-10- deficientmouse,wheremechanisms to keepimmune activation in check were already compromised [5&]. The findings of this study therefore had direct relevance to human inflammatory bowel diseases (IBDs), in which *B. wadsworthia* and other sulfur-reducing bacteria (SRB) have been found to be highly represented. This has led many to implicate SRB in causing IBD. The findings provided a clear demonstration of how functional foods can be, in this case, triggering the onset of disease on the background of host genetic susceptibility. Many of these triggering dietary components are highly represented in Western diets, therefore raising the possibility that the increased incidence and prevalence of IBD and other complex immune disorders are related to shifts in the human microbiome, caused by Westernizing influences such as diet, environment, and lifestyle.

Cholesterol metabolism may also affect the microbiota, a process again intimately linked to bile acid metabolism. Walter et al. found in hamsters a dramatic reduction in the bacterial taxa *Coriobacteriaceae* and *Erysipelotrichaceae* that was associated with alterations in cholesterol metabolism caused by the addition of dietary plant sterol esters. Increases in host cholesterol metabolites were followed by dramatic and reproducible reductions in these taxa, displaying an almost perfect fit to a sigmoidal nonlinear model of bacterial inhibition [6&]. Thus, whereas excess of a particular bile acid may promote the growth of bile-tolerant pathobionts, excess cholesterol may contribute to this effect by inhibiting the microbes that would otherwise prevent the selection of potential pathobionts. In contrast to these studies that have mostly focused on overfed states, Hashimoto et al. [7&] examined the role of gut microbiota in causing intestinal inflammation associated with malnutrition, particularly amino acid malnutrition. Mice lacking the angiotensin 1 converting enzyme 2 (ACE2) have impaired uptake of neutral amino acids leading to tryptophan deficiency, which, in humans, can lead to pellagra. These mice display chronic intestinal inflammation and diarrhea, which implicated gut dysbiosis as a causative factor because transplantation of microbiota from ACE2 mutant mice into germ-free, wild-type mice resulted in colitis. This effect could be rescued by tryptophan supplementation. Kwashiorkor, another form of malnutrition, also appears to have dramatic effects on the human microbiome. Smith et al. [8&&] performed a longitudinal study of the microbiomes of 317 twin pairs born in Malawai with samples analyzed before and after treatment with ready-to-use therapeutic food (RUTF). In half of the individuals, both twins thrived, in 7%, both were malnourished and among the rest, one twin thrived, whereas the other developed kwashiorkor. In cases of discordance, this occurred equally in both fraternal and identical twins, suggesting that the development of kwashiorkor was not due to genetic differences. Therefore, the researchers proposed that an extragenetic factor, such as an altered microbiome, may be influencing the risk for disease. Indeed, the twins who developed kwashiorkor had a different microbiome compared to their healthy siblings. However, to determine whether the altered microbiome was a cause or a consequence of the malnutrition, the authors transferred the fecal microbiota from the malnourished or healthy twin into wild-type, germ-free mice. Interestingly, the kwashiorkor phenotype appeared transmissible in the recipient mice, and the most distinct microbial signature was characterized by the emergence of *Bilophila wadsworthia* and *Clostridium innocuum* with the traditional Malawian diet, which the authors proposed altered hepatic bile metabolism. *B. wadsworthia*, as previously shown, is linked to Th1-mediated intestinal inflammation, and *Clostridium innocuum* functions as an opportunist in immunocompromised hosts [9]. When mice were switched to the RUTF diet, there was a rapid change in the gut microbial structure, most notably, in favor of *Bifidobacteria*.

Taken together, these human and rodent data suggest that the overnutrition seen in Western societies and malnutrition seen in underdeveloped countries can both result in a dysbiosis that favors the growth of pathobionts and leads to intestinal inflammation, and in one case even atherosclerosis. This highlights the exquisite sensitivity of the microbiota to nutritional status and substrate availability, and offers the potential to selectively target harmful microbes through nutritional intervention.

1.4 DIETARY IMPRINTING OF THE DEVELOPING MICROBIOTA: IMPLICATIONS FOR HEALTHY AGING

How the gut microbiome changes over the course of one's life has been a subject of intense investigation. Most of these studies have focused on the microbiomes of infants and the elderly because longer prospective studies are either difficult to perform or infeasible. These studies have shown that diet has an important role in the assemblage of our gut microbiota, which may have lasting consequences that determine the states of health or disease. A remarkable example of this comes from a study that tracked the microbiota of an individual baby over the first 2.5 years of life with a diary of diet and health status [10]. The development of the gut microbiota was nonchaotic and nonrandom, building gradually over time but with discrete punctuations coinciding with changes in diet, antibiotics, or health. These punctuations were marked by abrupt shifts in abundance of particular microbes—perhaps the most notable shift in the microbial composition coming when the baby switched from breast milk to a full adult diet. In an extensive survey of the developing gut microbiome in individuals across cultures, Yatsunenko et al. [11&&] identified microbial gene signatures that distinguished Malawian and Amerindian infants from infants in the USA based largely on the content of the mother's breastmilk and the native diet onto which the infant was weaned. For example, microbial genes for foraging host-derived glycans, such as exo-a-sialidase and a-fucosidase, were significantly overrepresented in Malawian and Amerindian infants, compared with infants in the USA, and decreased over time as the infants were transitioned to the native vegetable-based diet. Conversely, microbial expression of a-fucosidase increased over time in U.S. infants as they were transitioned from breast milk to a Western diet high in readily absorbed sugars. Therefore, the functional microbiomes acquired by these infants were very likely determined initially by the maternal factors early in life, then adapted to the native diet, the long-term consequences of which have yet to be determined. Many other studies have looked at the impact of breast-feeding versus formula-feeding on inflammation and allergies, and they have underscored the relationship between infant feeding and later-life disease outcomes. Studies by Carlisle et al. [12&] in mice and Schwartz et al. [13&] in humans analyzed the taxonomic and metatranscriptomic differences in microbiota to better understand the impact of breast-feeding versus formula-feeding on host–microbiome interactions. Whereas there appears to be an increase in *Firmicutes* in maternal-fed mice, and *Proteobacteria* and *Bacteroides* in formula-fed mice, the opposite was found in human infants. At the metatranscriptomic and metagenomic level, however, both studies revealed consistent and distinct differences in the microbiota of breast-fed and formula-fed individuals, where microbial genes related to oxidative stress, gut structural integrity [12&], and immunity/defense genes in the host [13&] were highly represented in formula-fed hosts. These findings support the notion that the types of diet consumed early in life by individuals can profoundly affect the assemblage of gut microbial communities, but, ultimately, the functional profile of the microbial community determines the impact and long-term consequences in the host.

Whereas there are data to suggest that the healthy adult gut microbiome is relatively stable [14], that of the infant appears to be in flux. It now appears that the gut microbiome of elderly individuals may also be metastable. In a study of 178 individuals with an average age of 78 years old, Claesson et al. [15&&] found significant interindividual differences in the gut microbiota, which they felt were related to the composition and diversity of the diet. In their study, the diet was primarily determined by the living arrangements, that is, whether in a free-living community setting or in long-term residential care. The microbiota of individuals in long-stay care were significantly less diverse than that of community dwellers, and the authors found that the differences in the respective microbiota significantly correlated with the measures of frailty, comorbidity, nutritional status, markers of inflammation, and with metabolites in fecal water. These data therefore supported the interrelationship between diet, microbiota, and health status, but particularly underscored the role for diet-driven microbiota alterations in varying rates of health decline upon aging. Together, the emerging evidence supports the notion that the diets consumed at different stages of life can greatly influence health status through their effects on the gut microbiome, and in turn impact on the host. From these data, a compelling case for dietary intervention, aimed at reshaping the gut microbiome, can be made to restore intestinal, metabolic, and immune homeostasis.

1.5 CONCLUSION

The data presented highlight the important role of diet on intestinal microbial assembly and homeostasis. Modern society has shown us the effects of overconsumption apparent in the growing worldwide trend in obesity and diabetes, but overconsumption may have much more subtle effects on the intestinal milieu before overt pathologies become apparent. Whether a specific dietary fat or a metabolite of L-carnitine, for example, overconsumption of either led first to a state of chronic inflammation—in one instance leading to colitis and in the other leading to atherosclerosis. In the developing world, issues of malnutrition persist and often have secondary effects of diarrhea and intestinal inflammation, but it has been unclear as to the cause of the secondary effects. It now appears that dysbiosis of the microbiota is a key culprit. A better understanding of the adult microbiome has led us to question whether we may be able to change the course of disease by altering the succession of microbial communities in infancy. An individual's earliest nutrient exposure, whether by breast or by formula, and continuing onto introduction of solid foods, creates a profoundly different course of microbial assembly. We are only beginning to understand how these differences may prime the immune system and affect the health later in life.

Strategies to target specific microbial populations and individual pathobionts through dietary interventions are attractive and attainable means by which we may take control of our health.

REFERENCES AND RECOMMENDED READING

Papers of particular interest, published within the annual period of review, have been highlighted as:
& of special interest
&& of outstanding interest

1. Chow J, Mazmanian SK. A pathobiont of the microbiota balances host colonization and intestinal inflammation. Cell Host Microbe 2010; 7:265–276.
2. &Koeth R, Wang Z, Levison BS, et al. Intestinal microbiota metabolism of L-carnitine, a nutrient in red meat, promotes atherosclerosis. Nat Med 2013; 19:576–585.

A new mechanism by which microbial metabolism of a specific dietary component may promote atherosclerosis by producing a proinflammatory byproduct, trimethylamine oxide, in humans.

3. Wang Z, Klipfell E, Bennett BJ, et al. Gut flora dependent metabolism of dietary phosphatidylcholine contributes to cardiovascular disease. Nature 2011; 472:57–63.
4. Wu GD, Chen J, Hofmann C, et al. Linking long-term dietary patterns with gut microbial enterotypes. Science 2011; 334:105–108.
5. &Devkota S, Wang Y, Musch MW, et al. Dietary-fat-induced taurocholic acid production promotes pathobiont expansion and colitis in IL10-/- mice. Nature 2012; 487:104–107.

The first elucidated mechanism by which a single dietary factor can precipitate intestinal inflammation by influencing the growth of a single microbe.

PART II

MICROBIOME'S ROLE IN OBESITY

CHAPTER 2

GUT MICROBIOTA: IN SICKNESS AND IN HEALTH

M. JOSÉ HUERTAS and CARMEN MICHÁN

At birth, the human colon is rapidly colonized by a vast amount of gut microbes that affect host physiology and metabolism because of their ability to ferment nutrients and secrete bioactive compounds (de Vos, 2013). Lately, different reports are exploring their potential use for the treatment of a wide variety of diseases, although the clinical use of the gut microbiota is not all that innovative, since detailed faecal therapies for the treatment of abdominal pains were documented by Ming dynasty Chinese doctors, over 1000 years ago (Zhang et al., 2012). Researchers are now working on how faecal micro-organisms contribute to diseases, particularly in the context of obesity and other related metabolic disorders or ageing.

Several publications analyse the differences in composition and/or activity of the gut microbiota of slim vs. fat individuals, proposing that only few bacterial genera are associated with obesity, swelling and associated

This chapter was originally published under the Creative Commons Attribution License. Huertas MJ and Michán C. Gut Microbiota: In Sickness and In Health. Microbial Biotechnology *7,2 (2014); 88–89. doi:10.1111/1751-7915.12106.*

metabolic disorders, both in humans and rodents. But the main difficulty in determining these relationships is the fluctuation of microbial community configuration among unrelated individuals. We highlight an article published in *Science* (Ridaura et al., 2013) because of its smart approach. The authors describe the transplantation of faecal microbiota from several pairs of human twins, an obese and a slim one, into germ-free mice. The rodents that received the obese twin's faecal microbiota noticeably increased their adipose mass compared with the receptors of the slim twin's microbiota. Furthermore, cohousing of mice harbouring 'obese' microbiota along with mice harbouring a 'slim' one, prevented high body mass and obesity in the first group, which the authors attributed to a directional transfer of microbes. Also, this invasion of beneficial bacteria seems to depend on food intake because obesity was not prevented when obese mice harbouring a 'slim' microbiota ate a high-fat/low-fibre diet (Ridaura et al., 2013).

The importance of diet on the establishment of the gut flora meets the results of a long-term study on intestinal microbiota published in *Environmental Microbiology* showing that, although adults gut microbiota profiles are unique and mostly stable, diet, together with the use of antibiotics, intestinal transit and lifestyle clearly alter their proportions (Rajilić-Stojanović et al., 2013). These authors designed a comprehensible and highly reproducible phylogenetic microarray, the human intestinal tract chip, to analyse faecal samples of young adults gathered for several years and identifying subject-specific microbiota profiles preserved over time. They also showed how changes in environmental conditions are associated with changes in the abundance of certain species/genera of this microbiota. The challenge now is to link specific metabolic disorders to their corresponding gut microbiota alterations.

This question has also been addressed in a *Nature* article that reports the correlation between diversity of gut microbial genes, metabolic markers (e.g., body weight, fat mass, glucose and lipid metabolism, inflammation) and susceptibility to lose weight upon dietary restrictions (Cotillard et al., 2013). Using a quantitative metagenomics approach, Cotillard et al. proposed a bimodal distribution of microbial genes: low gene count (LGC) and high gene count (HGC). Individuals with a LGC showed increased weight, adiposity, insulin resistance and inflammatory diseases over time compared with HGC individuals. Additionally, and in agreement with the work by (Rajilić-Stojanović et al., 2013), individuals with a LGC also exhibited specific microbial genera known to be linked to in-flammatory diseases or altered gut barrier function. The authors concluded that individuals with LGC exhibited metabolic disorders and suggested that microbial gene wealth may be enhanced by dietary intervention. In the near future, these parameters may be used as biomarkers for the prognosis of obesity-related diseases.

Another current issue is the relationship between gut microbiota and human ageing that Harald Brüssow has recently reviewed in *Microbial Biotechnology*, in view of the classic book *The Prolongation of Life* by Metchnikoff (1907), and the ELDERMET project that pursues health im-provement of elderly people via modification of their gut flora (Brüssow, 2013a). All the reviewed studies show constraints that prevent from draw-ing a clear conclusion: small samples, high inter-individual variability, changing nutritional habits among populations and/or along life or detect-ing the presence of bacteria but not their viability. Nevertheless, the decay of gut microbiota in elderly people seems to be more related with poor diet habits and lack of exercise, than with ageing itself. All of that work will facilitate targeted modifications on the microbiome structure—maybe via specific food intake—that will help to improve gut communities in the elderly as suggested by (http://eldermet.ucc.ie/). Complementary to this report and also in *Microbial Biotechnology*, Prof. Brüssow presents an inquisitive review of the different health concepts (Brüssow, 2013b), and discusses whether it can be measured with the appropriate tools. The author also examines the concept of ageing—not only in humans—and how our current knowledge may be biased by short-lived animal studies. Although so far our life expectancy keeps growing, biological systems are not perfect, and so they will probably come to a point where accumulated errors will no longer allow life, particularly on complex organisms. If the focus is not set on increasing our life expectancy, but rather on improving the quality of our ageing, it would be a better choice, and the study of the gut microbiota will undoubtedly contribute to that improvement.

Faecal communities are crucial for health not only in adults or seniors, but also in children, because besides their common functions, they play an important role in the development of their immune system (Jost et al., 2012). Neonates' initial colonization depends both on transference from their mothers and on their environment, either during birth or through close contact. Benefits from breastfeeding include the acquisition of probiotic bacteria, but also of other anaerobic microbes that have not been extensively investigated yet. Jost and co-workers have published a very revealing paper in *Environmental Microbiology* (Jost et al., 2013), establishing the correlation between micro-organisms found in maternal faeces, breast milk and the gut of their corresponding neonates. The novelty of this report is that the authors not only address the presence of the micro-organisms but also their viability, dealing with one of the deficiencies commonly found in gut communities studies. Their results clearly show divergences between both approaches. Pyrosequencing assigns similar numbers to both mothers' milk and faeces bacteria, but when determining ribosomal ribonucleic acid or colony-forming unit counts, milk samples contain more than a million-fold less microbes than faecal ones. This report certainly supports the transference of living gut microbes from mothers to infants through breastfeeding, although the route between the mother's intestines and the breasts still remains unknown.

Where does all this research lead to? Maybe the clue is to be found in a recently published *Microbial Biotechnology* review by Willem de Vos where he highlights the need to understand how intestinal microbial communities work to develop effective biotechnological tools for targeted modification of gut flora (de Vos, 2013). He establishes the concept of minimal microbiome that can be defined as the smallest set of microbes and/or microbial functions necessary to develop a stable community. Systemic analysis of the interaction between intestinal microbes and the host are under way and will allow the prediction of the minimal synthetic microbiomes for the treatment of different diseases. Next-generation therapies against obesity, ageing and metabolic disorders could be based on the targeted implementation of these microbial communities.

REFERENCES

1.   Brüssow, H. (2013a) Microbiota and healthy ageing: observational and nutritional intervention studies. Microb Biotechnol 6: 326–334.
2.   Brüssow, H. (2013b) What is health? Microb Biotechnol 6: 341–348.

3. Cotillard, A., Kennedy, S.P., Kong, L.C., Prifti, E., Pons, N., Le Chatelier, E., et al. (2013) Dietary intervention impact on gut microbial gene richness. Nature 500: 585–588.

4. Jost, T., Lacroix, C., Braegger, C.P., and Chassard, C. (2012) New insights in gut microbiota establishment in healthy breast fed neonates. PLoS ONE 7: e44595.

5. Jost, T., Lacroix, C., Braegger, C.P., Rochat, F., and Chassard, C. (2013) Vertical mother-neonate transfer of maternal gut bacteria via breastfeeding. Environ Microbiol doi:10.1111/1462–2920.12238. [Epub ahead of print]

6. Metchnikoff, E. (1907) The prolongation of life: optimistic studies. New York, NY, USA: Putnam.

7. Rajilić-Stojanović, M., Heilig, H.G.H.J., Tims, S., Zoetendal, E.G., and de Vos, W.M. (2013) Long-term monitoring of the human intestinal microbiota composition. Environ Microbiol 15: 1146–1159.

8. Ridaura, V.K., Faith, J.J., Rey, F.E., Cheng, J., Duncan, A.E., Kau, A.L., et al. (2013) Gut microbiota from twins discordant for obesity modulate metabolism in mice. Science 341: 1241214.

9. de Vos, W.M. (2013) Fame and future of faecal transplantations – developing next-generation therapies with synthetic microbiomes. Microb Biotechnol 6: 316–325.

10. Zhang, F., Luo, W., Shi, Y., Fan, Z., and Ji, G. (2012) Should we standardize the 1700-year-old fecal microbiota transplantation? Am J Gastroenterol 107: 1755. author reply p 1755–1756.

CHAPTER 3

MICROBIAL REPROGRAMMING INHIBITS WESTERN DIET-ASSOCIATED OBESITY

THEOFILOS POUTAHIDIS, MARKUS KLEINEWIETFELD, CHRISTOPHER SMILLIE, TATIANA LEVKOVICH, ALISON PERROTTA, SIDDHESHVAR BHELA, BERNARD J. VARIAN, YASSIN M. IBRAHIM, JESSICA R. LAKRITZ, SEAN M. KEARNEY, ANTONIS CHATZIGIAGKOS, DAVID A. HAFLER, ERIC J. ALM MAIL, AND SUSAN E. ERDMAN

3.1 INTRODUCTION

The risk of developing obesity rises with a Westernized lifestyle. In industrialized and developing countries obesity contributes to increased mortality by predisposing to serious pathological conditions such as type 2 diabetes, cardiovascular disease, fatty liver, arthritis, asthma, and neoplasia [1]–[2]. Clinical and experimental data suggest that the white adipose tissue of obese organisms is in a low-grade, persistent state of chronic inflammation that exerts adverse systemic effects [2]–[3]. The most prominent inflammatory cell type of the obesity-associated inflammation is the

This chapter was originally published under the Creative Commons Attribution License. Poutahidis T, Kleinewietfeld M, Smillie C, Levkovich T, Perrotta A, Bhela S, Varian BJ, Ibrahim YM, Lakritz JR, Kearney SM, Chatzigiagkos A, Hafler DA, Alm EJ, and Erdman SE. Microbial Reprogramming Inhibits Western Diet-Associated Obesity. PLoS ONE 8,7 (2013). doi:10.1371/journal.pone.0068596.

adipose tissue macrophage. Macrophages are recruited and surround dead adipocytes, thus creating the so-called crown-like structures (CLS). These cells along with hypertrophic adipocytes are thought to be the key cells initiating the unique subclinical pro-inflammatory signaling cascade encountered in obesity [2], [4]–[5]. Macrophages, B and T lymphocytes, and up-regulated pro-inflammatory cytokines including TNF-α, IL-1, IL-6, IL-17, and monocyte chemoattractant protein-1 (MCP-1) have been reported to contribute to obesity-associated pathologies. In parallel, regulatory T cells down-regulate host inflammatory responses [2]–[3], [6]–[10].

It is well documented that "fast food" with high fat and salt content at relatively low cost is a major cause of the obesity epidemic in Western societies. Recent epidemiological research shows while dietary "fast food" contributes to obesity, eating yogurt surprisingly prevents age-associated weight gain, though the mechanism is unknown. It has been thought that slenderizing outcomes of yogurt are due to a probiotic bacteria-mediated mechanism [1]. Dietary probiotic consumption alters gut microbiota and may be an effective strategy not only for weight loss but also for preventing weight regain after loss [11]–[14]. Furthermore, alterations in the composition of gut microbiota may affect not only gut health but also distant tissues and overall health and longevity via immune-mediated mechanisms [15]–[20].

Using a mouse model of obesity we found that purified probiotic organisms alone prevented weight gain, and these protective effects were irrespective of the baseline diet. We show that this effect could be isolated to a single purified probiotic microbe, namely *Lactobacillus reuteri*. Importantly, eating *L. reuteri* bacteria acted without changing the existing gastrointestinal (GI) microbial composition in stool or level of calorie consumption; instead, the slenderizing microbial mechanism involved bacteria-triggered changes in the host immune system composition. The effect was in particular dependent on CD4$^+$ T cells and the presence of anti-inflammatory Il-10, as Il-10 deficient animals were resistant to *L. reuteri*-induced effects. Adoptive transfer of purified Il-10-competent *L. reuteri*-induced Foxp3$^+$ Treg cells was sufficient to rescue fat pathology and lessen body fat in naïve recipient animals. These data provide a mechanism whereby simple dietary manipulation can have major health impact, highlighting the utility of directly harnessing bacteria for public health initiatives.

3.2 RESULTS

3.2.1 EATING WESTERNIZED "FAST FOOD" STYLE DIET RESTRUCTURES THE GUT MICROBIOME AND ACCELERATES AGE-ASSOCIATED OBESITY IN MICE

Knowing that eating "fast food" contributes to age-associated weight gain in humans, we first used animal models to test specific roles for diet and the gastrointestinal (GI) tract microbiome in obesity. Genetically outbred Swiss mice were fed an ad libitum diet of Westernized chow mimicking typical human "fast food" diets that are high in fat and sugar, and low in fiber and vitamins B and D, that lead to age-associated obesity (Figure 1a). Abdominal fat examined histologically at five months of age revealed increased crown-like structures (CLS) (Figs. 1a and 1b) and a type of pyogranulomatous inflammation characteristic of obesity in humans [2]. Although both genders exhibited significant increases in fat pathology after Western chow, both CLS and pyogranulomatous inflammation lesions were more pronounced in male mice than in female mice when examined at five months of age (Fig. S1). Gastrointestinal tract microbial communities in mice changed within weeks after beginning Western diet formula (Fig. 1c; Fig. S1), showing that altered gut microbes may be associated with weight gain and obesity [1], [11].

3.2.2 SUBJECTS DINING ON WESTERNIZED "FAST FOOD"-STYLE DIET EXHIBIT TH17-BIASED IMMUNITY

It is well established that intestinal microbes modulate host health through activities of CD4+ T cells [21]–[22], at least in part through Il-6-dependent reciprocal functions of anti-inflammatory Foxp3+ Treg cells and pro-inflammatory Th17 cells [6], [23]. Thus, we examined T cell subpopulations and found that obese mice eating Western chow had increased frequencies of Il-

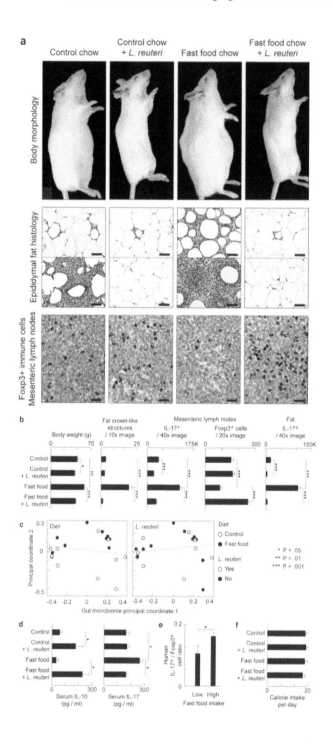

FIGURE 1: Eating probiotics blocks a gut microbiota-immunity-obesity axis. *L. reuteri* protects mice from Western diet-associated obesity. Data are shown in male outbred Swiss mice at the age of 5 months. Numerous crown-like structures (CLS) caused by adipocyte death-related inflammation, and focal pyogranulomatous inflammation (PGI) arise in abdominal fat of "fast food"-fed but not probiotic-fed animals. Probiotics increase anti-inflammatory Foxp3+ regulatory (Treg) cells and reduce pro-inflammatory Il17 protein to restore immune balance coinciding with a slender physique (a and b), without restructuring GI microbial communities (c). In the same mice, serum cytokine analysis shows that the pro-inflammatory Il-17-associated effect of obesity is systemic, and that *L. reuteri* negates this effect up-regulating the anti-inflammatory cytokine Il-10 (d). Humans frequently eating "fast food" also show an elevated ratio of pro-inflammatory IL17+/anti-inflammatory Foxp3+ Treg in peripheral blood cells compared to subjects never eating "fast food" (e). Probiotic-consuming slim mice chose similar calories when compared with obese animals, regardless of baseline diet, highlighting potential for translational medicine (f). Fat histology: Hematoxylin and eosin, Bars = 50 μm; MLN Immunohistochemistry: Diaminobenzidine chromogen, hematoxylin counterstain, Bars = 8.3 μm.

17 expressing cells which is in line with a previous report [6] (Fig. 1b and 1d). Importantly, when examining peripheral blood of human subjects frequently dining on "fast food" we found a similar pro-inflammatory Th17-biased profile (Fig. 1e).

3.2.3 DIETARY SUPPLEMENTATION WITH PROBIOTIC YOGURT INHIBITS OBESITY DUE TO WESTERNIZED "FAST FOOD" STYLE DIET

Recent epidemiological research shows eating "yogurt" prevents age-associated weight gain in humans [1]. To examine whether this epidemiologic observation could be modeled in genetically outbred experimental animals, and as a prelude to testing isolated microbes, we first examined the effect of a commercially available probiotic yogurt by feeding 0.8ml/mouse thrice weekly to Swiss mice eating either control or Westernized diets. Surprisingly, we discovered that feeding of probiotic yogurt together with either control chow (N = 5 mice/group; body weight of mice eating control diet = 37.42±4.711g versus control diet+yogurt = 24.9±4.995, $p < 0.05$), or with "fast food" style chow (fast food diet = 42.39±7.455 versus fast food diet+yogurt = 28.08±0.732, $p < 0.001$), entirely inhibited the age-associated fat pathology accumulation and body weight gain when examined upon necropsy at five months of age. Differences in body weight were attributable at least in part to intra-abdominal fat, which was significantly reduced in mice eating the probiotic yogurt (intra-abdominal fat of mice eating control diet = 1.692 ± 0.9036 g versus control diet+yogurt = 0.3067 ± 0.1684, $p < 0.05$; fast food diet = 3.06 ± 0.9737 versus fast food diet+yogurt = 0.5054 ± 0.2536, $p < 0.05$). These data showed that probiotic yogurt yielded significantly leaner animals regardless of dietary 'fast food.'

3.2.4 FEEDING OF PURIFIED LACTOBACILLUS REUTERI WAS SUFFICIENT TO INHIBIT WESTERN DIET OBESITY

To examine whether the effect of the yogurt was due to probiotic bacteria, or instead other compounds such as extra protein or vitamin D supplied in yogurt, we fed mice purified probiotic organism *Lactobacillus reuteri* ATCC 6475 cultivated as described elsewhere [24] using a dosage of 3.5×10^5 organisms/mouse/day in drinking water. Mice received the organisms as above in their drinking water starting at age 8 weeks and continuing for three months throughout the study until necropsy at age = five months. We found probiotic bacteria alone were sufficient for the slenderizing effect and entirely blocked development of abdominal fat pathology arising from ad libitum feeding of Western "fast food" chow (Figs. 1a and 1b). Abdominal fat (Fig. 2a) and subcutaneous fat (Fig. 2b) accumulations were significantly reduced in Swiss mice eating purified *L. reuteri* in combination with either control or Western diet (Fig. 2a–c). This was not a generic attribute of bacteria added to the drinking water, as mice consuming 3.5×10^5 *Escherichia coli* K12 organisms/mouse/day in drinking water did not develop the slender physique (Fig. S1). This protection from age-associated weight gain was sustained as evidenced by older Swiss mice at seven months and nine months of age (Fig. 2d) while consuming 3.5×10^5 *L. reuteri* organisms daily in their drinking water also starting at the age of 8 weeks. Similar outcomes were also achieved in inbred C57BL/6 strain mice eating special diets with or without *L. reuteri* supplementation (Figs. 3a). Taken together, these data demonstrate that purified lactic acid bacteria, in this case *L. reuteri* ATCC 6475 organisms alone, are sufficient for the anti-obesity effects of eating a probiotic yogurt formulation.

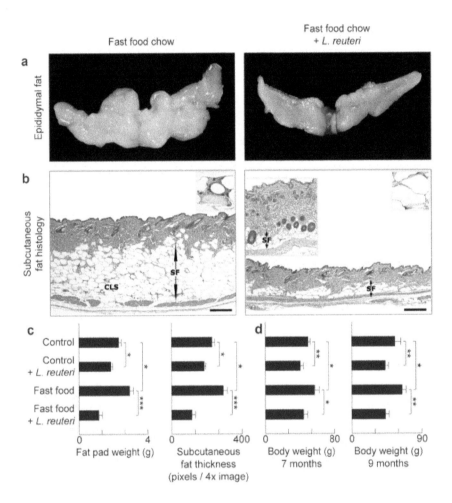

FIGURE 2: Dietary supplementation with *L. reuteri* protects from age-associated Western diet obesity. Specifically, the abdominal (epididymal) fat mass is significantly reduced in probiotic-consuming Swiss mice (a). The slenderizing effect of *L. reuteri* is also observed in the subcutaneous fat depot. The subcutaneous fat layer (SF) is significantly thicker and has many CLS (inset) in "fast food"-fed mice in contrast to mice eating the same diet and *L. reuteri*. There is thicker dermis and increased subcutaneous hair follicle profiles in the left inset of the "fast food"+probiotic skin image (b). Fad pad weight and subcutaneous fat thickness histomorphometric analyses show that probiotics protect from age-associated obesity irrespective of baseline diet (c). Eating probiotics benefits aged Swiss mice as well as the young animals, evident here from the body weight analysis of 7- and 9-months-old male and female mice (d). Skin histology: Hematoxylin and eosin, Bars = 250 μm.

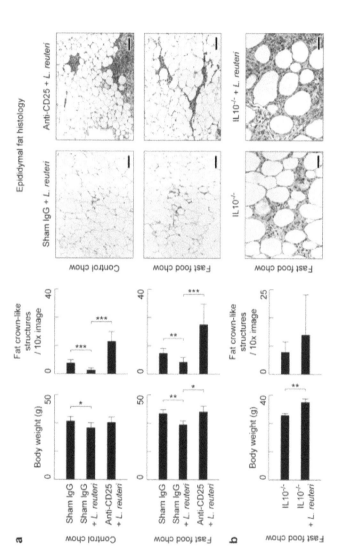

FIGURE 3: Mice exhibit an Interleukin 10-dependent Treg cell-mediated gut microbiota-immunity-obesity axis. Genetically-inbred C57BL/6 strain mice similarly benefit from probiotic protection against Western diet-associated obesity and fat pathology, including CLS and focal pyogranulomatous inflammation as shown here in males at 5 months of age (a). *Interleukin (Il)* 10-deficient C57BL/6 male mice eating Westernized chow failed to benefit from oral *L. reuteri* supplementation. Mice from both experimental groups were obese and had increased CLS that were often seen coalescing to form focally diffuse areas of adipocyte necrosis (b). Fat histology: Hematoxylin and eosin. Bars = 250 μm (a) and 100 μm (b).

3.2.5 EATING L. REUTERI DAILY DID NOT CHANGE THE EXISTING GUT MICROBIOME

Knowing that eating probiotics made mice slim, we next tested whether purified probiotic *L. reuteri* may act to change the microbial ecology in the gut. Using paired-end Illumina sequencing targeting the V4 region of the 16S rRNA gene on animal stools, it was found that daily intake of probiotic organisms did not change the existing gut microbiome profile (Fig. 1c). Thus, animals eating *L. reuteri* had a GI tract microbiome output that was not significantly different from their matched diet counterparts eating either regular chow or Western diet. Although probiotics didn't restructure resident microbiota communities, a pre-existing diverse microbial community was required for optimal slenderizing effects as illustrated by the fact that mice raised under germ-free conditions, and then fed L reuteri under general housing conditions, fail to benefit from eating probiotic organisms (Fig. S1h).

3.2.6 PROBIOTIC BACTERIA-CONSUMING SLIM MICE CHOSE SIMILAR CALORIES AS OBESE ANIMALS

Another possible explanation for significantly slimmer physiques after eating *L. reuteri* was reduced caloric intake when eating probiotic bacteria. In order to test this, we calculated daily "free choice" consumption of mouse chow in animals with *L. reuteri* bacteria added to their drinking water versus regular water controls. We found that *L. reuteri*-consuming slim mice chose similar calories to those of the regular-water drinking obese animals (Fig. 1f), in spite of large (p<0.001) body weight discrepancies.

3.2.7 PROBIOTIC MICROBES INHIBIT FAT PATHOLOGY BY AN IL-10-DEPENDENT MECHANISM

Recognizing that eating probiotics made mice thin without restructuring their microbial communities or reducing food intake, we hypothesized that probiotic organisms may protect from obesity by up-regulating anti-inflammatory immune activities; in particular, levels of anti-inflammatory cytokine IL-10. This reasoning was based upon data that interleukin-10 is pivotal in mounting immune tolerance to microbes along intestinal mucosal interfaces [25]–[26]. In support of this concept, it was found that the Swiss mice eating *L. reuteri* exhibited higher levels of IL-10 protein in serum than matched control mice (Fig. 1d). To test this further, we examined C57BL/6 strain mice with deletion of the *Il-10* gene and thus entirely lacking IL-10. Importantly, we found that *Il-10*-null animals eating Western chow with yogurt or Western chow with *L. reuteri* failed to benefit from probiotic bacteria and instead became obese (Fig. 3b). Likewise, C57BL/6 Rag2-deficient mice (that entirely lack functional lymphocytes) eating Westernized diets were unprotected from obesity after eating *L. reuteri* (N = 7 mice/group; body weight of mice eating Western diet = 42.94±1.19 g versus Western diet+*L. reuteri* = 41.78±1.45, p = 0.1 not significant). Taken together these data indicated that probiotic microbes acted to inhibit fat pathology by an IL-10-dependent adaptive immune cell mechanism.

3.2.8 PROBIOTIC-TRIGGERED PROTECTION FROM FAT PATHOLOGY IS TRANSFERABLE TO NAÏVE HOSTS VIA PURIFIED CD4⁺ T CELLS

Based upon our earlier work [27], and that of others [7], [28]–[30], we postulated that probiotic organisms such as *L. reuteri* protected from obesity by IL-10-mediated induction of lymphocytes [21]–[22]. To test whether probiotic-triggered lymphocytes were sufficient for reduced fat pathology we used adoptive transfer of purified CD4⁺ T cells into naïve syngeneic C57BL/6 Rag2-deficient mice. For these experiments, cell donors were fed supplementary probiotic yogurt or ate only baseline diets, and exhibited fat pathology typical for that treatment. We found that Rag2-null recipients of cells from donor mice eating the probiotic bacteria had reduced abdominal fat pathology when compared with recipients of cells from untreated control mice (Fig. 4). Moreover, subcutaneous fat was significantly reduced in regular-chow Rag2-knockout recipients of cells from L reuteri-consuming mice (Fig. 4a). Importantly, these protective effects required

IL-10-competency in cell donor mice (Fig. 4b–c). These data showed that the microbe-imbued protection from obesity resided in IL-10-dependent functions of CD4[+] T cells, confirming the findings of Feuerer et al (2009) who observed that protective IL-10-dependent Treg cells are associated inversely with adiposity [31].

3.2.9 FEEDING OF PURIFIED L. REUTERI RESTORES FOXP3+ TREG/TH17 BALANCE

Based upon earlier work by DiGiacinto et al (2005), we postulated that probiotic organisms protect from obesity by IL-10-mediated induction of anti-inflammatory Treg cells [21]–[22], [28]. We tested whether feeding of *L. reuteri* may restore host immunity from a diet-induced pro-inflammatory Th17 bias towards a beneficial anti-inflammatory Treg cell dominated immunity. We found that slim mice eating Westernized chow plus probiotic *L. reuteri* showed significantly increased anti-inflammatory Foxp3[+] Treg cells and also lower levels of IL-17A protein within abdominal lymph tissues when compared with mice feeding on Westernized "fast food"–style chow alone (Figs. 1a and 1b). Further, humans frequently eating "fast food" displayed a pro-inflammatory Th17-dominant phenotype when compared with control subjects who exhibited more Foxp3[+] cells and fewer Th17 cells in the peripheral blood (Fig. 1e). These data are in line with an earlier study showing the importance of anti-inflammatory Treg for prevention of adiposity and insulin resistance in mouse models [31]. Thus feeding *L. reuteri* specifically induced Foxp3[+] Treg cells and restored the Treg/Th17 balance observed in lean animals.

3.2.10 L. REUTERI INDUCED EFFECTS ARE DEPENDENT ON ACTIVE IMMUNE REGULATION BY FOXP3+ TREG CELLS

To test whether probiotic-triggered Foxp3[+] regulatory T cells were the key population and sufficient for reduced fat pathology in Western diet-fed mice, we used adoptive transfer of purified CD4[+]Foxp3[+] Treg cells delivered by intraperitoneal injection into naïve syngeneic C57BL/6 Rag2-

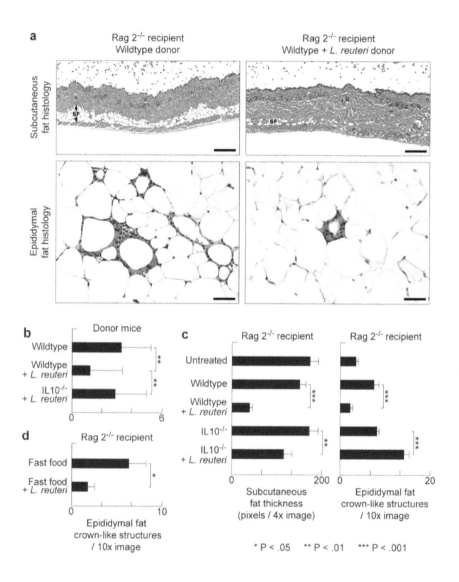

FIGURE 4: Diet-associated fat pathology is transferable to naïve animals using purified T-lymphocytes. Adoptive transfer of purified CD4+ cells from C57BL/6 wild type donor mice eating probiotics into C57BL/6 Rag2-null mice was sufficient to significantly reduce recipient body fat depots such as subcutaneous fat, as well as ameliorate abdominal fat pathology (a). Control diet-fed mice used as donors for lymphocyte transfer experiments showed IL10-dependent *L.reuteri* benefits including significantly less CLS in their abdominal fat (b). This immune-mediated protection requires Il10, as adoptive transfer of CD4+ cells from probiotic-fed Il10-deficient donors did not protect the recipient mice from

obesity and associated fat pathology (c). Purified wild type CD4$^+$ FoxP3+ Treg cells from mice eating *L. reuteri* were sufficient for beneficial effects in Rag2-null recipient mice rescuing them from obesity-associated pathology (d). Skin and fat histology: Hematoxylin and eosin. Bars skin = 250 μm, edididymal fat = 50 μm.

deficient mice. For these experiments, cell donors were green fluorescent protein (gfp)-Foxp3 transgenic C57BL/6 mice that had received *L. reuteri* in their drinking water, in addition to Western-style chow. We found significantly reduced abdominal fat pathology in recipients of *L. reuteri*-treated cells when compared with cells from donors eating Western diet alone (Fig. 4d). These adoptive transfer model data showed that probiotic-mediated protection from obesity resided in functions of Foxp3+ regulatory T cells. In line with these observations, selectively depleting Tregs by targeting CD25 [32] showed similar effects. We found eight-week-old Swiss mice eating *L. reuteri* and also simultaneously treated with anti-CD25 antibody rapidly developed morbid obesity, sluggish demeanor, and profound abdominal fat pathology during the ensuing three months (Fig. 5a); whereas control animals eating *L. reuteri* and treated with sham isotype matched IgG had reduced fat pathology and slender outcomes (Figs. 5a and 5b). Requirements for CD25$^+$ cells for slenderizing benefits of *L. reuteri* were also evident in abdominal fat weights that were significantly increased after CD25 depletion (Fig. 5c). A role for CD25 in controlling inflammatory cytokines was displayed in peripheral blood in this model (Fig. 1d). Thus, dietary supplementation with *L. reuteri* seems to restore beneficial balanced Th17/Treg host immunity, even in individuals otherwise suffering from a pro-inflammatory immunity and chronic inflammation when dining on Westernized "fast food"-style diets (Fig. 6).

3.3 DISCUSSION

We devised an animal model to examine the mechanisms of diet [i.e., "fast food" or "yogurt"] previously shown to impact obesity in humans [1]. Genetically outbred mice consuming "fast food" mimicked adiposity patterns in people [1] and displayed enteric microbial similarities with

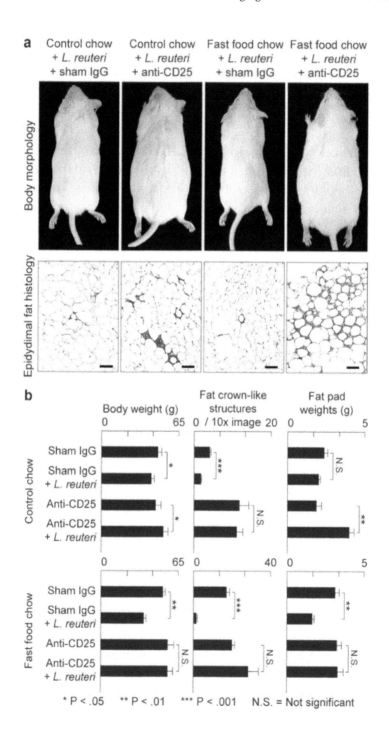

FIGURE 5: Anti-obesity protection of oral probiotics in outbred Swiss mice requires CD25$^+$ immune cells. Depletion of CD4$^+$CD25$^+$ Treg cells entirely inhibits probiotic-induced protection from age-associated obesity and abdominal fat pathology (a). Probiotics protect from weight gain unless mice were simultaneously treated with anti-CD25 antibody, in which case animals rapidly became obese. Frequency of prototype crown-like structures was increased in abdominal fat after depletion of CD25$^+$ cells but not in sham IgG-treated control animals (b). Fat histology: Hematoxylin and eosin. Bars = 100 μm.

other models and humans [11]. Mice eating yogurt—a food item most strongly linked with lean physique in human subjects [1]—were leaner than matched control animals. We demonstrate that a purified lactic acid microbe was sufficient to mediate this effect. Importantly, we show that 1) this lean outcome was achievable even while dining on Westernized chow, 2) eating probiotic microbes did not significantly change the established control or Westernized diet microbiome in stool, 3) *L. reuteri* consumption did not significantly alter the caloric intake even though mice were significantly slimmer, and 4) lean outcomes involved microbe-triggered CD4$^+$ Foxp3$^+$ regulatory T cells, dependent on IL-10. These observations led us to propose a circular mechanistic model where both lactic acid organisms and the resident GI microbiome [1], [11] affect host immunity [21]–[22], which in turn affects obesity [31], which impact host immunity, and so forth. Once initiated, adiposity may then become a self-sustaining condition.

Consuming Westernized "fast food"-style chow rapidly re-structured the murine microbiome coincident with increased IL-17 protein levels and developing obesity in our mouse models [11]. In our human subjects, a Th17 biased profile also emerged when eating fast food, matching that seen in animals eating the Western chow. Although the New Western diet for mice was selected specifically to mimic human "fast food", the 'potato chip' diet of humans also includes high salt and other factors not included in mouse chow. Nonetheless, these mice exhibited elevated levels of Il-17A, whether a result of the diet, or microbes, or from the obesity itself [6]. Following this line of reasoning, the insertion of dietary probiotics may break this inflammatory-adiposity cycle. Although a Th17 pro-inflammatory bias has been clearly linked with obesity, there's evidence of a dichotomy in effects of IL-17A in adipogenesis [6], [33]–[34]. One

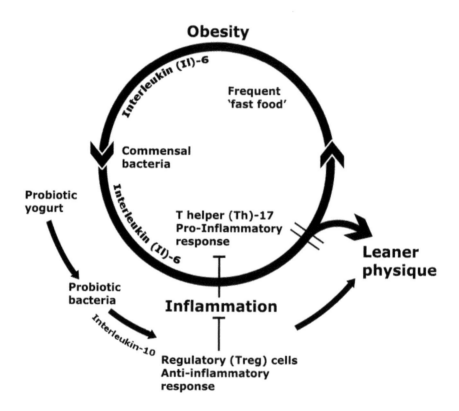

FIGURE 6: Proposed mechanistic overview. In order to explain the "fast food" versus "yogurt" age-associated weight disparity observed in human subjects, we propose that Western-style dietary habits alter gut microbiota fueling an IL-6 driven, IL-17-dominant, systemic smoldering inflammatory milieu, ultimately leading to a vicious circle of obesity and inflammation. On the other hand, individuals consuming probiotic yogurt enrich their gut with probiotic bacteria that stimulate the anti-inflammatory arm of the immune system. Potent IL-10-associated Treg responses in these individuals rescue them from the inflammation-obesity cycle, thus increasing likelihood of a leaner physique.

possible explanation for this might be the recently uncovered heterogeneity amongst Th17 cells [35]–[37]. As a result, such complex immune feedback mechanisms are difficult to interrupt without untoward consequences to the host, making pro-inflammatory molecules TNF-α, IL-6 and IL-17 [8], [38]–[40] challenging targets in this process. These constraints are perhaps best overcome by directly harnessing bacteria that apparently induce global immune homeostasis that may serve public health initiatives.

In contrast with microbiome changes induced by eating "fast food", consuming yogurt or purified probiotic bacteria in the form of *L. reuteri* did not significantly alter the existing gut microbiome as measured in stool in the present or other studies [41]. However, feeding of this lactic acid microbe *did* recapitulate leaner physique recently observed in a large epidemiological survey of human subjects when eating yogurt [1], and in line with recent work by others [42]–[47]. However, in separate epidemiological studies, the presence of *L. reuteri* in human guts has been associated with obesity [48]–[49]. Whether this discrepancy reflects the wide genomic variation of *L. reuteri* strains or differences [50] in host-microbial interactions warrants further investigation. A health-protective role for *L. reuteri* in host metabolism, as displayed in the present study, offers mutually beneficial gut symbiont-host relationship and co-evolution [51].

Interestingly, feeding probiotic yogurt or the purified *L. reuteri* bacteria to our mice did not alter their caloric intake, and also revealed benefits to general demeanor, skin and hair coat, and reproductive performance coincident with elevated plasma levels of oxytocin [52]. Oxytocin, a neuropeptide hormone associated with reproduction and social bonding, has also been linked with dietary satiety [53]–[54]. Hypothalamic hormones such as oxytocin conceptually intersect microbes with social and physical fitness in evolutionary success. Studies are underway to more explicitly test the impact of a microbial – hypothalamic – immune axis upon obesity.

We postulate that microbes contained in probiotic yogurt impart immune homeostasis that maintains systemic health [21]–[22]. One specific aspect of this paradigm is reciprocal activities of pro-inflammatory Th-17 and anti-inflammatory Treg cells [23]. Diet and microbe-induced failure of tolerance unifies these data with prior work involving inflammation, obesity, and cancer [8], [55]–[58]. These data agree with Feuerer et al (2009) who discovered IL-10-dependent Treg arise inversely with adiposity and insulin resistance [31]. Along mucosal surfaces, IL-10 facilitates immune tolerance [59] and recruitment of Treg cells to skew host immunity away from pro-inflammatory IL-17. Diverse disorders such as asthma and auto-immune diseases associated with Westernized living are widely believed to result from insufficient levels of IL-10 and insufficient immune cali-bration essential for sustained systemic health [60]. Westernized diets are also low in vitamin D, a nutrient that normally works together with IL-10 to enforce immune tolerance and protect against inflammatory disorders [61]–[63] and some types of cancer [64].

Feeding of palatable probiotic organisms offers potentially potent, cost-effective and practical options for public weight management. Appar-ent requirements for other beneficial resident commensal microbes may be further tested using gnotobiotic models [41], [65]–[66]. Such microbial re-programming may ultimately target other diseases linked with obesity and inflammation such as diabetes [2], cancer [8], and multiple sclerosis [15] for healthful longevity to combat a growing Westernized "fast food" public health crisis.

3.4 EXPERIMENTAL PROCEDURES

3.4.1 ANIMALS

Genetically outbred CD-1 mice (Charles River; Wilmington, MA), inbred *wild type* or *Interleukin 10-deficient* C57BL/6 strain mice (Jackson Labs, Bar Harbor, ME), plus inbred *Rag2-deficient* C57BL/6 strain mice and outbred Swiss Webster mice (Taconic; Germantown, NY) were housed and handled in Association for Assessment and Accreditation of Laborato-ry Animal Care (AAALAC)-accredited facilities with diets, experimental methods, and housing as specifically approved by the Institutional Animal Care and Use Committee. The MIT CAC (IACUC) specifically approved the studies as well as the housing and handling of these animals. Mice were bred in-house to achieve experimental groups. The experimental de-sign was to expose mice to diets starting at age = eight weeks, and then continue the treatment for 12 weeks until euthanasia using carbon dioxide at five months of age, unless otherwise specified (Fig. S1). Each experiment included 5–15 animals per group with two replications (total N = 10–30 mice per group). For microbiome analyses, fresh stools were collected twice weekly and stored in RNA-later at −20C for later testing. Other tissues were collected upon necropsy.

3.4.2 HUMAN SUBJECTS AND SPECIMEN COLLECTION

The PhenoGenetic Cohort of Brigham and Women's Hospital including 1200 healthy control subjects provided subject recruitment and sample collection, in compliance with the Declaration of Helsinki with local ethics committee approval before initiation, and written informed consent from all subjects. The Brigham and Womens Institutional Review Board (IRB): Partners Human Research Committee specifically approved the studies. Subjects had the following characteristics: female/male sex ratio was 60:40%; race distribution was 14% African American, 12% Asian American, 68% white, and 6% Hispanic; mean age was 24.3 y (range, 18–50 y); mean body mass index was 22.5 (range, 13–50). Blood samples were processed on the day of collection. Dietary and lifestyle behaviour was assessed by questionnaire on day of the visit. Total N = 23 for high fast food intake, and N = 26 for low fast food intake.

3.4.3 SPECIAL DIETS FOR ANIMALS

Mice of 6–8 wks were placed on experimental diets: control AIN-76A (Harlan-Teklad Madison WI), and a Westernized diet with high fat and low fiber with substandard levels of Vitamin D (TD.96096; Harlan-Teklad) starting at 8 weeks of age until euthanasia at 5 months of age. Subgroups were supplemented with commercially available vanilla probiotic yogurt (0.8 ml/mouse 3X weekly) containing a microbial cocktail including *S. thermophilus, L. bulgaricus, L. acidophilus, Bifidobacterium bifidus, L. casei*, and *L. rhamnosus* during this same time. Separate groups of animals received a purified preparation of an anti-inflammatory strain of *Lactobacillus reuteri* ATCC 6475 cultivated as described elsewhere [24] using a dosage of 3.5×10^5 organisms/mouse/day, or a sham *E. coli* K12 3.5×10^5

organisms/mouse/day in drinking water. Drinking water was replaced at least weekly. Viability of *L. reuteri* organisms in drinking water was assessed using standard aerobic plate culture methods and determined to be too numerous to count (TNTC) at day one and less than ten colonies by day seven.

3.4.4 STOOL MICROBIOME ANALYSES

Genomic DNA was extracted from stool samples using the Qiagen QIAamp DNA Stool Mini Kit. Samples for paired-end Illumina sequencing were constructed using a two-step PCR amplicon approach targeting the V4 region of the 16S rRNA gene (U515F and E786R) as described in [67] and reads were quality filtered and clustered into operational taxonomic units (OTUs) at 97% nucleotide identity. Principal coordinates analysis is based on the Jensen-Shannon divergence between samples, and differences in microbiome composition were tested for significance using an empirical p-value estimated by permutation. Data presented in Fig. 1 were from stool collected at 5 days after onset of treatments.

3.4.5 HUMAN T CELL ISOLATION AND STIMULATION

Peripheral blood mononuclear cells (PBMC) were separated by Ficoll-Paque PLUS (GE Healthcare, Piscataway, NJ) gradient centrifugation. Untouched CD4$^+$ T cells were isolated from PBMC by negative selection via the CD4$^+$ T cell isolation kit II (Miltenyi Biotec, Auburn, CA). CD4$^+$ T cells were cultured in serum-free X-Vivo 15 medium (BioWhittaker, Walkersville, MD) and stimulated for 4 h with PMA (50 ng/ml) and ionomycin (250 ng/ml; Sigma-Aldrich) with GolgiPlug (BD Biosciences). Stimulated cells, with dead cells excluded by LIVE/DEAD cell kit (Live Technologies), were fixed and made permeable according to manufacturer's instructions (Fix/Perm; eBioscience) and were stained with anti-IL17A (eBio64DEC17; eBioscience, San Diego, CA) and anti-FOXP3 (206D; BioLegend, San Diego CA) for 30–45 min. Data were acquired on a LSR II (BD Biosciences, San Jose, CA) and analyzed with FlowJo software (TreeStart, Ashland OR) and GraphPad Prism (GraphPad Software, La Jolla, CA).

3.4.6 ADOPTIVE TRANSFER OF T CELLS INTO RECIPIENT MICE

$CD4^+$ lymphocytes isolated from wild type or IL-10-deficient C57BL/6 mice using magnetic beads (Dynal/Invitrogen; Carlsbad CA) are sorted by hi-speed flow cytometry (MoFlow2) to obtain purified populations of $CD4^+$ lymphocytes and determined to be ~96% pure as previously described elsewhere [16]. Syngeneic $Rag2^{-/-}$ recipient mice were then injected intraperitoneally with 3×10^5 $CD4^+$ cells as previously described. For separate assays, purified populations of $CD4^+$ lymphocytes were collected as above from transgenic C57BL/6 mouse donors expressing green fluorescent protein (gfp)-Foxp3, and then further purified sorting gfp+ expression to achieve purified populations of $CD4^+$ $FoxP3^+$ TREG lymphocytes injected intraperitoneally at 3×10^5 cells/mouse into C57BL/6 $Rag2^{-/-}$ recipient mice.

3.4.7 DEPLETION OF $CD25^+$ CELLS

Mice were treated with anti-CD25 antibody (clone PC-61; Bio- Express, West Lebanon, NH) at 150 ug per mouse intraperitoneally 3X weekly for 12 weeks. Treated mice were compared to mice receiving sham isotype antibody alone. Depletion of $CD25^+$ cells was confirmed by undetectably low fractions of $CD25^+$ cells in spleens of mice treated with anti-CD25 antibody compared to sham-treated controls using flow cytometry. Depletion was confirmed by absence of $Foxp3^+$ cells in spleen.

3.4.8 DETECTION OF SYSTEMIC CYTOKINE PROTEIN EXPRESSION

Serum cytokine levels of six animals per group were analyzed using the Bioplex assay system (BioRad, Hercules, CA) according to the manufacturers protocol. Samples were analyzed in duplicate on a Bio-Plex 200 system (BioRad, Hercules, CA). Statistical analysis was performed using 2-tailed student's t-test; a p-value <0.05 was considered statistically significant.

3.4.9 HISTOPATHOLOGY AND IMMUNOHISTOCHEMISTRY

For histologic evaluation, formalin-fixed tissues were embedded in paraffin, cut at 5 µm, and stained with hematoxylin and eosin. Lesions were analyzed and quantified by a pathologist blinded to sample identity. Foxp3 and Il-17 were labeled immunohistochemically in mouse tissue. Immunohistochemistry and morphometric assessment of Il-17+ and FoxP3+ cells in mesenteric lymph nodes and abdominal fat were as previously described [16].

3.4.10 STATISTICAL ANALYSES

The Mann-Whitney U test was used for body weight, diet, calorie consumption, and histomorphometry. A p-value <0.05 was statistically significant.

REFERENCES

1. Mozaffarian D, Hao T, Rimm EB, Willett WC, Hu FB (2011) Changes in diet and lifestyle and long-term weight gain in women and men. N Engl J Med 364: 2392–2404. doi: 10.1056/NEJMoa1014296
2. Shoelson SE, Herrero L, Naaz A (2007) Obesity, inflammation, and insulin resistance. Gastroenterology 132: 2169–2180. doi: 10.1053/j.gastro.2007.03.059

3.   Lumeng CN, Saltiel AR (2011) Inflammatory links between obesity and metabolic disease. J Clin Invest 121: 2111–2117. doi: 10.1172/JCI57132
4.   Cinti S, Mitchell G, Barbatelli G, Murano I, Ceresi E, et al. (2005) Adipocyte death defines macrophage localization and function in adipose tissue of obese mice and humans. J Lipid Res 46: 2347–2355. doi: 10.1194/jlr.M500294-JLR200
5.   West M (2009) Dead adipocytes and metabolic dysfunction: recent progress. Curr Opin Endocrinol Diabetes Obes 16: 178–182. doi: 10.1097/MED.0b013e3283292327
6.   Winer S, Paltser G, Chan Y, Tsui H, Engleman E, et al. (2009) Obesity predisposes to Th17 bias. Eur J Immunol 39: 2629–2635. doi: 10.1002/eji.200838893
7.   Winer S, Chan Y, Paltser G, Truong D, Tsui H, et al. (2009) Normalization of obesity-associated insulin resistance through immunotherapy. Nat Med 15: 921–929. doi: 10.1038/nm.2001
8.   Park EJ, Lee JH, Yu GY, He G, Ali SR, et al. (2010) Dietary and genetic obesity promote liver inflammation and tumorigenesis by enhancing IL-6 and TNF expression. Cell 140: 197–208. doi: 10.1016/j.cell.2009.12.052
9.   Winer DA, Winer S, Shen L, Wadia PP, Yantha J, et al. (2011) B cells promote insulin resistance through modulation of T cells and production of pathogenic IgG antibodies. Nat Med 17: 610–617. doi: 10.1038/nm.2353
10. Deiuliis J, Shah Z, Shah N, Needleman B, Mikami D, et al. (2011) Visceral adipose inflammation in obesity is associated with critical alterations in tregulatory cell numbers. PLoS One 6: e16376. doi: 10.1371/journal.pone.0016376
11. Turnbaugh PJ, Ley RE, Mahowald MA, Magrini V, Mardis ER, et al. (2006) An obesity-associated gut microbiome with increased capacity for energy harvest. Nature 444: 1027–1031. doi: 10.1038/nature05414
12. Santacruz A, Marcos A, Warnberg J, Marti A, Martin-Matillas M, et al. (2009) Interplay between weight loss and gut microbiota composition in overweight adolescents. Obesity (Silver Spring) 17: 1906–1915. doi: 10.1038/oby.2009.112
13. Kallus SJ, Brandt LJ (2012) The intestinal microbiota and obesity. J Clin Gastroenterol 46: 16–24. doi: 10.1097/MCG.0b013e31823711fd
14. Vrieze A, Van Nood E, Holleman F, Salojarvi J, Kootte RS, et al.. (2012) Transfer of intestinal microbiota from lean donors increases insulin sensitivity in individuals with metabolic syndrome. Gastroenterology 143: 913–916 e917.
15. Berer K, Mues M, Koutrolos M, Rasbi ZA, Boziki M, et al. Commensal microbiota and myelin autoantigen cooperate to trigger autoimmune demyelination. Nature 479: 538–541. doi: 10.1038/nature10554
16. Erdman SE, Rao VP, Olipitz W, Taylor CL, Jackson EA, et al. (2010) Unifying roles for regulatory T cells and inflammation in cancer. Int J Cancer 126: 1651–1665. doi: 10.1002/ijc.24923
17. Claesson MJ, Jeffery IB, Conde S, Power SE, O'Connor EM, et al. (2012) Gut microbiota composition correlates with diet and health in the elderly. Nature 488: 178–184. doi: 10.1038/nature11319
18. Maynard CL, Elson CO, Hatton RD, Weaver CT (2012) Reciprocal interactions of the intestinal microbiota and immune system. Nature 489: 231–241. doi: 10.1038/nature11551

19. Flint HJ, Scott KP, Louis P, Duncan SH (2012) The role of the gut microbiota in nutrition and health. Nat Rev Gastroenterol Hepatol 9: 577–589. doi: 10.1038/nrgastro.2012.156

20. Hooper LV, Littman DR, Macpherson AJ (2012) Interactions between the microbiota and the immune system. Science 336: 1268–1273. doi: 10.1126/science.1223490

21. Powrie F, Maloy KJ (2003) Immunology. Regulating the regulators. Science 299: 1030–1031. doi: 10.1126/science.1082031

22. Lee YK, Mazmanian SK (2010) Has the microbiota played a critical role in the evolution of the adaptive immune system? Science 330: 1768–1773. doi: 10.1126/science.1195568

23. Bettelli E, Carrier Y, Gao W, Korn T, Strom TB, et al. (2006) Reciprocal developmental pathways for the generation of pathogenic effector TH17 and regulatory T cells. Nature 441: 235–238. doi: 10.1038/nature04753

24. Saulnier DM, Santos F, Roos S, Mistretta TA, Spinler JK, et al. (2011) Exploring metabolic pathway reconstruction and genome-wide expression profiling in Lactobacillus reuteri to define functional probiotic features. PLoS One 6: e18783. doi: 10.1371/journal.pone.0018783

25. Chaudhry A, Samstein RM, Treuting P, Liang Y, Pils MC, et al. (2011) Interleukin-10 signaling in regulatory T cells is required for suppression of Th17 cell-mediated inflammation. Immunity 34: 566–578. doi: 10.1016/j.immuni.2011.03.018

26. Rubtsov YP, Rasmussen JP, Chi EY, Fontenot J, Castelli L, et al. (2008) Regulatory T cell-derived interleukin-10 limits inflammation at environmental interfaces. Immunity 28: 546–558. doi: 10.1016/j.immuni.2008.02.017

27. Sakaguchi S, Miyara M, Costantino CM, Hafler DA (2010) FOXP3+ regulatory T cells in the human immune system. Nat Rev Immunol 10: 490–500. doi: 10.1038/nri2785

28. Di Giacinto C, Marinaro M, Sanchez M, Strober W, Boirivant M (2005) Probiotics ameliorate recurrent Th1-mediated murine colitis by inducing IL-10 and IL-10-dependent TGF-beta-bearing regulatory cells. J Immunol 174: 3237–3246.

29. Wang Y, Li J, Tang L, Charnigo R, de Villiers W, et al. (2010) T-lymphocyte responses to intestinally absorbed antigens can contribute to adipose tissue inflammation and glucose intolerance during high fat feeding. PLoS One 5: e13951. doi: 10.1371/journal.pone.0013951

30. Ilan Y, Maron R, Tukpah AM, Maioli TU, Murugaiyan G, et al. (2010) Induction of regulatory T cells decreases adipose inflammation and alleviates insulin resistance in ob/ob mice. Proc Natl Acad Sci U S A 107: 9765–9770. doi: 10.1073/pnas.0908771107

31. Feuerer M, Herrero L, Cipolletta D, Naaz A, Wong J, et al. (2009) Lean, but not obese, fat is enriched for a unique population of regulatory T cells that affect metabolic parameters. Nat Med 15: 930–939. doi: 10.1038/nm.2002

32. Shevach EM (2002) CD4+ CD25+ suppressor T cells: more questions than answers. Nat Rev Immunol 2: 389–400. doi: 10.1038/nri821

33. Ahmed M, Gaffen SL (2010) IL-17 in obesity and adipogenesis. Cytokine Growth Factor Rev 21: 449–453. doi: 10.1016/j.cytogfr.2010.10.005

34. Zuniga LA, Shen WJ, Joyce-Shaikh B, Pyatnova EA, Richards AG, et al. (2010) IL-17 regulates adipogenesis, glucose homeostasis, and obesity. J Immunol 185: 6947–6959. doi: 10.4049/jimmunol.1001269

35. Zielinski CE, Mele F, Aschenbrenner D, Jarrossay D, Ronchi F, et al. (2012) Pathogen-induced human TH17 cells produce IFN-gamma or IL-10 and are regulated by IL-1beta. Nature 484: 514–518. doi: 10.1038/nature10957

36. Lee MN, Roy M, Ong SE, Mertins P, Villani AC, et al.. (2012) Identification of regulators of the innate immune response to cytosolic DNA and retroviral infection by an integrative approach. Nat Immunol.

37. Esplugues E, Huber S, Gagliani N, Hauser AE, Town T, et al. (2011) Control of TH17 cells occurs in the small intestine. Nature 475: 514–518. doi: 10.1038/nature10228

38. Balkwill F, Mantovani A (2001) Inflammation and cancer: back to Virchow? Lancet 357: 539–545. doi: 10.1016/S0140-6736(00)04046-0

39. Naugler WE, Sakurai T, Kim S, Maeda S, Kim K, et al. (2007) Gender disparity in liver cancer due to sex differences in MyD88-dependent IL-6 production. Science 317: 121–124. doi: 10.1126/science.1140485

40. Baltgalvis KA, Berger FG, Pena MM, Davis JM, Muga SJ, et al. (2008) Interleukin-6 and cachexia in ApcMin/+ mice. Am J Physiol Regul Integr Comp Physiol 294: R393–401. doi: 10.1152/ajpregu.00716.2007

41. McNulty NP, Yatsunenko T, Hsiao A, Faith JJ, Muegge BD, et al. (2011) The impact of a consortium of fermented milk strains on the gut microbiome of gnotobiotic mice and monozygotic twins. Sci Transl Med 3: 106ra106. doi: 10.1126/scitranslmed.3002701

42. Kim SW, Park KY, Kim B, Kim E, Hyun CK (2013) Lactobacillus rhamnosus GG improves insulin sensitivity and reduces adiposity in high-fat diet-fed mice through enhancement of adiponectin production. Biochem Biophys Res Commun 431: 258–263. doi: 10.1016/j.bbrc.2012.12.121

43. Oksaharju A, Kooistra T, Kleemann R, van Duyvenvoorde W, Miettinen M, et al.. (2012) Effects of probiotic Lactobacillus rhamnosus GG and Propionibacterium freudenreichii ssp. shermanii JS supplementation on intestinal and systemic markers of inflammation in ApoE*3Leiden mice consuming a high-fat diet. Br J Nutr: 1–9.

44. Kang JH, Yun SI, Park HO (2010) Effects of Lactobacillus gasseri BNR17 on body weight and adipose tissue mass in diet-induced overweight rats. J Microbiol 48: 712–714. doi: 10.1007/s12275-010-0363-8

45. Naito E, Yoshida Y, Makino K, Kounoshi Y, Kunihiro S, et al. (2011) Beneficial effect of oral administration of Lactobacillus casei strain Shirota on insulin resistance in diet-induced obesity mice. J Appl Microbiol 110: 650–657. doi: 10.1111/j.1365-2672.2010.04922.x

46. Axling U, Olsson C, Xu J, Fernandez C, Larsson S, et al. (2012) Green tea powder and Lactobacillus plantarum affect gut microbiota, lipid metabolism and inflammation in high-fat fed C57BL/6J mice. Nutr Metab (Lond) 9: 105. doi: 10.1186/1743-7075-9-105

47. Fak F, Backhed F (2012) Lactobacillus reuteri prevents diet-induced obesity, but not atherosclerosis, in a strain dependent fashion in Apoe$^{-/-}$ Mice. PLoS One 7: e46837. doi: 10.1371/journal.pone.0046837

48. Million M, Maraninchi M, Henry M, Armougom F, Richet H, et al. (2012) Obesity-associated gut microbiota is enriched in Lactobacillus reuteri and depleted in Bifido-

bacterium animalis and Methanobrevibacter smithii. Int J Obes (Lond) 36: 817–825. doi: 10.1038/ijo.2011.153

49. Million M, Angelakis E, Maraninchi M, Henry M, Giorgi R, et al.. (2013) Correlation between body mass index and gut concentrations of Lactobacillus reuteri, Bifidobacterium animalis, Methanobrevibacter smithii and Escherichia coli. Int J Obes (Lond).

50. Frese SA, Benson AK, Tannock GW, Loach DM, Kim J, et al. (2011) The evolution of host specialization in the vertebrate gut symbiont Lactobacillus reuteri. PLoS Genet 7: e1001314. doi: 10.1371/journal.pgen.1001314

51. Walter J, Britton RA, Roos S (2011) Host-microbial symbiosis in the vertebrate gastrointestinal tract and the Lactobacillus reuteri paradigm. Proc Natl Acad Sci U S A 108 Suppl 14645–4652. doi: 10.1073/pnas.1000099107

52. Levkovich T, Poutahidis T, Smillie C, Varian BJ, Ibrahim YM, et al. (2013) Probiotic bacteria induce a 'glow of health'. PLoS One 8: e53867. doi: 10.1371/journal.pone.0053867

53. Tauber M, Mantoulan C, Copet P, Jauregui J, Demeer G, et al. (2011) Oxytocin may be useful to increase trust in others and decrease disruptive behaviours in patients with Prader-Willi syndrome: a randomised placebo-controlled trial in 24 patients. Orphanet J Rare Dis 6: 47. doi: 10.1186/1750-1172-6-47

54. Camerino C (2009) Low sympathetic tone and obese phenotype in oxytocin-deficient mice. Obesity (Silver Spring) 17: 980–984. doi: 10.1038/oby.2009.12

55. Erdman SE, Poutahidis T, Tomczak M, Rogers AB, Cormier K, et al. (2003) CD4+ CD25+ regulatory T lymphocytes inhibit microbially induced colon cancer in Rag2-deficient mice. Am J Pathol 162: 691–702. doi: 10.1016/S0002-9440(10)63863-1

56. Erdman SE, Sohn JJ, Rao VP, Nambiar PR, Ge Z, et al. (2005) CD4+CD25+ regulatory lymphocytes induce regression of intestinal tumors in ApcMin/+ mice. Cancer Res 65: 3998–4004. doi: 10.1158/0008-5472.CAN-04-3104

57. Gounaris E, Blatner NR, Dennis K, Magnusson F, Gurish MF, et al. (2009) T-regulatory cells shift from a protective anti-inflammatory to a cancer-promoting proinflammatory phenotype in polyposis. Cancer Res 69: 5490–5497. doi: 10.1158/0008-5472.CAN-09-0304

58. Salama P, Phillips M, Grieu F, Morris M, Zeps N, et al. (2009) Tumor-infiltrating FOXP3+ T regulatory cells show strong prognostic significance in colorectal cancer. J Clin Oncol 27: 186–192. doi: 10.1200/JCO.2008.18.7229

59. Kullberg MC, Jankovic D, Feng CG, Hue S, Gorelick PL, et al. (2006) IL-23 plays a key role in Helicobacter hepaticus-induced T cell-dependent colitis. J Exp Med 203: 2485–2494. doi: 10.1084/jem.20061082

60. Rook GA (2009) Review series on helminths, immune modulation and the hygiene hypothesis: the broader implications of the hygiene hypothesis. Immunology 126: 3–11. doi: 10.1111/j.1365-2567.2008.03007.x

61. Chang SH, Chung Y, Dong C (2010) Vitamin D suppresses Th17 cytokine production by inducing C/EBP homologous protein (CHOP) expression. J Biol Chem 285: 38751–38755. doi: 10.1074/jbc.C110.185777

62. Maslowski KM, Mackay CR (2011) Diet, gut microbiota and immune responses. Nat Immunol 12: 5–9. doi: 10.1038/ni0111-5

63. Litonjua AA, Weiss ST (2007) Is vitamin D deficiency to blame for the asthma epidemic? J Allergy Clin Immunol 120: 1031–1035. doi: 10.1016/j.jaci.2007.08.028

64. Harris DM, Go VL (2004) Vitamin D and colon carcinogenesis. J Nutr 134: 3463S–3471S.

65. Muegge BD, Kuczynski J, Knights D, Clemente JC, Gonzalez A, et al. (2011) Diet drives convergence in gut microbiome functions across mammalian phylogeny and within humans. Science 332: 970–974. doi: 10.1126/science.1198719

66. Faith JJ, McNulty NP, Rey FE, Gordon JI (2011) Predicting a human gut microbiota's response to diet in gnotobiotic mice. Science 333: 101–104. doi: 10.1126/science.1206025

67. Caporaso JG, Lauber CL, Walters WA, Berg-Lyons D, Lozupone CA, et al. (2011) Global patterns of 16S rRNA diversity at a depth of millions of sequences per sample. Proc Natl Acad Sci U S A 108 Suppl 14516–4522. doi: 10.1073/pnas.1000080107

There are several supplemental files that are not available in this version of the article. To view this additional information, please use the citation information cited on the first page of this chapter.

INCREASED GUT PERMEABILITY AND MICROBIOTA CHANGE ASSOCIATE WITH MESENTERIC FAT INFLAMMATION AND METABOLIC DYSFUNCTION IN DIET-INDUCED OBESE MICE

YAN Y. LAM, CONNIE W. Y. HA, CRAIG R. CAMPBELL, ANDREW J. MITCHELL, ANUWAT DINUDOM, JAN OSCARSSON, DAVID I. COOK, NICHOLAS H. HUNT, IAN D. CATERSON, ANDREW J. HOLMES, AND LEN H. STORLIEN

4.1 INTRODUCTION

Visceral adiposity is strongly related to metabolic dysfunction including insulin resistance and systemic inflammation [1]–[3]. The deleterious metabolic effect of visceral fat is a consequence, in large part, of increased production of pro-inflammatory cytokines [4]. Adipose-derived immune factors primarily originate from cells in the stromal-vascular fraction of fat depots [5], [6]. Specifically, macrophage infiltration has been identified as a major determinant of the metabolic effect of adipose tissue. The abundance of macrophages in visceral fat was negatively correlated with

This chapter was originally published under the Creative Commons Attribution License. Lam YY, Ha CWY, Campbell CR, Mitchell AJ, Dinudom A, Oscarsson J, Cook DI, Hunt NH, Caterson ID, Holmes AJ, and Storlien LH. Increased Gut Permeability and Microbiota Change Associate with Mesenteric Fat Inflammation and Metabolic Dysfunction in Diet-Induced Obese Mice. PLoS ONE 7,3 (2012). doi:10.1371/journal.pone.0034233.

insulin sensitivity of obese individuals, whereas no such relationship was observed with subcutaneous fat [7]. The primary driver of the macrophage infiltration and pro-inflammatory profile of visceral fat, however, remains largely unknown.

Evidence is now persuasive that the gut may play an important role in inducing adipose inflammation and metabolic disorders. In patients with Crohn's disease, the inflamed gut is associated with an expanded mesenteric fat depot characterized by an increased infiltration of immune cells [8]. A causal relationship between gut inflammation and mesenteric fat dysfunction (notably a relative expansion in size and an increase in expression of macrophages and immune factors) has been demonstrated in animal models of experimental colitis [9], [10]. Impaired gut barrier function, along with gut inflammation, have also been observed in both genetic [11] and dietary [12], [13] models of obesity.

Finally, there is an emerging body of literature demonstrating an association between altered gut microbiota profile and obesity in humans (see [14] and [15] for a recent review) which, from pioneering work on rodents [12], [16], [17], appears to be causative. The cross-linkage between gut microbiota, metabolic dysfunction and the immune system is best illustrated in Toll-like receptor-5 knockout mice which develop spontaneous colitis, insulin resistance, hyperlipidemia and increased visceral fat deposition [18]. Importantly, all of these deleterious effects can be ameliorated by antibiotic administration, implicating gut microbiota change as causative and suggesting a feedback loop from the innate immune system to gut inflammation and microbiota profile.

Taken together the case can be made, see [19], that obesogenic diets induce gut dysfunction, which may lead to the stimulation of contiguous fat by an adverse microbial load and subsequently results in visceral fat inflammation and systemic metabolic dysregulation.

The aim of the present study, therefore, was to characterize the relationship between gut health, visceral fat dysfunction and metabolic dysregulation in diet-induced obese mice. We showed that a prolonged high saturated fat feeding induced inflammation and impaired barrier function in the gut which associated with specific alterations in microbiota profile. This, together with a distinct pro-inflammatory nature of the mesenteric fat contiguous with the gut but not of depots more remote, implicates the gut in the genesis of visceral adipose inflammation and systemic metabolic dysfunction.

4.2 METHODS

4.2.1 ETHICS STATEMENT

All procedures were approved by the University of Sydney Animal Ethics Committee (approval number K00/2-2010/3/5225).

4.2.2 ANIMALS

Female C57BL/6J mice were obtained from the Australian Animal Resources Centre (Perth, Australia), group-housed (2–4 mice per cage) and kept with regulated temperature (18–22°C) and humidity (~50%) with a 12 h light/dark cycle. Starting at 16 weeks of age, the mice were fed either a control (10% kcal from fat) or a high saturated fat diet (HFD; 60% kcal from fat, of which 34% was saturated fat) ad libitum with free access to water for 8 or 12 weeks. For each mouse fresh stools (1 pellet per day) were collected on 3 consecutive days in the week before termination for gut microbiota profiling. At termination mice were anesthetized after a 4 h fast. Blood was taken by heart puncture and serum was stored at −80°C. After flushing with ice-cold bicarbonate buffer [20], segments of proximal colon (immediately below the cecum) were taken for assessment of gut permeability and gene expression (see below). Mesenteric, epididymal, perirenal and subcutaneous fat samples were taken for immunohistochemical staining and gene expression analysis, as was liver for the latter measurements.

4.2.3 BIOCHEMICAL ANALYSES

Blood glucose was measured using a glucometer (Accu-Chek Performa, Roche, Mannheim, Germany). Serum concentrations of insulin, adiponectin and serum amyloid A3 were measured using assays from Millipore

(Billerica, MA, USA). Liver was homogenized in isopropanol. Liver triglycerides and serum concentrations of alanine transaminase and triglycerides were measured using kits from Horiba ABX (Montpellier, France) and the assays were performed on the ABX Pentra 400 (Horiba ABX). Serum concentrations of interleukin (IL)-1β, IL-10, monocyte chemotactic protein (MCP)-1, tumor necrosis factor (TNF)-α, IL-6, IL-12p40 and plasminogen activator inhibitor (PAI)-1 were determined using commercially available cytokine kits and the xMAP® technology (Luminex Corporation, Austin, TX, USA). The data were analyzed with a four- or five-parametric curve fitting using the Bio-Plex Manager Software (version 5.0, Life Science Research, Hercules, CA, USA).

4.2.4 ASSESSMENT OF GUT PERMEABILITY

Gut permeability was measured as described by Wang et al [21] with minor modifications. The segments of proximal colon for gut permeability measurement were opened along the mesenteric border and mounted in the Ussing chamber with an aperture of 0.3 cm^2. The chamber was connected to a VCC MC6 amplifier, controlled and monitored using the Acquire & Analyze software (V2.3.177 Physiologic Instruments, San Diego, CA, USA). Experiments were carried out under current-clamp (open-circuit) conditions as described previously [22]. Segments of colon were incubated in oxygenated (95% O$_2$; 5% CO$_2$) bicarbonate buffer at 37°C [20]. Tissue was equilibrated for 15 min, thereafter a 3 μA current pulse was applied across the intestinal wall every 6 sec for 30 min. The transepithelial potential was measured and recorded by the Acquire & Analyze software, and the change in potential induced by the current pulse was used to calculate transepithelial resistance according to Ohm's Law.

4.2.5 QUANTITATIVE REAL-TIME PCR

RNA was extracted from homogenized tissue using TRI reagent (Sigma-Aldrich, St Louis, MO, USA) and isolated by phenol/chloroform extraction. Total RNA (200 ng) was reverse transcribed to cDNA using BioScript™ (Bioline, London, UK) and random hexamers (Applied Biosystems, Carlsbad, CA, USA). Primer sequences for sterol regulatory element binding protein (SREBP)-1c [23], peroxisome proliferator-activated receptor (PPAR)-γ [23], proglucagon [24], zona occludens (ZO)-1 [25], occludin [26] and IL-10 [27] have been published elsewhere. Primers for SCD1, TNF-α and IL-6 were purchased from Qiagen (Valencia, CA, USA). mRNA expression was quantified by RT-qPCR using the Rotorgene™ 3000 Real Time Thermal Cycler (Qiagen). Fluorescence data were analyzed using the Rotor-Gene 6 software (version 6.0, Qiagen). mRNA expression was normalized to RPL-19 [24], UBC [28] and 18S rRNA [29] for colon, adipose tissue and liver respectively and reported as arbitrary units.

4.2.6 IMMUNOHISTOCHEMICAL STAINING

Fat samples were fixed in formalin overnight and embedded in paraffin. Sections of 10 µm thickness were treated with 10 µg/ml proteinase K (Sigma-Aldrich) at room temperature for antigen retrieval. Endogenous peroxidase and biotin signals were minimized using 0.3% (v/v) hydrogen peroxide and avidin/biotin block (Dako, Glostrup, Denmark) respectively. After incubating with 10% (v/v) normal horse serum to reduce non-specific staining, sections were incubated with purified anti-mouse F4/80 antibody (BioLegend, San Diego, CA, USA) for 1 h and subsequently with biotinylated rabbit anti-rat IgG antibody (Vector Laboratories, Burlingame, CA, USA) for 30 min at room temperature. The expression of F4/80 was detected using the VECTASTAIN® ABC Kit (Vector Laboratories) and the Liquid DAB+ Substrate Chromogen System (Dako). All sections were counterstained with hematoxylin. F4/80$^+$ cells were quantified by counting the number of adipocytes and F4/80$^+$ cells in 10 random areas at ×40 magnification and the abundance of F4/80$^+$ cells was normalized to 100 adipocytes [30]. Adipocyte size was determined by averaging the cross-sectional area of 5 adipocytes of each of the 10 selected ×40 magnification field using ImageJ (version 1.44p, National Institutes of Health, MD, USA).

4.2.7 GUT MICROBIOTA PROFILING

For each mouse three stool pellets (one per day) were pooled and homogenized in TE buffer (pH 7.5). DNA was extracted from 0.5 ml of homogenate using a bead beating method as described previously [31] and stored at −20°C. Metagenomic DNA (>500 ng from each mouse) was sent to Research and Testing Laboratories (Lubbock, USA) for bacterial tag-encoded FLX amplicon pyrosequencing (bTEFAP) of the V6–V9 region of the 16S rDNA. Modified versions of primers F939 (5′TTGAC-GGGGGCCCGCAC3′) and R1492 (5′ATTAGATACCCNGGTAG3′) incorporating domains for 454 sequencing and unique identification tags were used to allow the identification of sequences from individual sample. Amplicons were sequenced on a GS Pico Titer Plate using the Roche 454 FLX instrument with corresponding FLX titanium reagents (Roche Applied Science, Indianapolis, IN, USA).

bTEFAP raw data were processed using Mothur [32] unless stated otherwise. Parameters used to filter sequences for analysis were based upon published studies [33], [34]. Briefly, sequences from the raw 454 data were quality-filtered to exclude those with an average Phred score <30. Remaining sequence reads were binned into individual sample sets by the unique tags with sequences >200 nucleotides in length (excluding primers and tags) retained. The sequences were then screened to remove chimeras using chimera slayer within Mothur to give a final set of quality-filtered sequence reads for each sample. Taxonomic classifications were assigned using the naïve Bayesian algorithm with the Ribosomal Database Project (RDP) Training Set 6 as a reference database. No new data were generated from DNA sequencing. Nomenclature of all bacterial identification was based on Bergey's taxonomic outline. Within each sample the number of sequences for each bacterial taxonomic assignment is expressed as a percentage of the total reads retained after quality-filtering (relative abundance). To quantify the coverage and sampling effort of bTEFAP, RDP pyrosequencing pipeline was used to generate rarefaction curves of the sequences.

4.2.8 STATISTICAL ANALYSIS

Data are expressed as means ± SEM. Student's t-test, one-way or two-way ANOVA were used to compare data from different treatment groups. Corrections of p-values for multiple testing were performed using Bonferroni post hoc tests. Relationships between selected outcome variables were examined by Pearson's correlation. Statistical analyses were performed using the GraphPad Prism Program (version 5.01, GraphPad Software Inc., San Diego, CA, USA). Significance was accepted at $P<0.05$.

4.3 RESULTS

4.3.1 HIGH SATURATED FAT DIET INDUCED WEIGHT GAIN, SYSTEMIC INSULIN RESISTANCE AND INFLAMMATION

By the end of the 8- and 12-week feeding protocols, the body weights of HFD mice were 22% and 36% higher respectively than animals fed the control diet (27.3±0.7 g vs 22.4±0.5 g for controls; $P<0.001$ at 8 weeks and 30.1±1.1 g vs 22.2±0.4 g for controls; $P<0.001$ at 12 weeks). Eight and 12 week results were not different for all other outcome variables and were therefore combined for analyses. HFD mice had a higher insulin/glucose ratio (1.4-fold; $P = 0.020$; insulin 91.1±8.8 pmol/l vs 56.8±6.8 pmol/l for controls; glucose 10.9±0.3 mmol/l vs 9.4±0.5 mmol/l for controls) as a marker of insulin resistance (Figure 1A). Circulating levels of the acute phase inflammatory marker serum amyloid A3 were 2.3-fold ($P = 0.008$; Figure 1B) higher in HFD mice, but in contrast, those of adiponectin were decreased by 36% ($P = 0.011$; Figure 1C). Serum concentrations of tri-glycerides, IL-1β, IL-10, MCP-1, TNF-α, IL-6, IL-12p40 and PAI-1 were not different between the diet groups (data not shown).

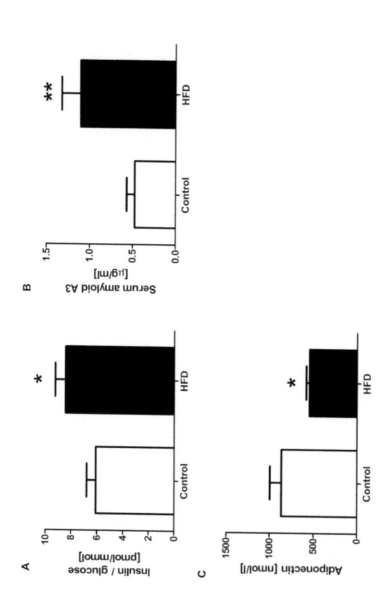

FIGURE 1: Serum biochemical analyses. Insulin/glucose ratio (A), concentrations of serum amyloid A3 (B) and adiponectin (C) in control and high saturated fat diet (HFD) fed mice (n = 15–16 per group). Data are shown as mean ± SEM. **P<0.01 and *P<0.05 compared to control.

A

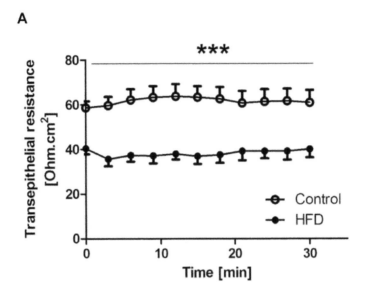

B

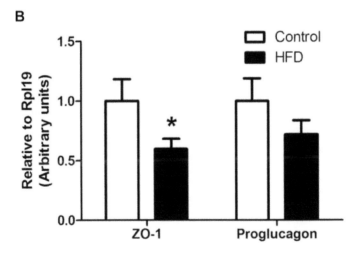

FIGURE 2: Effect of high saturated fat diet (HFD) on barrier function of proximal colon. A: Transepithelial resistance of mouse proximal colon was determined in the Ussing chamber by measuring the change in potential difference in response to 3 μA current generated across the tissue segment. B: mRNA levels of zona occludens (ZO)-1 and proglucagon were measured using RT-qPCR. Gene expression was normalized to RPL-19. Open circles/ bars = control; Closed circles/bars = HFD (n = 9–16 per group). Data are shown as mean ± SEM. ***P<0.001 and *P<0.05 compared to control.

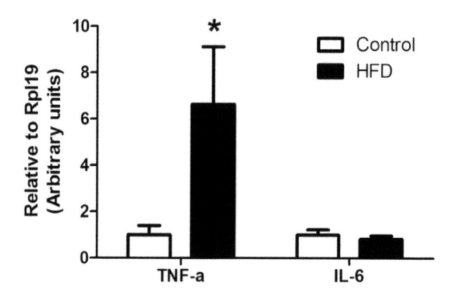

FIGURE 3: Effect of high saturated fat diet (HFD) on markers of inflammation in proximal colon. mRNA expression of indicated genes was measured by RT-qPCR as described in Figure 2. Open bars = control; Closed bars = HFD (n = 11–16 per group). Data are shown as mean ± SEM. *P<0.05 compared to control.

4.3.2 HIGH SATURATED FAT DIET INCREASED GUT PERMEABILITY AND INFLAMMATION

In the proximal colon, transepithelial resistance of HFD mice was reduced by 38% (37.4±2.6 Ohm.cm^2 vs 60.8±4.5 Ohm.cm^2 for controls; P<0.001; Figure 2A) as compared to controls. mRNA expression of ZO-1 and pro-glucagon were also reduced by 40% (P = 0.025) and 28% (P = 0.104) respectively in HFD mice (Figure 2B), whereas the mRNA levels of occlu-din were not different between the diet groups (data not shown). The colon tissue of the HFD treatment group had increased mRNA expression of TNF-α by 6.6-fold (P = 0.037) but that of IL-6 was unchanged (Figure 3).

4.3.3 HIGH SATURATED FAT DIET ALTERED GUT MICROBIOTA PROFILE

After quality-filtering a total of 246,694 sequences were obtained from 16 control and 16 HFD mice with a mean of 7,709 sequences per mouse (range 1,758–15,005; Table S1). The average number of reads for the control diet sample series was higher than that from HFD, however rarefaction analysis showed that taxonomic richness had plateaued in all samples at higher taxon level. Rarefaction curves at 95% sequence identity, considered to approximate genus level, showed that the rate of sampling was comparable across all samples and demonstrated sampling depth at this taxonomic resolution was comparable to previously reported studies (Figure S1) [35]–[37]. At the phylum level, HFD mice had more *Firmicutes* (73±1.5% vs 68±2.3% for controls; P = 0.041) and fewer *Bacteroidetes* (15±1.7% vs 19±1.3% for controls; P = 0.026) and thus a significantly higher *Firmicutes: Bacteroidetes* ratio (P = 0.019). HFD also induced significant shifts in fecal microbiota composition at the genus level of taxonomic resolution. Within members of the *Firmicutes*, notably there was a 75% decrease in *Lactobacillus* (P<0.001) and a 279% increase in *Oscillibacter* (P = 0.004) as compared to controls and these changes in abundance were closely associated with weight gain (Figure 4).

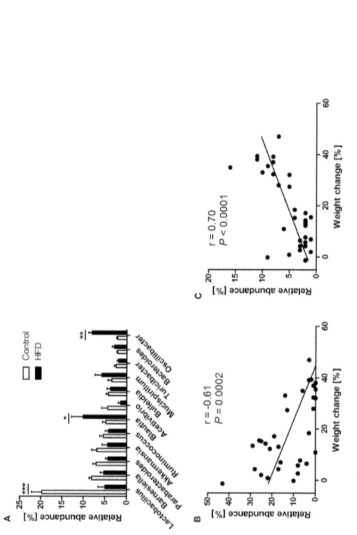

FIGURE 4: Gut microbiota composition in control and high saturated fat diet (HFD) fed mice. A: Relative abundance of main genera in fecal samples from control (open bars) and HFD (closed bars) mice (n = 16 per group). Data are shown as mean ± SEM. ***P<0.001, ** P<0.01 and *P<0.05 compared to control. Correlations between the abundance of *Lactobacillus* (B) and *Oscillibacter* (C) and weight changes. Gut microbiota profile was determined by metagenomic pyrosequencing from bacterial lineages in fecal samples.

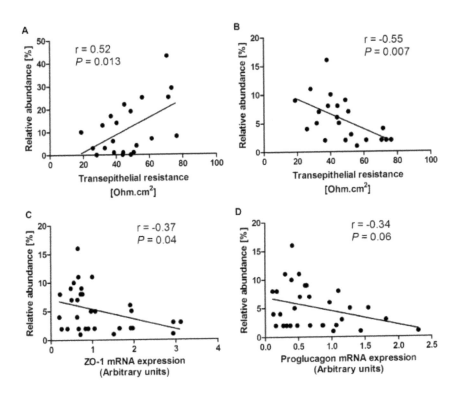

FIGURE 5: Correlations between *Lactobacillus* (A) and *Oscillibacter* (B–D) abundances and permeability parameters in proximal colon. Gut microbiota profile was determined as described in Figure 4 (n = 22–31). Transepithelia resistance and mRNA expression of zona occludens (ZO)-1 and proglucagon in proximal colon were measured as described in Figure 3.

Transepithelial resistance of the proximal colon was positively correlated with the abundance of *Lactobacillus* ($r = 0.52$; $P = 0.013$; Figure 5A) but negatively correlated with that of *Oscillibacter* ($r = -0.55$; $P = 0.007$; Figure 5B). Notably, increased *Oscillibacter* abundance was also associated with a reduction in the mRNA expression of ZO-1 ($r = -0.37$; $P = 0.039$; Figure 5C) and, although not statistically significant, a similar trend was observed with proglucagon ($r = -0.34$; $P = 0.061$; Figure 5D).

4.3.4 HIGH SATURATED FAT DIET INDUCED DEPOT-SPECIFIC INFLAMMATION AND ALTERED MORPHOLOGY IN ADIPOSE TISSUE

Representative immunohistochemical staining of the macrophage marker F4/80 in adipose tissue of control and HFD mice is shown in Figure 6A. The abundance of macrophages (F4/80+ cells) was similar across all fat depots in the control mice. HFD increased macrophage infiltration in mesenteric (58%; $P = 0.020$) and epididymal (71%; $P = 0.006$) fat but was without effect in perirenal and subcutaneous fat (Figure 6B). HFD increased adipocyte size in mesenteric (80%; $P<0.001$), epididymal (57%; $P = 0.008$), perirenal (104%; $P = 0.007$) and subcutaneous (103%; $P = 0.008$) fat (Figure 6C). In both diet groups, mesenteric fat was the depot with the smallest adipocytes (Figure 6C).

Compared to controls, HFD induced a 2.5-fold increase in the mRNA levels of both TNF-α ($P<0.001$; Figure 7A) and IL-6 ($P = 0.008$; Figure 7B) in the mesenteric fat. This depot had by far the highest expression of TNF-α and IL-6 in mice fed the control diet, with expression levels being very low, and unaffected by HFD, in epididymal, perirenal and subcutaneous depots (Figures 7A and B). HFD had no effect on the mRNA expression of SREBP-1c and PPAR-γ in adipose tissue. In both diet groups, the highest expression of PPAR-γ ($P<0.001$; Figure 7C) and SREBP-1c ($P = 0.003$; Figure 7D) were found in mesenteric and epididymal fat respectively.

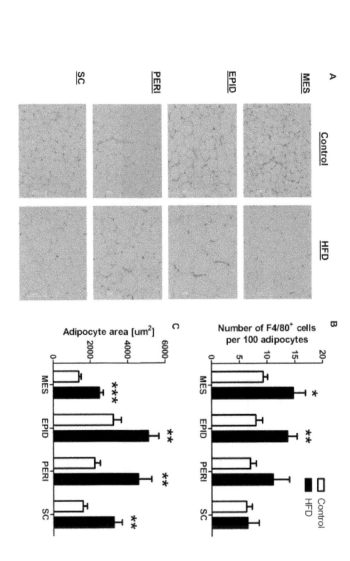

FIGURE 6: Effect of high saturated fat diet (HFD) on adipose macrophage infiltration and adipocyte size. A: Representative immunohistochemical staining of mesenteric (MES), epididymal (EPID), perirenal (PERI) and subcutaneous (SC) fat. Quantification of macrophage (F4/80+) infiltration (B) and adipocyte size (C). Tissues were fixed in formalin and embedded in paraffin. Sections were stained for F4/80 and counterstained with hematoxylin. Open bars = control; Closed bars = HFD (n = 4–10 per group). Data are shown as mean ± SEM. ***P<0.001, **P<0.01 and *P<0.05 compared to control.

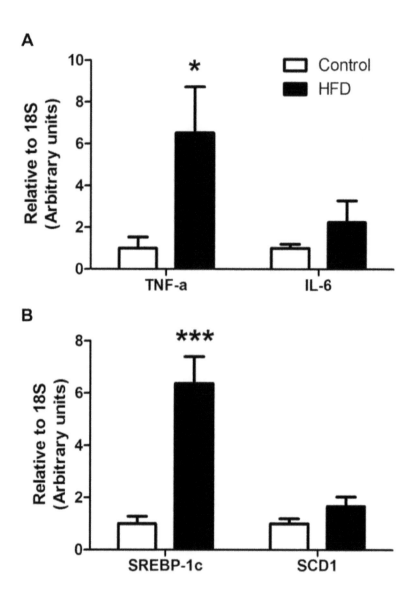

FIGURE 8: mRNA expression of genes involved in inflammation (A) and lipogenesis (B) in liver. mRNA levels of TNF-α, IL-6, SREBP-1c and SCD1 in control and high saturated fat diet (HFD) fed mice were measured using RT-qPCR. Gene expression was normalized to 18S. Open bars = control; Closed bars = HFD (n = 14–16 per group). Data are shown as mean ± SEM. ***P<0.001 and *P<0.05 compared to control.

4.3.5 HIGH SATURATED FAT DIET LED TO A PRO-INFLAMMATORY AND LIPOGENIC LIVER

As shown in Figure 8A, HFD-fed mice tended to have higher expression of pro-inflammatory factors in the liver, as evidenced by the increased TNF-α (6.5-fold; P = 0.018) and IL-6 (2.2-fold; P = 0.137) mRNA expression. Hepatic SREBP-1c (6.4-fold; P<0.001) and SCD1 (1.7-fold; P = 0.069) mRNA levels were also trended to be elevated in HFD mice (Figure 8B).

4.4 DISCUSSION

The present study aimed to determine the effect of a high, predominantly saturated, fat diet (HFD) on gut health and its relationship with metabolic dysfunction. HFD mice exhibited systemic inflammation, whole-body insulin resistance and liver inflammation. We showed that HFD increased gut permeability and altered gut microbiota profile. Importantly, we demonstrated a relationship between gut barrier function and the abundance of specific genera of the microbial community. Together with the evidence of inflammation in the proximal colon and the distinct pro-inflammatory nature of the contiguous mesenteric, but not other fat depots, the present results highlight gut dysfunction as a salient feature of diet-induced metabolic dysregulation.

Our data suggest that HFD initiates metabolic changes that impaired gut barrier function, as evidenced both by the decrease in transepithelial resistance and mRNA expression of ZO-1 in the proximal colon. Similar outcomes for other obesogenic diets on gut barrier function have also been reported. Cani et al [12] showed an increase in whole-gut permeability in HFD mice, an effect associated with a reduction in mRNA expression of tight-junction proteins including ZO-1. Little is known, however, about the barrier integrity of functionally distinct regions of the intestine in diet-induced models of obesity. The present study focused directly on the proximal colon, which is the part of the gut predicted to have the most intense microbial activity. Accordingly, loss of barrier integrity in the proximal colon has the potential to induce a disproportionate effect of gut microbiota on systemic metabolism.

The increased permeability of the proximal colon is postulated to participate in a feedback loop with inflammatory processes. In our study, and others using obesogenic diets, mice in the experimental groups had increased TNF-α mRNA expression [37] in the intestine. In an experimental model of colitis, the progressive increase in colonic permeability is associated with a corresponding reduction in ZO-1 protein expression [38]. There is also some evidence suggesting a direct effect of TNF-α on gut barrier integrity. Anti-TNF-α treatment improves gut barrier function in patients with Crohn's disease [39]. In Caco-2 cell cultures, TNF-α reduced transepithelial resistance and ZO-1 protein expression via a NFκB-dependent pathway [40]. The effect of TNF-α on NFκB activation also increased the expression and activity of myosin light chain kinase, which subsequently leads to disorganization of tight-junction proteins at the intestinal barrier [41]. It is worth noting that other cytokines upstream of NFκB, including IL-1β [42] and IFN-γ [43], also have been shown to decrease tight-junction function. The collective role of inflammatory pathways, rather than individual cytokines, therefore, appears to be critical in the regulation of gut barrier function.

The activity of the microbiota is a major determinant of gut health and a "poor" microbiota composition has been linked to obesity and metabolic dysfunction [44]. The shift in the ratio of *Firmicutes* and *Bacteroidetes* by obesogenic diets has been frequently reported, but not universally so. Here we observed a small, but significant shift towards an increased *Firmicutes: Bacteroidetes* ratio in the HFD mice. The most startling microbiota changes were observed within the *Firmicutes*, with a very strong association between changes in relative abundance of *Lactobacillus* and *Oscillibacter* and the two diet groups. Members of the genus *Lactobacillus* have been intensively investigated for probiotic properties and several strains have been shown to ameliorate gut inflammation [45] and enhance barrier function [46] in experimental models of gut dysfunction. A novel finding here is the positive correlation between the abundance of the indigenous *Lactobacillus* community (i.e. not administered probiotic strains) and barrier function of the proximal colon. However we did not observe a significant correlation between *Lactobacillus* content and mRNA expression of tight-junction proteins. The effect of probiotic *Lactobacillus* strains on tight-junction integrity is not entirely clear and appears to be strain-specific [47], [48]. In humans, administration of *L. plantarum* promoted localization of ZO-1 and occludin in the tight-junctions without necessarily affecting their transcriptional levels [49]. It is worth noting that the beneficial effect of *Lactobacillus* on gut health may not be restricted to the maintenance of barrier integrity, as there is some evidence suggesting that certain strains may alter the expression of defensin, an anti-microbial peptide, which is important for mucosal protection [50], [51].

The present study identified *Oscillibacter*-like organisms as a potentially important gut microbe that mediates HFD-induced gut dysfunction. This group, including *Oscillibacter* and *Oscillospira*, are very poorly represented in culture collections but have been consistently detected in the microbial community of humans [52], [53]. Recent data suggest that the abundance of *Oscillibacter* is diet-responsive in obese individuals [54] but to date little is known about its physiological role. The negative correlation between the abundance of *Oscillibacter* and parameters of barrier function in the proximal colon is intriguing. There is some in vitro evidence suggesting that metabolites from other gut microbes may modify the abundance of certain strains of *Oscillibacter* [55]. It is possible that *Oscillibacter* directly regulates components involved in the maintenance of gut barrier integrity, or its relationship with gut permeability may be a secondary effect consequent upon alterations in the overall composition of the microbial community. Characterization of the metabolic effect of *Oscillibacter* as well as its interactions with other microbes would be critical to elucidate its role in diet-induced metabolic dysfunctions.

We identified mesenteric fat as a metabolically distinct visceral fat depot with the most prominent pro-inflammatory nature. Our data showed that mesenteric fat has the highest mRNA expression of PPAR-γ and the smallest adipocyte size. This is in contrast to epididymal fat which had the biggest adipocytes and the highest mRNA content of SREBP-1c, a transcription factor that promotes lipogenesis. HFD mice had increased expression of TNF-α and IL-6 and macrophage infiltration in mesenteric fat [13], [56] and the role of TNF-α in the systemic dysmetabolism may be particularly critical [57]. Similar trends of depot-specific differences in the expression of pro-inflammatory cytokines have been reported previously in animal models of high-fat feeding [58], [59].

A range of non-adipocytes cells are known to contribute strongly to the pro-inflammatory secretory profile of adipose tissue [6]. Interestingly, the HFD-induced increase in macrophage infiltration was similar in mesenteric and epididymal fat, and yet only the former had a distinctly elevated expression of pro-inflammatory cytokines. A limitation of our study is that we used only F4/80 as a macrophage marker, which did not allow us to distinguish sub-populations of macrophages. The increased transcriptional expression of pro-inflammatory factors in the mesenteric fat may be a consequence of the preferential infiltration of macrophages with a pro-inflammatory phenotype [60]. Equally, the presence of lymph nodes in mesenteric [61], but not epididymal, fat implies that immune cells other than macrophages, e.g. B-cells, T-cells and Natural Killer cells, are likely to contribute to the secretory function of the mesenteric depot.

The increased macrophage infiltration and TNF-α expression in mesenteric fat of our HFD mice is consistent with results in rats with induced gut inflammation [9] and is likely to be a consequence of the 'leakage' of gut luminal content. Cenac et al [62] demonstrated the sequential occurrences of gut inflammation, impaired barrier function and bacterial translocation to the mesenteric lymph nodes in an experimental model of colitis. Similar metabolic sequelae of gut inflammation in obesity are yet to be reported. However, the recent report of bacterial translocation into the mesenteric fat of HFD mice [63] and of elevated circulating endotoxin levels in animal models of diet-induced obesity [12] and in obese and type 2 diabetic patients related to insulin resistance [64], [65] are consistent with our hypothesized role of the gut in metabolic dysfunction [19].

Mechanistic studies will be an important extension of the current work. We, and others, have shown that an obesogenic diet can induce gut dysfunction involving multiple feedbacks with immune and metabolic regulation. It remains unclear whether HFD-induced gut dysfunction is a specific effect of fatty acid subtype (e.g. saturated fatty acids are known to be pro-inflammatory) or is merely a consequence of energy overload. Elucidating the sequence of factors that initiates gut dysfunction will be important for the maintenance of optimal metabolic health. From the disease treatment perspective, the interactions and feedback mechanisms between the innate immune system and the microbiota profile and their effect on metabolic outcomes [18] imply that a combination of pharmaceutical interventions of immunomodulators (e.g. pro-resolving mediators that are critical in maintaining immunological homeostasis of mucosal surface [66]) and manipulation of microbiota (e.g. dietary supplementation of prebiotics, probiotics and resistant starches) may be novel gut-targeted approaches to ameliorate metabolic dysfunctions.

In summary, the current findings build on a literature now becoming compelling that the gut is a central player in the aetiology of diet-induced metabolic diseases.

REFERENCES

1. Miyazaki Y, Glass L, Triplitt C, Wajcberg E, Mandarino LJ, et al. (2002) Abdominal fat distribution and peripheral and hepatic insulin resistance in type 2 diabetes mellitus. Am J Physiol Endocrinol Metab 283: E1135–1143.
2. Sam S, Haffner S, Davidson MH, D'Agostino RB Sr, Feinstein S, et al. (2009) Relation of abdominal fat depots to systemic markers of inflammation in type 2 diabetes. Diabetes Care 32: 932–937.
3. Barbarroja N, Lopez-Pedrera R, Mayas MD, Garcia-Fuentes E, Garrido-Sanchez L, et al. (2010) The obese healthy paradox: is inflammation the answer? Biochem J 430: 141–149.
4. Lam YY, Janovska A, McAinch AJ, Belobrajdic DP, Hatzinikolas G, et al. (2011) The use of adipose tissue-conditioned media to demonstrate the differential effects of fat depots on insulin-stimulated glucose uptake in a skeletal muscle cell line. Obes Res Clin Pract 5: e43–e54.
5. Fain JN, Madan AK, Hiler ML, Cheema P, Bahouth SW (2004) Comparison of the release of adipokines by adipose tissue, adipose tissue matrix, and adipocytes from visceral and subcutaneous abdominal adipose tissues of obese humans. Endocrinology 145: 2273–2282.
6. Fain JN (2010) Release of inflammatory mediators by human adipose tissue is enhanced in obesity and primarily by the nonfat cells: a review. Mediators Inflamm 2010: 513948.
7. Cancello R, Tordjman J, Poitou C, Guilhem G, Bouillot JL, et al. (2006) Increased infiltration of macrophages in omental adipose tissue is associated with marked hepatic lesions in morbid human obesity. Diabetes 55: 1554–1561.
8. Bertin B, Desreumaux P, Dubuquoy L (2010) Obesity, visceral fat and Crohn's disease. Curr Opin Clin Nutr Metab Care 13: 574–580.
9. Thomaz MA, Acedo SC, de Oliveira CC, Pereira JA, Priolli DG, et al. (2009) Methotrexate is effective in reactivated colitis and reduces inflammatory alterations in mesenteric adipose tissue during intestinal inflammation. Pharmacol Res 60: 341–346.

10. Gambero A, Marostica M, Abdalla Saad MJ, Pedrazzoli J Jr (2007) Mesenteric adipose tissue alterations resulting from experimental reactivated colitis. Inflamm Bowel Dis 13: 1357–1364.

11. Brun P, Castagliuolo I, Di Leo V, Buda A, Pinzani M, et al. (2007) Increased intestinal permeability in obese mice: new evidence in the pathogenesis of nonalcoholic steatohepatitis. Am J Physiol Gastrointest Liver Physiol 292: G518–525.

12. Cani PD, Bibiloni R, Knauf C, Waget A, Neyrinck AM, et al. (2008) Changes in gut microbiota control metabolic endotoxemia-induced inflammation in high-fat diet-induced obesity and diabetes in mice. Diabetes 57: 1470–1481.

13. Li H, Lelliott C, Hakansson P, Ploj K, Tuneld A, et al. (2008) Intestinal, adipose, and liver inflammation in diet-induced obese mice. Metabolism 57: 1704–1710.

14. Turnbaugh PJ, Hamady M, Yatsunenko T, Cantarel BL, Duncan A, et al. (2009) A core gut microbiome in obese and lean twins. Nature 457: 480–484.

15. Diamant M, Blaak EE, de Vos WM (2011) Do nutrient-gut-microbiota interactions play a role in human obesity, insulin resistance and type 2 diabetes? Obes Rev 12: 272–281.

16. Membrez M, Blancher F, Jaquet M, Bibiloni R, Cani PD, et al. (2008) Gut microbiota modulation with norfloxacin and ampicillin enhances glucose tolerance in mice. FASEB J 22: 2416–2426.

17. Backhed F, Manchester JK, Semenkovich CF, Gordon JI (2007) Mechanisms underlying the resistance to diet-induced obesity in germ-free mice. Proc Natl Acad Sci U S A 104: 979–984.

18. Vijay-Kumar M, Aitken JD, Carvalho FA, Cullender TC, Mwangi S, et al. (2010) Metabolic syndrome and altered gut microbiota in mice lacking Toll-like receptor 5. Science 328: 228–231.

19. Lam YY, Mitchell AJ, Holmes AJ, Denyer GS, Gummesson A, et al. (2011) Role of the gut in visceral fat inflammation and metabolic disorders. Obesity (Silver Spring) 19: 2113–2120.

20. Gelbmann CM, Schteingart CD, Thompson SM, Hofmann AF, Barrett KE (1995) Mast cells and histamine contribute to bile acid-stimulated secretion in the mouse colon. J Clin Invest 95: 2831–2839.

21. Wang Q, Fang CH, Hasselgren PO (2001) Intestinal permeability is reduced and IL-10 levels are increased in septic IL-6 knockout mice. Am J Physiol Regul Integr Comp Physiol 281: R1013–1023.

22. Lee IH, Dinudom A, Sanchez-Perez A, Kumar S, Cook DI (2007) Akt mediates the effect of insulin on epithelial sodium channels by inhibiting Nedd4-2. J Biol Chem 282: 29866–29873.

23. Pachikian BD, Neyrinck AM, Cani PD, Portois L, Deldicque L, et al. (2008) Hepatic steatosis in n-3 fatty acid depleted mice: focus on metabolic alterations related to tissue fatty acid composition. BMC Physiol 8: 21.

24. Cani PD, Possemiers S, Van de Wiele T, Guiot Y, Everard A, et al. (2009) Changes in gut microbiota control inflammation in obese mice through a mechanism involving GLP-2-driven improvement of gut permeability. Gut 58: 1091–1103.

25. Holmes JL, Van Itallie CM, Rasmussen JE, Anderson JM (2006) Claudin profiling in the mouse during postnatal intestinal development and along the gastrointestinal tract reveals complex expression patterns. Gene Expr Patterns 6: 581–588.

26. Volynets V, Spruss A, Kanuri G, Wagnerberger S, Bischoff SC, et al. (2010) Protective effect of bile acids on the onset of fructose-induced hepatic steatosis in mice. J Lipid Res 51: 3414–3424.

27. Li P, Lu M, Nguyen MT, Bae EJ, Chapman J, et al. (2010) Functional heterogeneity of CD11c-positive adipose tissue macrophages in diet-induced obese mice. J Biol Chem 285: 15333–15345.

28. Zeyda M, Gollinger K, Kriehuber E, Kiefer FW, Neuhofer A, et al. (2010) Newly identified adipose tissue macrophage populations in obesity with distinct chemokine and chemokine receptor expression. Int J Obes (Lond) 34: 1684–1694.

29. Sachithanandan N, Fam BC, Fynch S, Dzamko N, Watt MJ, et al. (2010) Liver-specific suppressor of cytokine signaling-3 deletion in mice enhances hepatic insulin sensitivity and lipogenesis resulting in fatty liver and obesity. Hepatology 52: 1632–1642.

30. Aron-Wisnewsky J, Tordjman J, Poitou C, Darakhshan F, Hugol D, et al. (2009) Human adipose tissue macrophages: m1 and m2 cell surface markers in subcutaneous and omental depots and after weight loss. J Clin Endocrinol Metab 94: 4619–4623.

31. Thompson CL, Wang B, Holmes AJ (2008) The immediate environment during postnatal development has long-term impact on gut community structure in pigs. ISME J 2: 739–748.

32. Schloss PD, Westcott SL, Ryabin T, Hall JR, Hartmann M, et al. (2009) Introducing mothur: open-source, platform-independent, community-supported software for describing and comparing microbial communities. Appl Environ Microbiol 75: 7537–7541.

33. Costello EK, Lauber CL, Hamady M, Fierer N, Gordon JI, et al. (2009) Bacterial community variation in human body habitats across space and time. Science 326: 1694–1697.

34. Kumar PS, Brooker MR, Dowd SE, Camerlengo T (2011) Target region selection is a critical determinant of community fingerprints generated by 16S pyrosequencing. PLoS One 6: e20956.

35. Dowd SE, Sun Y, Wolcott RD, Domingo A, Carroll JA (2008) Bacterial tag-encoded FLX amplicon pyrosequencing (bTEFAP) for microbiome studies: bacterial diversity in the ileum of newly weaned Salmonella-infected pigs. Foodborne Pathog Dis 5: 459–472.

36. Huse SM, Dethlefsen L, Huber JA, Mark Welch D, Relman DA, et al. (2008) Exploring microbial diversity and taxonomy using SSU rRNA hypervariable tag sequencing. PLoS Genet 4: e1000255.

37. Ding S, Chi MM, Scull BP, Rigby R, Schwerbrock NM, et al. (2010) High-fat diet: bacteria interactions promote intestinal inflammation which precedes and correlates with obesity and insulin resistance in mouse. PLoS One 5: e12191.

38. Poritz LS, Garver KI, Green C, Fitzpatrick L, Ruggiero F, et al. (2007) Loss of the Tight Junction Protein ZO-1 in Dextran Sulfate Sodium Induced Colitis. Journal of Surgical Research 140: 12–19.

39. Suenaert P, Bulteel V, Lemmens L, Noman M, Geypens B, et al. (2002) Anti-tumor necrosis factor treatment restores the gut barrier in Crohn's disease. Am J Gastroenterol 97: 2000–2004.

40. Ma TY, Iwamoto GK, Hoa NT, Akotia V, Pedram A, et al. (2004) TNF-α-induced increase in intestinal epithelial tight junction permeability requires NF-κB activation. American Journal of Physiology - Gastrointestinal and Liver Physiology 286: G367–G376.

41. Ye D, Ma I, Ma TY (2006) Molecular mechanism of tumor necrosis factor-alpha modulation of intestinal epithelial tight junction barrier. Am J Physiol Gastrointest Liver Physiol 290: G496–504.

42. Al-Sadi R, Ye D, Said HM, Ma TY (2010) IL-1[beta]-Induced Increase in Intestinal Epithelial Tight Junction Permeability Is Mediated by MEKK-1 Activation of Canonical NF-[kappa]B Pathway. The American Journal of Pathology 177: 2310–2322.

43. Youakim A, Ahdieh M (1999) Interferon-γ decreases barrier function in T84 cells by reducing ZO-1 levels and disrupting apical actin. American Journal of Physiology - Gastrointestinal and Liver Physiology 276: G1279–G1288.

44. Vrieze A, Holleman F, Zoetendal EG, de Vos WM, Hoekstra JB, et al. (2010) The environment within: how gut microbiota may influence metabolism and body composition. Diabetologia 53: 606–613.

45. Xia Y, Chen H-Q, Zhang M, Jiang Y-Q, Hang X-M, et al. (2011) Effect of Lactobacillus plantarum LP-Onlly on gut flora and colitis in interleukin-10 knockout mice. Journal of Gastroenterology and Hepatology 26: 405–411.

46. Forsyth CB, Farhadi A, Jakate SM, Tang Y, Shaikh M, et al. (2009) Lactobacillus GG treatment ameliorates alcohol-induced intestinal oxidative stress, gut leakiness, and liver injury in a rat model of alcoholic steatohepatitis. Alcohol 43: 163–172.

47. Anderson RC, Cookson AL, McNabb WC, Park Z, McCann MJ, et al. (2010) Lactobacillus plantarum MB452 enhances the function of the intestinal barrier by increasing the expression levels of genes involved in tight junction formation. BMC Microbiol 10: 316.

48. Oliveira M, Bosco N, Perruisseau G, Nicolas J, Segura-Roggero I, et al. (2011) Lactobacillus paracasei Reduces Intestinal Inflammation in Adoptive Transfer Mouse Model of Experimental Colitis. Clin Dev Immunol 2011: 807483.

49. Karczewski J, Troost FJ, Konings I, Dekker J, Kleerebezem M, et al. (2010) Regulation of human epithelial tight junction proteins by Lactobacillus plantarum in vivo and protective effects on the epithelial barrier. Am J Physiol Gastrointest Liver Physiol 298: G851–859.

50. Schlee M, Harder J, Koten B, Stange EF, Wehkamp J, et al. (2008) Probiotic lactobacilli and VSL#3 induce enterocyte beta-defensin 2. Clin Exp Immunol 151: 528–535.

51. Paolillo R, Romano Carratelli C, Sorrentino S, Mazzola N, Rizzo A (2009) Immunomodulatory effects of Lactobacillus plantarum on human colon cancer cells. International Immunopharmacology 9: 1265–1271.

52. Mondot S, Kang S, Furet JP, Aguirre de Carcer D, McSweeney C, et al. (2011) Highlighting new phylogenetic specificities of Crohn's disease microbiota. Inflamm Bowel Dis 17: 185–192.

53. Claesson MJ, O'Sullivan O, Wang Q, Nikkila J, Marchesi JR, et al. (2009) Comparative analysis of pyrosequencing and a phylogenetic microarray for exploring microbial community structures in the human distal intestine. PLoS One 4: e6669.

54. Walker AW, Ince J, Duncan SH, Webster LM, Holtrop G, et al. (2011) Dominant and diet-responsive groups of bacteria within the human colonic microbiota. ISME J 5: 220–230.

55. Salazar N, Gueimonde M, Hernandez-Barranco AM, Ruas-Madiedo P, de los Reyes-Gavilan CG (2008) Exopolysaccharides produced by intestinal Bifidobacterium strains act as fermentable substrates for human intestinal bacteria. Appl Environ Microbiol 74: 4737–4745.

56. Terra X, Pallarés V, Ardèvol A, Bladé C, Fernández-Larrea J, et al. (2011) Modulatory effect of grape-seed procyanidins on local and systemic inflammation in diet-induced obesity rats. The Journal of Nutritional Biochemistry 22: 380–387.

57. Cawthorn WP, Sethi JK (2008) TNF-alpha and adipocyte biology. FEBS Lett 582: 117–131.

58. Adapala VJ, Buhman KK, Ajuwon KM (2011) Novel anti-inflammatory role of SLPI in adipose tissue and its regulation by high fat diet. J Inflamm (Lond) 8: 5.

59. Kim OY, Lee SM, Do H, Moon J, Lee KH, et al. (2011) Influence of Quercetin-rich Onion Peel Extracts on Adipokine Expression in the Visceral Adipose Tissue of Rats. Phytother Res.

60. Lumeng CN, Bodzin JL, Saltiel AR (2007) Obesity induces a phenotypic switch in adipose tissue macrophage polarization. J Clin Invest 117: 175–184.

61. Pond CM (2005) Adipose tissue and the immune system. Prostaglandins Leukot Essent Fatty Acids 73: 17–30.

62. Cenac N, Coelho AM, Nguyen C, Compton S, Andrade-Gordon P, et al. (2002) Induction of intestinal inflammation in mouse by activation of proteinase-activated receptor-2. Am J Pathol 161: 1903–1915.

63. Amar J, Chabo C, Waget A, Klopp P, Vachoux C, et al. (2011) Intestinal mucosal adherence and translocation of commensal bacteria at the early onset of type 2 diabetes: molecular mechanisms and probiotic treatment. EMBO Mol Med 3: 559–572.

64. Lassenius MI, Pietilainen KH, Kaartinen K, Pussinen PJ, Syrjanen J, et al. (2011) Bacterial endotoxin activity in human serum is associated with dyslipidemia, insulin resistance, obesity, and chronic inflammation. Diabetes Care 34: 1809–1815.

65. Creely SJ, McTernan PG, Kusminski CM, Fisher M, Da Silva NF, et al. (2007) Lipopolysaccharide activates an innate immune system response in human adipose tissue in obesity and type 2 diabetes. Am J Physiol Endocrinol Metab 292: E740–747.

66. Campbell EL, Serhan CN, Colgan SP (2011) Antimicrobial aspects of inflammatory resolution in the mucosa: a role for proresolving mediators. J Immunol 187: 3475–3481.

There are several supplemental files that are not available in this version of the article. To view this additional information, please use the citation information cited on the first page of this chapter.

CHAPTER 5

BACTEROIDES UNIFORMIS CECT 7771 AMELIORATES METABOLIC AND IMMUNOLOGICAL DYSFUNCTION IN MICE WITH HIGH-FAT-DIET INDUCED OBESITY

PAOLA GAUFFIN CANO, ARLETTE SANTACRUZ, ÁNGELA MOYA, AND YOLANDA SANZ

5.1 INTRODUCTION

Obesity is considered a major health issue due to its increasing prevalence and associated co-morbidities (e.g. type 2 diabetes, fatty liver and cardiovascular disease) affecting both the developed and the developing world [1]–[2]. This disorder is the result of a long-term positive energy imbalance and is associated with a chronic state of low grade inflammation and immune dysfunction [3]–[5].

This chapter was originally published under the Creative Commons Attribution License. Cano PG, Santacruz A, Moya A, and Sanz Y. Bacteroides uniformis *CECT 7771 Ameliorates Metabolic and Immunological Dysfunction in Mice with High-Fat-Diet Induced Obesity.* PLoS ONE *7,7 (2012). doi:10.1371/journal.pone.0041079.*

The microbiota of the human gastrointestinal tract has been considered as an organ that contributes to human physiological diversity by encoding additional metabolic capacities and regulating gene expression of pathways involved in host nutrient metabolism [6]. Animal studies indicate that colonisation of adult germ-free mice with a distal gut microbial community harvested from conventionally raised mice influences energy-balance by increasing both nutrient digestion and absorption, and adiposity [7]. This effect is mediated by different mechanisms, including microbial fermentation of dietary polysaccharides that are otherwise indigestible by the host, subsequent intestinal absorption of monosaccharides and short-chain fatty acids, conversion of these metabolites to more complex lipids in the liver; and microbial regulation of host genes that promote lipid accumulation in adipocytes [8].

In humans, the gut microbiota composition is also thought to play a role in energy balance, as inferred from observational studies reporting associations between obesity or weight loss and shifts in gut microbiota composition. It has been reported that 80–90% of bacterial phylotypes are members of two phyla, namely Bacteroidetes (including the genera *Bacteroides* and *Prevotella*) and Firmicutes (including the genera *Clostridium*, *Enterococcus*, *Lactobacillus* and *Ruminococcus*), followed by the phyla Actinobacteria (including the genus *Bifidobacterium*) and Proteobacteria (including *Helicobacter* and *Escherichia*) [9]–[10]. Therefore, relative proportions of Firmicutes and Bacteroides are considered good indicators of major changes in intestinal microbiota constitution. So far, most studies have reported associations between obesity and reduced proportions of the phylum Bacteroidetes [11] which, in some cases, were accompanied by increased proportions of Actinobacteria [6] or Firmicutes [12], as also observed in mice [9], [13]. In addition, weight loss in obese human subjects subjected to dietary or surgical interventions has been associated with increases in Bacteroidetes [12] or in *Bacteroides* spp., *Bacteroides-Prevotella* spp. or *Bacteroides* fragilis group [14]–[17]. Nevertheless, few observational studies have found no associations between weight-loss or obesity and numbers of *Bacteroides* spp. or *Bacteroides-Prevotella* spp. [18]–[19], reported opposite associations between obesity, and the relative proportion of Bacteroidetes to Firmicutes [19] or the numbers of *Prevotella*ceae, a subgroup of Bacteroidetes [20]. These discrepancies could partly be explained by differences in the analytical techniques used since, for example, real-time PCR or FISH target only specific groups of Bacteroidetes and underestimate some members of this phylum present in faecal samples [21]. By contrast, DNA sequence analyses of the phylum Bacteroidetes can cover up to 46 species of bacteria belonging to seven different genera of the order *Bacteroidales* [6], encompassing a taxonomic unit that is too broad to assess its possible implication in obesity [21].

In this study, we hypothesised that modification of the gut microbiota structure by increasing numbers of specific *Bacteroides* spp. could contribute to restoring obesity-related metabolic and immune dysfunction. To obtain direct evidence of the role of *Bacteroides* spp. in obesity and thus confirm such a hypothesis, we have evaluated in vitro the immunologic properties of different intestinal *Bacteroides* spp. on macrophages. Furthermore, we have assessed the effect of the selected strain (*B. uniformis* CECT 7771) on metabolic and immune parameters of mice with high-fat-diet induced obesity.

5.2 METHODS

5.2.1 BACTERIAL STRAIN AND CULTURE CONDITIONS

The following *Bacteroides* spp. and strains from the IATA-CSIC and Spanish Culture Collection (CECT) were studied: *Bacteroides dorei* SS1, *Bacteroides ovatus* SU2, *Bacteroides distasonis* CAY3, *Bacteroides uniformis* CECT 7771 (or CY1), *Bacteroides thetaiotaomicron* SAC4, *Bacteroides fragilis* SX3, *Bacteroides caccae* SV3 and *Bacteroides finegoldii* SX2. These strains were isolated from stools of healthy infants (mean age 5.7 years, range 1.0–10.8 years). Briefly, fresh stool samples were diluted (1:10 [w/v]) in phosphate-buffered saline (PBS) solution (130 mM sodium chloride, 10 mM sodium phosphate, pH 7.2) and homogenised. Then, aliquots of serial dilutions in PBS and aliquots were plated on Schaedler Agar (Scharlau, Barcelona, Spain) supplemented with kanamycin (100 mg/L), vancomycin (7.5 mg/L) and vitamin K (0.5 mg/L) and incubated under anaerobic conditions at 37 °C for 48 hours. Individual colonies were isolated from the highest dilution plate from each subject and their cellular morphology and Gram-staining characteristics were examined. The isolated clones were identified at species level by sequencing of amplified 16S rDNA regions with the primers 27f and 1401r as previously described [22]. The PCR products obtained were purified using the GFXtm PCR DNA and Gel Band DNA Purification Kit (GE Healthcare, Buckinghamshire, UK) for DNA sequencing. DNA sequencing was carried out by an ABI PRISM-3130XL Genetic Analyser (Applied Biosystems, California, USA). The closest relatives of the partial 16S rRNA gene sequences were sought in GenBank using the Basic Local Alignment Search Tool (BLAST) algorithm, and sequences with more than 97% similarity were considered as belonging to the same species. All new data has been deposited in GenBank (Accession numbers: JX183979, JX262250, JX183978, JX183977, JX183984, JX183983, JX183981 and JX183982, respectively).

For experimental purposes, the bacterial strains were grown in Brain Heart Infusion Broth (BH) (Scharlab, SL- Barcelona, Spain) at 37 °C in microaerophilic conditions (AnaeroGen; Oxoid, Basingstoke, UK). Cells were harvested by centrifugation (6,000 g for 15 min), washed twice in phosphate buffered saline (PBS, 130± sodium chloride, 10 mM sodium phosphate, pH 7.4), and re-suspended in PBS plus 15% glycerol for in vitro trials and in 10% skimmed milk for animal trials. Aliquots of these suspensions were frozen in liquid nitrogen and stored at -80°C until used. The number of live cells after freezing and thawing was determined by colony-forming unit (CFU) counting on BH agar after 48 h incubation. For the strain tested, more than 90% cells were alive upon thawing and no significant differences were found during storage time (2 months). One fresh aliquot was thawed for every new experiment to avoid variability in the viability of cultures.

5.2.2 EFFECT OF BATEROIDES STRAINS ON INDUCTION OF CYTOKINE PRODUCTION BY MACROPHAGES

To evaluate the immunological properties of different *Bacteroides* strains, the RAW 264 macrophage cell line, obtained from the American Type Culture Collection (Rockville, MD, USA), was cultured overnight in 24-well flat-bottom polystyrene microtiter plates (Corning, Cultek, Madrid,

Spain) at a concentration of 1×10^5 cells per ml in Dulbeco's Modified Eagles Medium (DMEM) (SigmaTM– St. Louis, MO/USA). Media were changed before stimulation and, then, cells were incubated in the presence of 100 µl of a cell suspension (1×10^7 cfu/ml) of each *Bacteroides* strain for 24 h. Purified LPS from *Salmonella enterica* serotype Typhimurium (Sigma Chemical Co, Madrid, Spain) was used at a concentration of 1 µg/ml as a positive control. Non-stimulated Raw 264.7 cells were also evaluated as controls of basal cytokine production. The cell culture supernatants were collected and stored at $-20°C$ until used for cytokine determination. TNF-α and IL-10 were quantified by ELISA Ready SET Go! Kit (BD Bioscience, San Diego, CA, USA). Every parameter was assayed in triplicate in two independent experiments.

TABLE 1: Oligonucleotide primers used in this study.

Target bacterial groups	Primers (name)	Sequence (5'–3')	Size (pb)	Annealing Tmp (°C)	References
Total bacteria	HDA 1, HDA 2	TGGCTCAGGACGAAC-GCTGGCGGCCCTACTGCT-GCCTCCCGTAGGAGT	200	59	[26]
Bifidobacterium spp.	BiFid F, BiFid R	CTCCTGGAAAC-GGGTGGGGTGTTCTTCCC-GATATCTACA	550	55	[26, 27]
Bacteroides spp.	Bfra F, Bfra R	ATA GCC TTT CGA AAG RAA GAT CCA GTA TCA ACT GCA ATT TTA	287	55	[26, 27]
Clostridium coccoides group	Ccoc F, Ccoc R	AAA TGA CGG TAC CTG ACT AA CTT TGA GTT TCA TTC TTG CGA A	440	50	[26, 27]
Clostridium leptum group	Clep F, Clep R3	GCA CAA GCA GTG GAG T CTT CCT CCG TTT TGT CAA	239	50	[26, 27]
Enterobacteriaceae	Entero 1, Entero 2	CATTGACGTTACCCG-CAGAAGAAGCCTCTAC-GAGACTCAAGCTTGC	195	63	[28]
Lactobacillus group	Lac 1, Lac 2	AGCAGTAGGGAATCTTC-CAATTYCACCGCTACA-CATG	340	61	[29, 30]

5.2.3 ANIMALS, DIETS AND EXPERIMENTAL DESIGN

Animal experiments were carried out in strict accordance with the recommendations in the Guide for the Care and Use of Laboratory Animals of University of Valencia (Central Service of Support to Research [SCSIE], University of Valencia, Spain) and the protocol was approved by its Ethic Committee (approval ID A1245740259386). Adult (age 6–8 week) male wild-type C57BL-6 mice were purchased from Harlan Laboratories. During the adaptation period (7 days), six animals were housed in each stainless-steel cage in a temperature-controlled (23 °C) room with a 12-h light/dark cycle and 40–50% relative humidity. Then, mice were randomly divided into four groups (n = 6–8 mice per group) as follows: (1) a control group, receiving a standard diet (SD); (2) an obese group, receiving a high-fat diet (HFD); (3) a group receiving a SD and a daily dose of 5.0×10^8 CFU *B. uniformis* CECT 7771 by gavage; and (4) an obese group receiving the HFD and a daily dose of 5.0×10^8 CFU *B. uniformis* CECT 7771 by oral gavage. To induce obesity, mice were switched from the SD (CA.170481-AIN-76A Purified Diet-Rats/Mice, Harlan Laboratories, Madison, WI 53744-4220) administered during the adaptation period to all mice, to a HFD (TD.06414 - Adjusted Calories Diet - 60/Fat, Harlan Laboratories, Madison, WI 53744-4220) for 7 weeks. The HFD provided 18.4% kcal as protein, 21.3% kcal as carbohydrate and 60.3% kcal as fat (5.1 kcal/g), whereas the SD provided 18.8% kcal as protein, 68.8% kcal as carbohydrate and 12.4% kcal as fat (3.8 kcal/g). Therefore, there was an increase in fat at expenses of a reduction in carbohydrates in the HFD. Mice had free access to feed and sterile water.

Body weight was measured once a week and, at the end of study, animals were fasted for 16 h, anaesthetised, bled by aortic puncture and sacrificed by cervical dislocation. To analyse the metabolic parameters, blood samples were collected in tubes containing EDTA and centrifuged to obtain plasma that was stored at -20°C. Stools were collected at the end of the experimental period (7 weeks) for microbiological analyses. The liver, white adipose (perirenal and epididymal) and small intestinal tissues were excised and rinsed with saline solution, and sections were fixed in 10% neutral formalin buffered solution for histological analysis. The white adipose deposits (perirenal and epididymal) were previously weighed. Liver sections were also used for lipid extraction and quantification as described below.

5.2.4 HISTOLOGY OF LIVER, WHITE ADIPOSE TISSUES AND SMALL INTESTINE

Paraffin-embedded tissues were sectioned to a thickness of 4–5 µm and fixed to glass slides. Slides were deparaffinised and stained with haematoxylin-eosin. The severity of steatosis was determined in 100 hepatocytes of two liver tissue sections per mouse and scored as follows: grade 0 when fat was not detected in hepatocytes; grade 1 when fat occupied less than 30% of hepatocytes; grade 2 when fat occupied between 30 and 60% of hepatocytes; grade 3, when fat occupied more than 60% of hepatocytes.

Adipocyte cell sizes were measured in 100 cells of two sections of epididymal adipose tissue per mouse [23]. Adipocyte cell sizes were expressed as area ranges using the following ranges: <2000, 2000–4000, 4000–6000 and 6000–7000 µm².

The ratio of fat micelles to enterocyte was determined in 100 cells from two sections of small intestinal tissue of each mouse by counting ten 100X light microscope fields. All parameters were measured in a NIKON Eclipse 90i Microscopic, using the NIS Elements BR 2.3 basic research software (Kingston, Surrey, KT2 5PR, England). All histological analyses were conducted by an experienced histologist in a blind fashion.

5.2.5 ANALYSIS OF SERUM AND LIVER BIOCHEMICAL PARAMETERS AND GLUCOSE TOLERANCE

Biochemical parameters were quantified in plasma using enzymatic assay kits for glucose (Glucose Liquid Kit; Química Analítica Aplicada SA, Spain), cholesterol (Cholesterol Liquid kit, Química Analítica Aplicada SA, Spain) and triglycerides (Triglyceride Liquid kit, Química Analítica Aplicada SA, Spain). Serum leptin concentration was determined by enzyme-linked immunosorbent assay (ELISA) (BD Bioscience, San Diego,

CA, USA). Serum insulin was determined by Ultrasensitive Mouse Insulin ELISA (Mercondia AB, Sweden, 2010).

Triglycerides and cholesterol were also quantified in liver. Lipids were extracted by homogenising the tissue with 2:1 chloroform-methanol (v/v) making a 20-fold dilution, and filtering the homogenate through a nylon filter (Cell Strainer 40 micrometros Nylon.BD Falcon; BD BIOSCIENCIES). Non-lipidic substances were eliminated by adding 5-volumes of $CaCl_2$ solution (5 mg/L) in water to the filtrate fraction. After centrifugation (4,000 g, for 5 minutes, at room temperature) the upper phase, containing all of the non-lipidic substances, was discarded. This process was repeated three times. Extracted lipids were dried under vacuum (Concentrator Plus 5301, Eppendorf Inc., NY, USA) and then triglyceride and total cholesterol concentrations were determined as described above.

Oral glucose tolerance tests were performed in vivo after 6 weeks of treatment. Food was removed 2 h after the onset of the daylight cycle and, after a 4-h fasting period, glucose was administered orally at a dose of 2 g/kg and blood samples were taken with heparinised capillary tubes from the tail vein before and 15, 30, 60, 90 and 120 minutes after glucose administration. Plasma glucose levels were analysed with glucose test strips (Ascensia Esyfill, Bayer, Tarrytown, NY; USA) and a glucometer (Ascensia VIGOR, Bayer Tarrytown, NY; USA), with a detection level ranging from 30 to 550 mg glucose/dl.

5.2.6 ISOLATION AND ASSESSMENT OF CYTOKINE PRODUCTION BY PERITONEAL MACROPHAGES

Peritoneal cells were collected by washing the peritoneal cavity of different groups of mice, with 5 ml of sterile cold DMEM (Sigma), containing 10% inactivated (56°C for 30 min) foetal bovine serum (FBS) (Gibco, Barcelona, Spain), 100 µg/ml streptomycin and 100 U/ml penicillin (SigmaTM– St. Louis, MO/USA). Isolated macrophages were plated in flasks (Corning, Cultek, Madrid, Spain) at a concentration of 1×10^6 cells per ml in DMEM and incubated for 2 h at 37°C in an atmosphere containing 5% CO_2. Non-adhered cells were washed out with warm PBS. To evaluate differences in the response to a common stimulus, macrophages from different mouse groups were incubated in the presence of purified LPS from *Salmonella enterica* serotype Typhimurium (Sigma Chemical Co, Madrid, Spain) at a concentration of 1 µg/ml. Non-stimulated peritoneal macrophages were also evaluated as controls of basal cytokine production. To evaluate microbiota-related immune properties of faecal samples, macrophages from control mice were incubated in the presence of faecal samples (30 µl of 10-fold dilution) from the different mouse groups for 24 h. Stool samples used as stimuli were collected from six mice of each experimental group at the end of the study, diluted 10-fold in PBS and homogenised for 3 min. Macrophage culture supernatants were collected and stored at −20°C until used for cytokine determination. TNF-α and IL-10 were quantified by ELISA Ready SET Go! Kit (BD Bioscience, San Diego, CA, USA). Each parameter was assayed in triplicate in two independent experiments.

TABLE 2: Effect of different *Bacteroides* strains on cytokine production by RAW264.7 macrophages.

Bacteriodes strains	Cytokine production	
	TNF-α (pg/ml)	IL-10 (pg/ml)
DEMEN	491.2 (112.1)[a,b']	97.2 (10.8)[a,a']
LPS	1425.4 (77.6)[b,a']	162.3 (37.6)[a,a']
B. dorei SS1	3765.5 (150.0)[b, b',a"]	215.8 (12.5)[b,a',b"]
B. ovatus SU2	4515.7 (211.3)[b,b'b"]	271.5 (8.1)[b,b',b"]
B. distasonis CAY3	4462.4 (173.9)[b,b',b"]	215.8 (9.7)[b,a',b"]
B. uniformis CECT 7771	2998.4 (50.4)[b,b',a"]	341.3 (13.5)[b,b',a"]
B. thetaiotaomicron SAC4	2931.2 (464.5)[b,b',a"/]	109.2 (3.0)[a,a',b"]
B. fragilis SX3	6657.3 (278.3)[b,b',b"]	81.2 (14.6)[a,a',b"]
B. caccae SV3	11622.0 (818.3)[b,b',b"]	171.7 (12.9)[b,a',b"]
B. finegoldii SX2	6535.8 (62.2)[b,b',b"]	83.5 (17.4)[a,a',b"]

Purified lipopolysaccharide (1 mg/ml) (LPS) from S.enterica *serotype. Typhimurium was used as a positive control. Non-stimulated cells were also evaluated as controls of basal cytokine levels (DEMEN). Results are expressed as mean (SD) of duplicate measures determined in three independent experiments. Significant differences were established at P < 0.05 by applying ANOVA and post hoc Tukey's test. Means in the same columns with different letters were significantly different in relation to non-stimulated cells (a-b) or to LPS (a'-b') or to* B. uniformis *CECT 7771 (a"-b")*

5.2.7 BACTERICIDAL ACTIVITY OF PERITONEAL MACROPHAGES

The bactericidal activity of peritoneal macrophages was analysed according to Vieira et al. [24] Cells were washed with serum-free DMEM and nitroblue tetrazolium (NBT – SigmaTM– St. Louis, MO/USA) at 0.5 mg/ml together with a bacterial extract (Stimulant, No. 840-15-SigmaTM– St. Louis, MO/USA) in an equivalent concentration of McFarland Scale 2 in Lab-tek chamber slide w/cover (Nalge Nunc International, USA). After 1 h of incubation at 37 °C in 5% CO_2 atmosphere, the cells were washed with PBS, then fixed with 4% paraformaldehyde and observed in a NIKON Eclipse 90i Microscope, using the NIS Elements BR 2.3 basic research software (Kingston, Surrey, KT2 5PR, England). One hundred cells were counted per mouse and the percentage of NBT positive cells was determined. This measurement was taken in triplicate, in two independent experiments.

5.2.8 ISOLATION AND CYTOKINE PRODUCTION BY BONE MARROW-DERIVED DENDRITE CELLS (DC)

DCs were generated from bone marrow as described previously [25]. Cells were seeded at a concentration of 1×10^6 (90–94% DCs) in 1 ml of culture medium without rm GM-CSF in 24-well plates (Corning, Cultek, Madrid, Spain) and incubated in the presence of faeces (30 µl) from the respective mouse group at 37°C under 5% CO_2 for 24 h. Purified LPS from *S. enterica* serotype Typhimurium (Sigma Chemical Co, Madrid, Spain) was used at a concentration of 1 µg/ml as a positive control. Non-stimulated DCs were also evaluated as controls of basal cytokine production. Stool samples were obtained and prepared as described above. The cell culture supernatants were collected and stored at −20°C until used for cytokine determination (TNF-α and IL-10) as described above. Every parameter was assayed in triplicate, in two independent experiments.

5.2.9 INTERACTIONS BETWEEN DCS AND CD4+ T LYMPHOCYTES

CD4+ T lymphocytes were isolated from mouse spleens, which were excised, suspended in complete medium and passed through a stainless steel wire mesh. The obtained crude cell suspension was washed once. CD4+ T cells were immune-magnetically isolated by positive selection with "CD4+ (L3T4) microbeads" (Miltenyi Biotec GmbH, Bergisch Gladbach, Germany), following the manufacturer's instructions. CD4+ T cells (purity exceeded 95%) were used for mixed lymphocyte reaction.

Isolated DCs were incubated for 24 h in the presence of 1 µg/ml LPS from *S. Typhimurium* (Sigma Chemical Co, Madrid, Spain). Aliquots of mature DCs from different mouse groups were plated in triplicate with allogeneic CD4+ T cells (TL) at 1:1, 1:2, and 1:4 TL/DC cell ratios, in 0.2 ml culture medium in 96-well flat-bottomed plates (Corning, Cultek, Madrid, Spain) at 37 °C for 72 h. Lymphocyte proliferation was measured with the cell proliferation ELISA BrdU-colorimetric assay (Roche, Diagnostic, Germany). Individual cultures of DCs and TL stimulated with or without ConA, used as mitogen, were used as controls.

5.2.10 SAMPLES AND MICROBIAL ANALYSIS BY QUANTITATIVE PCR (QPCR)

Stool samples were weighed, diluted 1:5 (w/v) in PBS (pH 7.2), homogenised by shaking in a vortex and stored at -20 °C till analysed. One aliquot of this dilution was used for DNA extraction using the QIAamp DNA stool Mini kit (Qiagen, Hilden, Germany). Specific primers (Table 1) [26]–[30] targeting different bacterial genera and species were used to characterise the composition of the microbiota by qPCR using LightCycler® 480 SYBR Green I Master (Roche, USA) with a an ABI PRISM 7000-PCR sequence detection system (Applied Biosystems, UK), as described previously [14].

5.2.11 STATISTICAL ANALYSES

Statistical analyses were carried out using SPSS 11.0 software (SPSS Inc., Chicago, IL, USA). Data of biochemical parameters were normally distributed and significant differences were determined by applying One-Way Anova with pos hoc Tukey's test. Remaining data were non-normally distributed and the differences were determined by applying the Mann-Whitney U tests. In every case, P-values <0.05 were considered statistically significant.

5.3 RESULTS

5.3.1 BACTEROIDES *STRAIN SELECTION BASED ON IN VITRO ABILITY TO INDUCE CYTOKINE PRODUCTION*

Results in Table 2 show the ability of different *Bacteroides* strains to induce cytokine production by Raw264.7 macrophages. All strains induced the production of significantly higher amounts of the pro-inflammatory cytokine TNF-α than the non-stimulated cells and LPS-stimulated macrophages, although the magnitude of this effect was strain-dependent. The strains *B. dorei* SS1, *B. uniformis* CECT 7771 and *B. thetaiotaomicron* SAC4 induced the lowest TNF-α production. Different bacterial strains also induced anti-inflammatory cytokine IL-10 production above basal levels to different extents, except for *B. thetaiotaomicron* SAC4, *B. fragilis* SX3 and *B. finegoldii* SX2 whose effects were not significant. *B. uniformis* CECT 7771 induced the highest IL-10 levels compared to the other *Bacteroides* strains under study. Therefore, this strain was selected for its greater anti-inflammatory properties.

5.3.2 BODY WEIGHT GAIN, ADIPOSE TISSUE WEIGHT AND BIOCHEMICAL PARAMETERS IN OBESE MICE

Body weight gain and total adipose tissue weight of mice after a 7-week intervention are shown in Table 3. The time course body weight gain over the intervention period is also shown in Figure 1. HFD-fed mice

TABLE 3: Biometric parameters and serum and liver biochemistry in mice fed either a high-fat diet (HFD) or standard diet (SD), supplemented or not with *B. uniformis* CECT 7771.

Outcome measure	Experimental Groups								P-value HFD vs. SD	P-value (SD+B vs. SD)	P-value (HFD+B vs HFD)
	SD		HFD		SD+B		HFD+B				
	Mean	sd	Mean	sd	Mean	sd	Mean	sd			
Biometric parameters											
Body weight gain (%)	24.21	3.34	36.19	1.55	23.61	3.17	30.33	0.92	0.007*	0.890	0.005*
Adipose tissue (g)/100 g body weight	0.06	0.04	0.15	0.03	0.03	0.02	0.14	0.04	0.016*	0.150	0.423
Serum parameters											
Cholesterol (mg/dl)/	120.00	13.67	176.02	14.91	128.22	11.91	143.97	17.29	<0.001*	0.222	0.003*
Triglyceride (mg/dl)	130.31	11.56	156.99	27.47	129.77	13.94	118.21	10.04	0.041*	0.937	0.004*
Glucose (mg/dl)	219.81	26.41	485.92	140.63	372.41	13.50	233.52	30.62	0.001*	0.237	0.002*
Insulin (µg/l)	0.57	0.47	1.59	0.09	0.69	0.05	0.92	0.14	0.018*	0.892	0.018*
Leptin (ng/ml)	8.07	1.12	18.28	4.28	6.80	1.23	12.98	3.24	<0.001*	0.048	0.014*
Liver lipids											
Cholesterol (mg/g)	29.94	4.08	35.51	4.35	29.22	6.32	27.48	6.39	0.029*	0.801	0.024*
Triglyceride (mg/g)	22.93	13.03	45.99	11.53	31.36	4.76	34.17	9.51	<0.001*	0.142	0.039*

*ST: standard diet group (control) (n=6); SD+B: standard diet group receiving a daily dose of 5.0 x 10⁸ CFU B. uniformis CECT 7771 by gavage for 7 weeks (n=6); HFD: high fat diet group (n=6); HFD+B: high fat diet group receiving a daily dose of 5.0 x 10⁸ CFU B. uniformis CECT 7771 by gavage during 7 weeks (n=6). Body composition and biochemical parameters were determine after 7 weeks of intervention. Adipose tissue included epididymal and perirenal white adipose tissues. Values are expressed as means and standard deviation (sd). *Significant differences were established at P<0.050.*

experienced significant greater weight gain compared to SD-fed mice from the first 4 weeks of treatment till the 7th week. The weights of total adipose tissues were also statistically significantly greater in obese mice than in lean mice. The administration of *B. uniformis* CECT 7771 significantly reduced body weight gain in HFD-fed mice by the end of the intervention, but did not significantly modify total adipose tissue weight (Table 3, Figure 1). No mice died and all of them remained healthy throughout the study.

Serum concentrations of biochemical and hormonal parameters of metabolic relevance are shown in Table 3. The HFD induced a significant increase in all serum parameters analysed compared to SD-fed mice. The administration of *B. uniformis* CECT 7771 significantly reduced serum glucose, insulin, triglycerides and cholesterol concentrations in HFD-fed mice but not in SD-fed mice. In HFD-fed mice *B. uniformis* CECT 7771 reduced cholesterol levels by 18% and triglyceride levels by 25%. *B. uniformis* CECT 7771 administration also significantly lowered fasting glucose levels (Table 3) and improved glucose tolerance, reducing the maximum peak and the area under the curve during the oral glucose tolerance test (Figure 2). The increased serum leptin concentrations induced by the HFD were significantly reduced by the administration of *B. uniformis* CECT 7771 (Table 3).

The specific concentrations of cholesterol and triglycerides present in total lipids extracted from the liver were also analysed (Table 3). The HFD induced a significant increase in both parameters compared to levels in SD-fed mice, while the administration of *B. uniformis* CECT 7771 significantly reduced triglycerides and cholesterol concentrations in the liver of HFD-fed mice (Table 3).

5.3.3 HEPATIC STEATOSIS, ADIPOCYTE SIZE, AND FAT ABSORPTION BY ENTEROCYTES IN OBESE MICE

Figure 3 shows the effects on hepatic steatosis of the administration of *B. uniformis* CECT 7771 to SD- or HFD-fed mice. The bacterial strain significantly reduced steatosis in HFD-fed animals, and also reduced lipid accumulation in the liver of SD-fed mice.

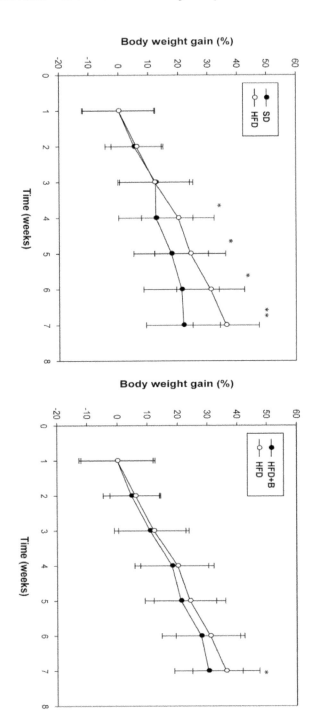

FIGURE 1: Time course of relative body weight gain in control mice and mice with high fat diet-induced obesity, administered or not *B. uniformis* CECT 7771. SD: standard diet group (control) (n = 6); HFD: high fat diet group (n = 6); HFD+B: high fat diet group receiving a daily dose of 5.0×10⁸ CFU *B. uniformis* CECT 7771 by gavage for 7 weeks (n = 6).

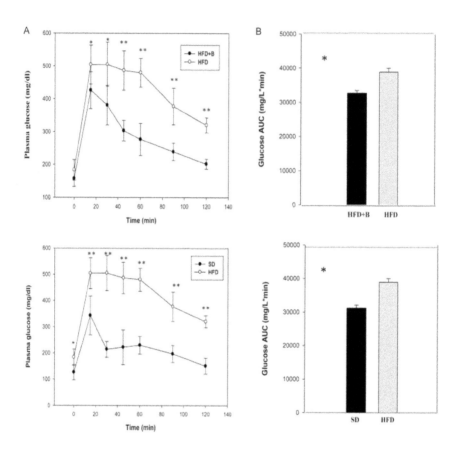

FIGURE 2: Glucose tolerance in control mice and mice with high fat diet-induced obesity, administered or not *B. uniformis* CECT 7771. SD: standard diet group (control) (n = 6); HFD: high fat diet group (n = 6); HFD+B: high fat diet group receiving a daily dose of 5.0×10⁸ CFU *B. uniformis* CECT 7771 by gavage for 7 weeks (n = 6). A: Plasma glucose profile following 2 g/kg glucose oral challenge after 4 h fasting; B: Mean area under the curve measured between 0 and 120 min after glucose administration.

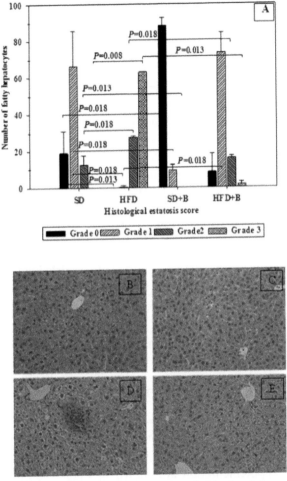

FIGURE 3: Determination of hepatic steatosis (hepatic histology) in control mice and mice with high fat diet-induced obesity, administered or not *B. uniformis* CECT 7771. SD: standard diet group (control) (n = 6); SD+B: standard diet group receiving a daily dose of 5.0×10^8 CFU *B. uniformis* CECT 7771 by gavage for 7 weeks (n = 6); HFD: high fat diet group (n = 6); HFD+B: high fat diet group receiving a daily dose of 5.0×10^8 CFU *B. uniformis* CECT 7771 by gavage for 7 weeks (n = 6).The fat vacuoles were measured in 100 hepatocytes of two liver tissue sections per mouse and scored for the severity of steatosis according to the following criteria: For grade-0 steatosis, no fatty hepatocytes; grade-1 steatosis, fat occupying less than 30% of the hepatocyte; grade-2 steatosis, fat occupying less than 30 to 60% of the hepatocyte; grade-3 steatosis, fat occupying more than 60% of the hepatocyte. Photomicrographs 20X of representative HE-stained slides are shown. (B) SD group, (C) SD+P group, (D) HFD group and (F) HFD+P group. Data are expressed as means ± SD and statistically significant differences are established at P<0.05.

The administration of *B. uniformis* CECT 7771 to SD mice significantly increased the number of hepatocytes with no steatosis (0-grade) and reduced those with steatosis grades 1 and 2. In HFD-fed animals, *B. uniformis* CECT 7771 administration contributed to increasing the number of hepatocytes with 0- and 1-grade steatosis and to reducing those with 2-and 3-grade steatosis.

The effects of the intervention on adipocyte size on epididimal adipose tissue are shown in Figure 4. HFD induced a significant increase in adipocyte size in the following ranges 2000–4000, 4000–6000 and 6000–7000 μm^2, and reduced those of size <2000 μm^2. The administration of *B. uniformis* CECT 7771 in SD-fed mice did not induce significant changes in adipocyte size, while a significant increase in the number of small adipocytes (<2000) was observed in HFD-fed mice.

The effects of the HFD and the administration of the bacterial strain on the number of fat micelles per enterocyte, which indicate dietary fat absorption, are shown in Figure 5. The HFD induced a significant increase in fat micelles in enterocytes, whereas the administration of *B. uniformis* CECT 7771 reduced these numbers. In the SD group, no significant changes were observed due to intervention with the aforementioned bacterium.

5.3.4 MACROPHAGE FUNCTIONALITY

The results of cytokine production by LPS-stimulated peritoneal macrophages from SD- and HFD-fed mice with and without *B. uniformis* CECT 7771 supplementation are shown in Figure 6. Obesity induced by a HFD led to a decrease in cytokine TNF-α production by peritoneal macrophages stimulated with LPS compared to macrophages of SD-fed mice (Figure 6A). The administration of *B. uniformis* CECT 7771 significantly increased the ability of LPS-stimulated macrophages to produce TNF-α in HFD-fed mice but not in SD-fed mice (Figure 6A). The HFD did not affect the ability of LPS-stimulated macrophages to produce the anti-inflammatory cytokine IL-10 and this feature was not modified by the administration of *B. uniformis* CECT 7771 (Figure 6A). The oxidative burst in peritoneal macrophage after uptake of a microbial extract was also studied to analyse effects on phagocytosis function

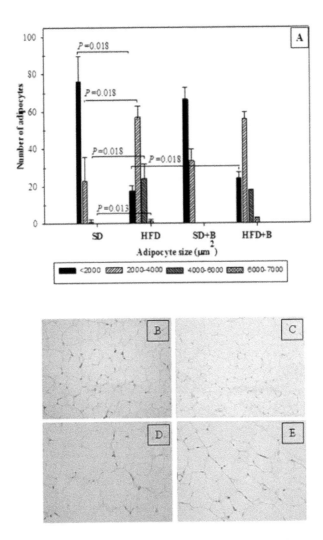

FIGURE 4: Distribution of adipocyte size in epididymal adipose tissue in control mice and mice with high fat diet-induced obesity, administered or not *B. uniformis* CECT 7771. SD: standard diet group (control) (n = 6); SD+B: standard diet group receiving a daily dose of 5.0×10^8 CFU *B. uniformis* CECT 7771 by gavage for 7 weeks (n = 6); HFD: high fat diet group (n = 6); HFD+B: high fat diet group receiving a daily dose of 5.0×10^8 CFU *B. uniformis* CECT 7771 by gavage for 7 weeks (n = 6). Adipocyte cell sizes were expressed as area ranges and were the following: <2000, 2000–4000, 4000–6000 and 6000–7000 μm². Data are expressed as means ± SD and statistically significant differences are established at P<0.05. Photomicrographs 20X of representative HE-stained slides are shown. (B) SD group, (C) SD+B group, (D) HFD group and (E) HFD+B group.

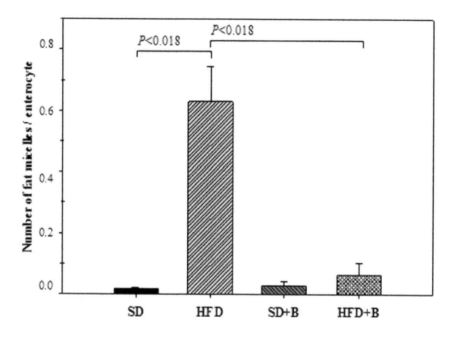

FIGURE 5: Number of fat micelles per enterocyte in control mice and mice with high fat diet-induced obesity, administered or not *B. uniformis* CECT 7771. SD: standard diet group (control) (n = 6); SD+B: standard diet group receiving a daily dose of 5.0×10^8 CFU *B. uniformis* CECT 7771 by gavage for 7 weeks (n = 6); HFD: high fat diet group (n = 6); HFD+B: high fat diet group receiving a daily dose of 5.0×10^8 CFU *B. uniformis* CECT 7771 by gavage for 7 weeks (n = 6). The relation fat micelles/enterocyte was determined in 100 cells from two sections of the small intestine of each mouse by counting ten 100X light microscope fields. Data are expressed as means ± SD and statistically significant differences are established at P<0.05.

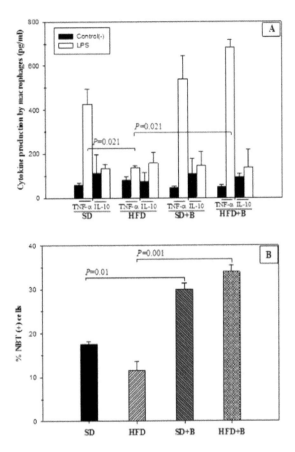

FIGURE 6: Cytokine production in LPS-stimulated peritoneal macrophages and phagocytosis function of control mice and mice with high-fat diet induced obesity, administered or not *B. uniformis* CECT 7771. SD: standard diet group (control) (n = 6); SD+B: standard diet group receiving a daily dose of 5.0×10^8 CFU *B. uniformis* CECT 7771 by gavage for 7 weeks (n = 6); HFD: high fat diet group (n = 6); HFD+B: high fat diet group receiving a daily dose of 5.0×10^8 CFU *B. uniformis* CECT 7771 by gavage for 7 weeks (n = 6). In the cytokine production study, peritoneal macrophages were stimulated with purified lipopolysaccharide (LPS) from S. enterica serotype Typhimurium (Figure 6A). Non-stimulated peritoneal macrophages were evaluated as controls of basal cytokine levels. In the phagocytosis study (Figure 6B), evidence of oxygen-radical production by macrophages was determined by the NBT test after in vitro interaction with a bacterial extract. Figure 6A: TNF- α and IL-10 cytokines produced by LPS-stimulated macrophages; Figure 6B: % NBT (+) cells. Data are expressed as mean and standard deviation of duplicate measurements determined in two independent experiments. Statistically significant differences of data are established at P<0.05.

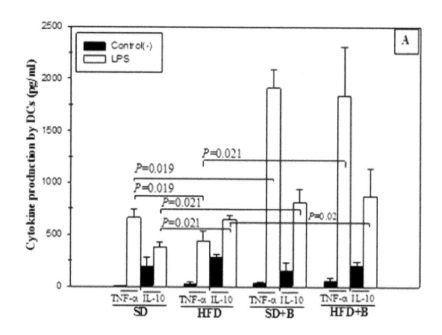

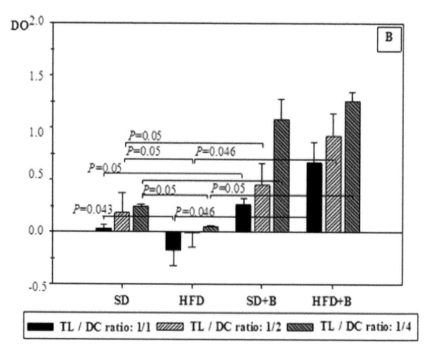

FIGURE 7: Influence of LPS stimuli on cytokine production and activation of T-lymphocyte proliferation by dendritic cells (DCs) generated from control mice and mice with high-fat diet induced obesity, administered or not *B. uniformis* CECT 777. SD: standard diet group (control) (n = 6); SD+B: standard diet group receiving a daily dose of 5.0×10^8 CFU *B. uniformis* CECT 7771 by gavage for 7 weeks (n = 6); HFD: high fat diet group (n = 6); HFD+B: high fat diet group receiving a daily dose of 5.0×10^8 CFU *B. uniformis* CECT 7771 by gavage for 7 weeks (n = 6). In the cytokine production study, DCs were stimulated with purified lipopolysaccharide (LPS) from *S. enterica* serotype Typhimurium (Figure 7A). Non-stimulated DCs were evaluated as controls of basal cytokine levels. In the lymphocyte proliferation study (Figure 7B), matured DCs were used for priming a T-cell proliferative response at the following LT/CD ratios: 1:1, 1:2, 1:4. Lymphocyte proliferation was measured with the cell proliferation ELISA BrdU-colorimetric assay. Figure 7A: TNF-α and IL-10 cytokines produced by LPS-stimulated CDs; Figure 7B: Lymphocyte proliferation. Data are expressed as means ± SD of duplicate measures determined in two independent experiments. Statistically significant differences of data are established at P<0.05.

(Figure 6B). The results indicated that the oral administration of *B. uniformis* CECT 7771 stimulated this function in macrophages in both SD- and HFD-fed mice (Figure 6B).

5.3.5 DENDRITIC CELL (DC) FUNCTIONALITY

The results of cytokine production by LPS-stimulated DC from SD- and HFD-fed mice, with and without *B. uniformis* CECT 7771 supplementation are shown in Figure 7A. The administration of *B. uniformis* CECT 7771 to obese and lean mice increased the ability of DC to produce TNF-α in response to LPS stimulation, which was significantly reduced by the HFD (Figure 7A). In HFD-fed mice, IL-10 production by LPS-stimulated DCs was significantly increased. The administration of *B. uniformis* CECT 7771 increased IL-10 values even more in HFD-fed mice and also stimulated this cytokine production in SD-fed mice (Figure 7A).

The results of the influence of HFD-induced obesity and oral administration of *B. uniformis* CECT 7771 on the ability of matured DCs to priming a T cell proliferative response are shown in Figure 7B. DCs from SD-fed mice were able to induce a significant increase in T cell proliferation in comparison to T cells alone (data not shown) in all the examined DC:T cell ratios. The HFD impaired the capacity of DCs to induce a T cell proliferation response, but this function was restored by *B. uniformis* CECT 7771 administration, and the strongest effects were obtained at 1:4 DC:T ratio. This effect was also significant for SD-fed mice.

5.3.6 MICROBIOTA COMPOSITION AND INFLAMMATORY PROPERTIES

The composition of the faecal microbiota in SD- and HFD-fed mice is shown in Table 4. The HFD led to reductions in the gene copy numbers of most of the bacterial groups analysed, including *Lactobacillus*, *C. coccoides* and *C. leptum* groups and the genus *Bifidobacterium*. This diet also caused increases in gene copy numbers of members of the *Enterobacteriaceae* family. In HFD-fed mice, *B. uniformis* CECT 7771 administration increased the gene copy numbers of the genera *Bacteroides* and *Bifidobacterium* and the group *C. coccoides* and reduced those of members of the *Enterobacteriaceae* family, partially restoring the alteration of the microbiota associated with the HFD. In SD fed mice, the administration of the strain led to an increase in the gene copy numbers of total bacteria the genera *Bacteroides* and *Bifidobacterium* and the group *C. leptum*. The numbers of the *C. coccoides* group followed the same trend, but the differences were not significant.

To evaluate whether these changes in the microbiota could modify the inflammatory signals coming from the gut in the different mouse groups, the ability of faecal samples to induce the production of cytokines by immunocompetent cells in vitro was evaluated (Figure 8A and 8B). Stool samples from HFD-fed mice induced a higher production of TNF-α than those from SD-fed mice by macrophages (Figure 8A) and DCs (Figure 8B), indicating that the HFD induced an increase in the pro-inflammatory signals coming from the gut. The administration of *B. uniformis* CECT 7771 significantly reduced the production of this pro-inflammatory cytokine in macrophages stimulated with stools from both mouse groups (Figure 8A), and in DCs stimulated with stools from the HFD group. Therefore, this bacterial strain seems to have ability to reduce the inflammatory

TABLE 4: Microbiota composition of stool samples from different mouse groups analysed by quantitative PCR[a].

Bacterial group	Experimental groups						
	SD	HFD		SD+B		HFD+B	
	[a]Median (IQR)	[a]Median (IQR)	p-value[b]	[a]Median (IQR)	p-value[c]	[a]Median (IQR)	p-value[d]
Total bacteria	10.8 (10.6–11.1)	10.5 (10.3–10.8)	0.092	11.4 (11.3–11.6)	0.010*	11.0 (10.7–11.2)	0.629
Lactobacillus group	9.9 (9.4–10.5)	9.4 (9.2–9.5)	0.040*	9.6 (9.3–9.8)	0.470	9.7 (9.5–10.1)	0.936
Bacteroides spp.	8.4 (8.3–8.6)	8.7 (8.3–9.0)	0.6674	9.3 (9.1–9.5)	0.004*	9.0 (8.8–9.3)	0.016*
Bifidobacterium spp.	7.1 (6.8–7.2)	6.0 (5.9–6.3)	0.004*	8.1 (7.9–8.3)	0.013*	7.5 (7.0–7.7)	0.004*
C. leptum group	8.4 (8.3–8.6)	7.6 (7.5–7.7)	0.004*	9.6 (9.4–9.8)	0.004*	8.5 (8.1–8.7)	0.936
C. coccoides group	9.1 (8.6–9.3)	8.4 (8.2–8.5)	0.016*	9.9 (9.4–10.0)	0.054	9.6 (9.4–9.7)	0.036*
Enterobacteriaceae	7.3 (7.2–7.7)	8.1 (7.8–8.2)	0.019*	8.1 (7.6–8.2)	0.052	7.9 (7.5–8.0)	0.029*

SD: standard diet group (control) (n=6); SD+B: standard diet group receiving a daily dose of 5.0 x 10⁸ CFU B. uniformis CECT 7771 by gavage for 7 weeks (n=6); HFD: high fat diet group (n=6); HFD+B: high fat diet group receiving a daily dose of 5.0 x 10⁸ CFU B. uniformis CECT 7771 by gavage during 7 weeks (n=6).

[a]Data are expressed as median of log gene copy numbers of each bacterial group per gram of stools.

[b]Significant differences in log gene copy numbers of specific bacterial groups between SD and HFD mouse groups.

[c]Significant differences in log gene copy numbers of specific bacterial groups between SD and SD+B mouse groups.

[d]Significant differences in log gene copy numbers of specific bacterial groups between HFD and HFD+B mouse groups.

[e]Significant differences were established at P < 0.005 by using Mann-Whitney U-test.

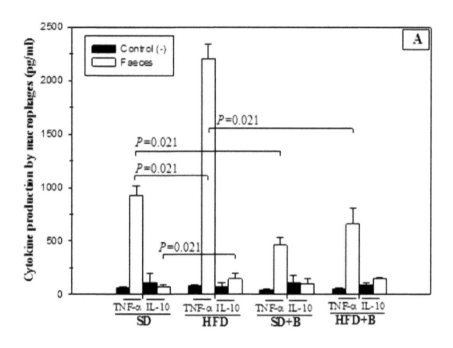

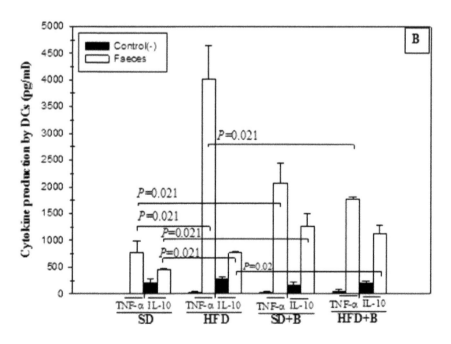

FIGURE 8: Influence of stool samples from mice fed standard diet or high-fat diet, supplemented or not with *B. uniformis* CECT 7771, on cytokine production by peritoneal macrophages and dendritic cells (DCs) from control mice. SD: standard diet group (control) (n = 6); SD+B: standard diet group receiving a daily dose of 5.0×10^8 CFU *B. uniformis* CECT 7771 by gavage for 7 weeks (n = 6); HFD: high fat diet group (n = 6); HFD+B: high fat diet group receiving a daily dose of 5.0×10^8 CFU *B. uniformis* CECT 7771 by gavage for 7 weeks (n = 6). In the cytokine production study, peritoneal macrophages (Figure 8A) and DCs (Figure 8B) were stimulated with stool stimuli. Non-stimulated peritoneal macrophages and DCs were evaluated as controls of basal cytokine levels. Figure 8A: TNF- α and IL-10 cytokines produced by stool-stimulated peritoneal macrophages; Figure 8B: TNF- α and IL-10 cytokines produced by stool-stimulated CDs. Data are expressed as means ± SD of duplicate measures determined in two independent experiments. Statistically significant differences of data are established at $P<0.05$.

properties of the gut content, although confirmatory studies measuring additional inflammatory markers in the gut would be required to draw definitive conclusions.

In macrophages (Figure 8A) and DCs (Figure 8B), stool samples of HFD-fed mice induced significantly higher production of the anti-inflammatory cytokine IL-10 than those from SD-fed mice, which could be due to the activation of regulatory mechanisms to counteract other inflammatory signals inducing also TNF-α. Stool samples from both SD and HFD mouse groups administered *B. uniformis* CECT 7771 induced a significant increase in IL-10 production by DCs, suggesting an increase in the anti-inflammatory signals emanating from the gut (Figure 8B). These *B. uniformis* CECT 7771-related effects were not detected in macrophages (Figure 8A).

5.4 DISCUSSION

This study has provided direct evidence of the metabolic and immune effects of *B. uniformis* CECT 7771 in a murine model of diet-induced obesity. Previous scientific research was controversial and had only established associations between either a lean phenotype or weight loss with increased intestinal numbers of the phylum Bacteroidetes phylum, or the groups *Bacteroides-Prevotella* or *Bacteroides fragilis* [9], [11]–[20]. The selection of the specific strain tested was based on its lower inflammatory potential in vitro on macrophages compared to strains belonging to other intestinal *Bacteroides* spp. This trait could be relevant in the context of obesity since it is considered a chronic inflammatory disorder, largely mediated by macrophage infiltration in the adipose tissue [31]–[33]. Our study demonstrated that *B. uniformis* CECT 7771 induced low TNF-α production and the highest IL-10 production in comparison with other strains of *Bacteroides* spp. Our recent studies also demonstrated that the prevalence of *B. uniformis* CECT 7771 in the gut of infants is favoured by breast-feeding [22] and breast-feeding seems to protect against later development of obesity as compared to formula feeding [34]–[35]. Considering these data altogether led us to hypothesise that the oral administration of *B. uniformis* CECT 7771 could exert beneficial effects in an obesity model as reported in this study.

In our mouse obesity model, *B. uniformis* CECT 7771 administration induced significant modifications in total body weight gain by the end of intervention, although differences in adipose tissue weight were not significant, probably due to the limited duration of the trial. However, *B. uniformis* CECT 7771 increased the number of small adipocytes in obese mice, which could precede fat weight reduction. In contrast, colonisation of germ-free mice by *B. thetaiotaomicron* and *Methanobrevibacter smithii* augmented de novo lipogenesis and adiposity [36]. In this context, it was proposed that gut colonisation by the conventional microbiota or by specific commensal bacteria (e.g. *B. thetaiotaomicron*) provides the hydrolases necessary to utilise complex polysaccharides and the resulting products are absorbed or metabolised to short-chain fatty acids. Subsequently, the latter are delivered to the liver and converted to triacylglycerols and, then, part of these de novo synthesised lipids are deposited in adipocytes [37]–[38]. In addition, it was considered that the gut microbiota could reduce the fasting-induced adipose factor (Fiaf, also known as angiopoietin-like protein-4), a secreted lipoprotein lipase (LPL) inhibitor [8], promoting storage of fatty acids released by the LPL in the host adipose tissue, but this mechanism was not confirmed in a latter study [39]. Although the animal models used in our and previous studies are not comparable, the results suggest that different *Bacteroides* spp. might exert different effects on energy balance and lipid storage.

In obese subjects there is also an increased flux of free fatty acids to the liver due to their excessive accumulation in the adipose tissue and to the inability of insulin to suppress lipolysis in adipocytes due to insulin resistance, which leads to steatosis or fatty liver disease [40]–[41]. In our study, the administration of *B. uniformis* CECT 7771 significantly reduced steatosis in obese animals and, interestingly, also reduced liver cholesterol and triglyceride accumulation. In obese mice, liver steatosis and adipocyte hypertrophy is reported to be related to an increased energy input via intestinal lipid absorption, which is transported in the form of chylomicrons to peripheral tissues [42]. Therefore, we also analysed the number of fat micelles per enterocyte, which partly represents fat absorbed from the diet. *B. uniformis* CECT 7771 administration significantly reduced the fat micelles in enterocytes, particularly in obese mice, indicating that this is a mechanism by which this bacterial strain exerts a positive effect on liver steatosis and serum lipids. Other studies also demonstrated that specific lactobacilli or bifidobacterial strains might reduce the absorption of dietary fat, but this is the first evidence that a *Bacteroides* strain exerts this effect depending on the diet [40], [42], [43]. However, the involvement of other mechanisms, such as reduction of endogenous biosynthesis or reduction of lipid uptake by hepatocytes, cannot be disregarded [44].

Dyslipidaemia is also a frequent feature of obese subjects, with the most common being hypertriclyceridaemias and hypercholesterolaemias [45], [46], which are also induced by HFD in mice. In this study, HFD-fed mice showed higher values of serum cholesterol and triglyceride levels than SD-fed mice. *B. uniformis* CECT 7771 administration reduced serum cholesterol and triglyceride levels in HFD-fed mice. These effects could also be partially related to a reduction of dietary fat absorption and possibly to modulation of the expression of genes and proteins involved in lipid homeostasis in the gut and liver, as indicated previously.

Hyperglycaemia and insulin resistance are also frequently associated with obesity in humans [1]–[2]. This feature was also reproduced in our mice obesity model, which showed increased fasting glucose levels and reduced glucose tolerance. However, the administration of *B. uniformis* CECT 7771 significantly improved the response to an oral glucose challenge and reduced the fasting glycaemia in parallel to insulin, suggesting an improvement in glucose metabolism and insulin sensitivity. Comparisons between germ-free and conventional mice indicated that the commensal microbiota, as a whole, induced hyperglycaemia and insulin resistance [44] while administration of antibiotics causing a reduction in the intestinal bacterial load improved oral glucose tolerance in *ob/ob* and HFD-fed mice [47], [48]. The adverse effects attributed to the microbiota were related to a reduction of AMPK activity and, therefore, reduced insulin-stimulated glucose transport in muscles [38] and to a reduction of inflammatory signals coming from the gut, such as LPS from Gram-negative bacteria and its correlation with intestinal and plasma TNF-α levels [49]. Nevertheless, our present and previous studies indicated that intervention in the gut ecosystem with specific strains may improve diet-induced insulin sensitivity and glucose tolerance above the commensal microbiota effects [40].

Obesity often manifests with hyperleptinemia, associated with leptin resistance, leading to different central and peripheral adverse effects, including increased hunger and reduced energy expenditure as well as increased lipid accumulation [50]. *B. uniformis* CECT 7771 administration also led to reduced leptin levels in obese mice, which could be indicative of an improvement in leptin function or sensitivity, leading to lower leptin production [51]. These improved leptin levels could be related to improvements in glucose tolerance and reduced serum concentration since leptin favours insulin function [52]. In addition, the reduction of serum leptin levels could also be related to increases in smaller adipocytes and reduced liver steatosis in HFD-fed mice supplemented with the bacterial strain due to the role of leptin in fat accumulation in peripheral tissues [53].

Our study also showed that *B. uniformis* CECT 7771 administration improves immune function of macrophages and DCs, which is particularly important in obese mice. It is known that macrophage function is impaired in obesity, showing reduced phagocytic capacity and oxidative burst, which has been linked to increased susceptibility to infections of obese subjects [54], [55]. In our study, phagocytic function of macrophages was slightly reduced by the HFD, in accordance with others authors [56]. However, *B. uniformis* CECT 7771 administration stimulated the oxidative burst of macrophages in both HFD and SD-fed mice. Our study also demonstrates that *B. uniformis* CECT 7771 administration improved the ability of macrophages and DCs to produce cytokines in response to a pathogenic bacterial stimulus (LPS). *B. uniformis* CECT 7771 also restored the capacity of DCs to present antigens and stimulate T lymphocyte proliferation. A functional deficiency of DCs in *ob/ob* mice has also been described previously, suggesting that this damage could be generalised to the more frequent forms of obesity [41]. Altogether, our data indicates that *B. uniformis* CECT 7771 can improve innate and adaptive defence mechanisms against infections in diet-induced obesity.

This study also confirms that diet has a tremendous impact on the intestinal microbiota composition and supports the hypothesis that its modulation through the use of dietary strategies could ameliorate the metabolic and immune dysfunctions associated with imbalanced diets. The HFD reduced gene copy numbers of Gram-positive bacteria, including *Bifidobacterium* spp. and *C. coccoides* group, in accordance with previous studies [49]. Our study also demonstrates that the HFD increased the gene copy numbers of enterobacteria, while *B. uniformis* CECT 7771 slightly reduced these numbers and increased those of *C. coccoides* group, *Bifidobacterium* spp. and *Bacteroides* spp. Furthermore, the *B. uniformis* CECT 7771-related changes in microbiota contributed to reducing the gut inflammatory signals, which could affect other peripheral tissues involved in obesity. In this context, endotoxins (LPS) from enterobacteria, present in the gut, have been shown to play an important role in the development of insulin resistance and non-alcoholic fatty liver disease [57]. In *ob/ob* mice, reductions of intestinal *E. coli* numbers by antibiotic treatment were associated with the reduction of metabolic endotoxaemia and inflammatory status as well as with improvements in insulin resistance [58]. Another recent study also reported that positive effects of prebiotics (oligofructose and inulin mixture) on body weight and fat and related metabolic parameters could be due to their ability to increase numbers of both *bacteroides* and bifidobacteria in the gut microbiota of obese JCR:LA-cp rats [13]. These changes were related to modifying the expression of anorexigenic and orexigenic peptides, but the role of each bacterial group on such effects remains unclear.

In conclusion, the results support the hypothesis that the *B. uniformis* CECT 7771 modulates the metabolic and immune dysfunction induced by HFD at least in mice. The study provides direct evidence of the potential beneficial roles played by *B. uniformis* CECT 7771 in obesity, bringing us one step ahead of the mere associations inferred from previous observational studies. Therefore, the use of dietary strategies targeting the gut ecosystem may be an additional tool to control metabolic disorders. However, further studies are required to support this hypothesis and to reveal plausible mechanisms of action of the specific bacterial strain used in this preclinical study. Furthermore, safety issues should also be addressed before proposing the possible use of the strain tested in humans.

REFERENCES

1. Moreno LA, Mesana MI, Gonzalez-Gross M, Gil CM, Fleta J, et al. (2006) Anthropometric body fat composition reference values in Spanish adolescents. The AVENA Study. Eur J Clin Nutr 60: 191–196. doi: 10.1038/sj.ejcn.1602285
2. Badman MK, Flier JS (2007) The adipocyte as an active participant in energy balance and metabolism. Gastroenterology 132: 2103–2115. doi: 10.1053/j.gastro.2007.03.058
3. Sanz Y, Santacruz A, Gauffin P (2010) Gut microbiota in obesity and metabolic disorders. Proc Nutr Soc 69: 434–441. doi: 10.1017/S0029665110001813
4. Wolowczuk I, Verwaerde C, Viltart O, Delanoye A, Delacre M, et al. (2008) Feeding our immune system: impact on metabolism. Clin Dev Immunol 2008: 639803. doi: 10.1155/2008/639803
5. Verwaerde C, Delanoye A, Macia L, Tailleux A, Wolowczuk I (2006) Influence of high-fat feeding on both naive and antigen-experienced T-cell immune response in DO10.11 mice. Scand J Immunol 64: 457–466. doi: 10.1111/j.1365-3083.2006.01791.x
6. Turnbaugh PJ, Gordon JI (2009) The core gut microbiome, energy balance and obesity. J Physiol 587: 4153–4158. doi: 10.1113/jphysiol.2009.174136
7. Jumpertz R, Le DS, Turnbaugh PJ, Trinidad C, Bogardus C, et al. (2011) Energy-balance studies reveal associations between gut microbes, caloric load, and nutrient absorption in humans. Am J Clin Nutr 94: 58–65. doi: 10.3945/ajcn.110.010132
8. Backhed F, Ding H, Wang T, Hooper LV, Koh GY, et al. (2004) The gut microbiota as an environmental factor that regulates fat storage. Proc Natl Acad Sci U S A 101: 15718–15723. doi: 10.1073/pnas.0407076101
9. Ley RE, Backhed F, Turnbaugh P, Lozupone CA, Knight RD, et al. (2005) Obesity alters gut microbial ecology. Proc Natl Acad Sci U S A 102: 11070–11075. doi: 10.1073/pnas.0504978102
10. Eckburg PB, Bik EM, Bernstein CN, Purdom E, Dethlefsen L, et al. (2005) Diversity of the human intestinal microbial flora. Science 308: 1635–1638. doi: 10.1126/science.1110591
11. Armougom F, Henry M, Vialettes B, Raccah D, Raoult D (2009) Monitoring bacterial community of human gut microbiota reveals an increase in *Lactobacillus* in obese

patients and Methanogens in anorexic patients. PLoS One 4: e7125. doi: 10.1371/journal.pone.0007125

12. Ley RE, Turnbaugh PJ, Klein S, Gordon JI (2006) Microbial ecology: human gut microbes associated with obesity. Nature 444: 1022–1023. doi: 10.1038/4441022a

13. Parnell JA, Reimer RA (2011) Prebiotic fibres dose-dependently increase satiety hormones and alter Bacteroidetes and Firmicutes in lean and obese JCR:LA-cp rats. Br J Nutr. 1–13. doi: 10.1017/s0007114511003163

14. Santacruz A, Collado MC, Garcia-Valdes L, Segura MT, Martin-Lagos JA, et al. (2010) Gut microbiota composition is associated with body weight, weight gain and biochemical parameters in pregnant women. Br J Nutr 104: 83–92. doi: 10.1017/S0007114510000176

15. Santacruz A, Marcos A, Warnberg J, Marti A, Martin-Matillas M, et al. (2009) Interplay between weight loss and gut microbiota composition in overweight adolescents. Obesity (Silver Spring) 17: 1906–1915. doi: 10.1038/oby.2009.112

16. Nadal I, Santacruz A, Marcos A, Warnberg J, Garagorri M, et al. (2009) Shifts in clostridia, *bacteroides* and immunoglobulin-coating fecal bacteria associated with weight loss in obese adolescents. Int J Obes (Lond) 33: 758–767. doi: 10.1038/ijo.2008.260

17. Furet JP, Kong LC, Tap J, Poitou C, Basdevant A, et al. (2010) Differential adaptation of human gut microbiota to bariatric surgery-induced weight loss: links with metabolic and low-grade inflammation markers. Diabetes 59: 3049–3057. doi: 10.2337/db10-0253

18. Duncan SH, Lobley GE, Holtrop G, Ince J, Johnstone AM, et al. (2008) Human colonic microbiota associated with diet, obesity and weight loss. Int J Obes (Lond) 32: 1720–1724. doi: 10.1038/ijo.2008.155

19. Schwiertz A, Taras D, Schafer K, Beijer S, Bos NA, et al. (2010) Microbiota and SCFA in lean and overweight healthy subjects. Obesity (Silver Spring) 18: 190–195. doi: 10.1038/oby.2009.167

20. Zhang H, DiBaise JK, Zuccolo A, Kudrna D, Braidotti M, et al. (2009) Human gut microbiota in obesity and after gastric bypass. Proc Natl Acad Sci U S A 106: 2365–2370. doi: 10.1073/pnas.0812600106

21. Hoyles L, McCartney AL (2009) What do we mean when we refer to Bacteroidetes populations in the human gastrointestinal microbiota? FEMS Microbiol Lett 299: 175–183. doi: 10.1111/j.1574-6968.2009.01741.x

22. Sánchez E, De Palma G, Capilla A, Nova E, Pozo T, et al. (2011) Influence of environmental and genetic factors linked to celiac disease risk on infant gut colonization by *Bacteroides* species. Appl Environ Microbiol 77: 5316–23.23. doi: 10.1128/AEM.00365-11

23. Cariou B, van Harmelen K, Duran-Sandoval D, van Dijk TH, Grefhorst A, et al. (2006) The farnesoid X receptor modulates adiposity and peripheral insulin sensitivity in mice. J Biol Chem 281: 11039–11049. doi: 10.1074/jbc.M510258200

24. Vieira JM, Seabra SH, Vallim DC, Americo MA, Fracallanza SE, et al. (2009) *Bacteroides* fragilis induce necrosis on mice peritoneal macrophages: In vitro and in vivo assays. Biochem Biophys Res Commun 387: 627–632. doi: 10.1016/j.bbrc.2009.05.124

25. Ciccocioppo R, Rossi M, Pesce I, Ricci G, Millimaggi D, et al. (2008) Effects of gliadin stimulation on bone marrow-derived dendritic cells from HLA-DQ8 transgenic MICE. Dig Liver Dis 40: 927–935. doi: 10.1016/j.dld.2008.05.005

26. Matsuki T, Watanabe K, Fujimoto J, Miyamoto Y, Takada T, et al. (2002) Development of 16S rRNA-gene-targeted group-specific primers for the detection and identification of predominant bacteria in human feces. Appl Environ Microbiol 68: 5445–5451. doi: 10.1128/AEM.68.11.5445-5451.2002

27. Matsuki T, Watanabe K, Fujimoto J, Takada T, Tanaka R (2004) Use of 16S rRNA gene-targeted group-specific primers for real-time PCR analysis of predominant bacteria in human feces. Appl Environ Microbiol 70: 7220–7228. doi: 10.1128/AEM.70.12.7220-7228.2004

28. Malinen E, Rinttila T, Kajander K, Matto J, Kassinen A, et al. (2005) Analysis of the fecal microbiota of irritable bowel syndrome patients and healthy controls with real-time PCR. Am J Gastroenterol 100: 373–382. doi: 10.1111/j.1572-0241.2005.40312.x

29. Walter J, Hertel C, Tannock GW, Lis CM, Munro K, et al. (2001) Detection of *Lactobacillus*, Pediococcus, Leuconostoc, and Weissella species in human feces by using group-specific PCR primers and denaturing gradient gel electrophoresis. Appl Environ Microbiol 67: 2578–2585. doi: 10.1128/AEM.67.6.2578-2585.2001

30. Heilig HG, Zoetendal EG, Vaughan EE, Marteau P, Akkermans AD, et al. (2002) Molecular diversity of *Lactobacillus* spp. and other lactic acid bacteria in the human intestine as determined by specific amplification of 16S ribosomal DNA. Appl Environ Microbiol 68: 114–123. doi: 10.1128/AEM.68.1.114-123.2002

31. Ito A, Suganami T, Yamauchi A, Degawa-Yamauchi M, Tanaka M, et al. (2008) Role of CC chemokine receptor 2 in bone marrow cells in the recruitment of macrophages into obese adipose tissue. J Biol Chem 283: 35715–35723. doi: 10.1074/jbc.M804220200

32. Kanda H, Tateya S, Tamori Y, Kotani K, Hiasa K, et al. (2006) MCP-1 contributes to macrophage infiltration into adipose tissue, insulin resistance, and hepatic steatosis in obesity. J Clin Invest 116: 1494–1505. doi: 10.1172/JCI26498

33. Nguyen MT, Favelyukis S, Nguyen AK, Reichart D, Scott PA, et al. (2007) A subpopulation of macrophages infiltrates hypertrophic adipose tissue and is activated by free fatty acids via Toll-like receptors 2 and 4 and JNK-dependent pathways. J Biol Chem 282: 35279–35292. doi: 10.1074/jbc.M706762200

34. Arenz S, Ruckerl R, Koletzko B, von Kries R (2004) Breast-feeding and childhood obesity–a systematic review. Int J Obes Relat Metab Disord 28: 1247–1256. doi: 10.1038/sj.ijo.0802758

35. FAO/WHO/UNU (2007) Protein and amino acid requirements in human nutrition. World Health Organ Tech Rep Ser-Report of a Joint WHO/FAO/UNU Expert Consultation-WHO Technical Report Series 935: 1–265, back cover.

36. Samuel BS, Gordon JI (2006) A humanised gnotobiotic mouse model of host-archaeal-bacterial mutualism. Proc Natl Acad Sci U S A 103: 10011–10016. doi: 10.1073/pnas.0602187103

37. Collado MC, Isolauri E, Laitinen K, Salminen S (2008) Distinct composition of gut microbiota during pregnancy in overweight and normal-weight women. Am J Clin Nutr 88: 894–899.

38. Backhed F, Manchester JK, Semenkovich CF, Gordon JI (2007) Mechanisms underlying the resistance to diet-induced obesity in germ-free mice. Proc Natl Acad Sci U S A 104: 979–984. doi: 10.1073/pnas.0605374104

39. Fleissner CK, Huebel N, Abd El-Bary MM, Loh G, Klaus S, et al. (2010) Absence of intestinal microbiota does not protect mice from diet-induced obesity. Br J Nutr. 104(6): 919–929.

40. Ma X, Hua J, Li Z (2008) Probiotics improve high fat diet-induced hepatic steatosis and insulin resistance by increasing hepatic NKT cells. J Hepatol 49: 821–830. doi: 10.1016/j.jhep.2008.05.025

41. Boden G, She P, Mozzoli M, Cheung P, Gumireddy K, et al. (2005) Free fatty acids produce insulin resistance and activate the proinflammatory nuclear factor-kappaB pathway in rat liver. Diabetes 54: 3458–3465. doi: 10.2337/diabetes.54.12.3458

42. Hamad EM, Sato M, Uzu K, Yoshida T, Higashi S, et al. (2009) Milk fermented by *Lactobacillus* gasseri SBT2055 influences adipocyte size via inhibition of dietary fat absorption in Zucker rats. Br J Nutr 101: 716–724. doi: 10.1017/S0007114508043808

43. Li Z, Yang S, Lin H, Huang J, Watkins PA, et al. (2003) Probiotics and antibodies to TNF inhibit inflammatory activity and improve nonalcoholic fatty liver disease. Hepatology 37: 343–350. doi: 10.1053/jhep.2003.50048

44. Rabot S, Membrez M, Bruneau A, Gérard P, Harach T, et al. (2010) Germ-free C57BL/6J mice are resistant to high-fat-diet-induced insulin resistance and have altered cholesterol metabolism. FASEB J. 24(12): 4948–59. doi: 10.1096/fj.10-164921

45. Misra A (2000) Risk factors for atherosclerosis in young individuals. J Cardiovasc Risk 7: 215–229. doi: 10.1096/fj.10-164921

46. Porkka KV, Raitakari OT (1996) Serum lipoproteins in children and young adults: determinants and treatment strategies. Curr Opin Lipidol 7: 183–187. doi: 10.1097/00041433-199608000-00002

47. Cani PD, Amar J, Iglesias MA, Poggi M, Knauf C, et al. (2007) Metabolic endotoxemia initiates obesity and insulin resistance Diabetes. 56(7): 1761–72. doi: 10.2337/db07-1181

48. Membrez M, Blancher F, Jaquet M, Bibiloni R, Cani PD, et al. (2008) Gut microbiota modulation with norfloxacin and ampicillin enhances glucose tolerance in mice. FASEB J. 22(7): 2416–26. doi: 10.2337/db07-1181

49. Cani PD, Delzenne NM (2007) Gut microflora as a target for energy and metabolic homeostasis. Curr Opin Clin Nutr Metab Care 10: 729–734. doi: 10.1097/MCO.0b013e3282efdebb

50. El-Haschimi K, Pierroz DD, Hileman SM, Bjørbaek C, Flier JS (2000) Two defects contribute to hypothalamic leptin resistance in mice with diet-induced obesity. J Clin Invest. 105(12): 1827–32. doi: 10.2337/db07-1181

51. Jiang L, Wang Q, Yu Y, Zhao F, Huang P, et al. (2009) Leptin contributes to the adaptive responses of mice to high-fat diet intake through suppressing the lipogenic pathway. PLoS One: 3 4(9): e6884.

52. La Cava A, Matarese G (2004) The weight of leptin in immunity. Nat Rev Immunol. 4(5): 371–9).

53. Guo KY, Halo P, Leibel RL, Zhang Y (2004) Effects of obesity on the relationship of leptin mRNA expression and adipocyte size in anatomically distinct fat depots in mice. Am J Physiol Regul Integr Comp Physiol. 287(1): R112–9.

54. Smith AG, Sheridan PA, Harp JB, Beck MA (2007) Diet-induced obese mice have increased mortality and altered immune responses when infected with influenza virus. J Nutr 137: 1236–1243.

55. Amar S, Zhou Q, Shaik-Dasthagirisaheb Y, Leeman S (2007) Diet-induced obesity in mice causes changes in immune responses and bone loss manifested by bacterial challenge. Proc Natl Acad Sci U S A 104: 20466–20471. doi: 10.1073/pnas.0710335105

56. Zhou Q, Leeman SE, Amar S (2009) Signaling mechanisms involved in altered function of macrophages from diet-induced obese mice affect immune responses. Proc Natl Acad Sci U S A 106: 10740–10745. doi: 10.1073/pnas.0904412106

57. Solga SF, Diehl AM (2003) Non-alcoholic fatty liver disease: lumen-liver interactions and possible role for probiotics. J Hepatol 38: 681–687. doi: 10.1016/S0168-8278(03)00097-7

58. Membrez M, Blancher F, Jaquet M, Bibiloni R, Cani PD, et al. (2008) Gut microbiota modulation with norfloxacin and ampicillin enhances glucose tolerance in mice. FASEB J 22: 2416–2426. doi: 10.1096/fj.07-102723

SUPPLEMENTATION OF *LACTOBACILLUS CURVATUS* HY7601 AND *LACTOBACILLUS PLANTARUM* KY1032 IN DIET-INDUCED OBESE MICE IS ASSOCIATED WITH GUT MICROBIAL CHANGES AND REDUCTION IN OBESITY

DO-YOUNG PARK, YOUNG-TAE AHN, SE-HOON PARK, CHUL-SUNG HUH, SAE-ROM YOO, RINA YU, MI-KYUNG SUNG, ROBIN A. MCGREGOR, AND MYUNG-SOOK CHOI

6.1 INTRODUCTION

The gastrointestinal tract in an adult human contains approximately 10^{12} microorganisms per milliliter of luminal content and harbors approximately 500 to 1000 distinct bacteria species [1] collectively termed the microbiota. The gut microbiota plays an important role in the innate immune system and host metabolism[1]–[3]. There exists conflicting evidence whether the gut microbiota plays a role in obesity. Bäckhed et al. [4] observed that Germ-free (GF) B6 mice fed a chow diet appeared to be protected from excessive fat accumulation compared to conventional-

This chapter was originally published under the Creative Commons Attribution License. Park D-Y, Ahn Y-T, Park S-H, Huh C-S, Yoo S-R, Yu R, Sung M-K, McGregor RA, and Choi M-S. Supplementation of Lactobacillus curvatus *HY7601 and* Lactobacillus plantarum *KY1032 in Diet-Induced Obese Mice Is Associated with Gut Microbial Changes and Reduction in Obesity. PLoS ONE **8,**3 (2013). doi:10.1371/journal.pone.0059470.*

ized mice fed the same diet in both males and females. When GF animals were fed a Western-style, high-fat and sugar-rich diet, they appeared to be protected from diet-induced obesity [5]. However, another study reported that the absence of gut microbiota did not provide general protection from diet-induced obesity [6]. Mestdagh et al. [7] also reported that the total body fat content of GF C3H/Orl female mice fed a standard chow diet was not significantly different from that of conventional female mice fed the same diet. Therefore, the protection of GF mice from obesity appears to be dependent on diet and animal strain. Nevertheless, diet-induced obesity is reported to be associated with marked but reversible alterations in the mouse gut microbiota [8]. Hence the gut microbiota represents a therapeutic target with the potential to reverse existing obesity.

Probiotics consist of individual or multiple live bacteria species, which directly alter the gut microbiota, such as lactobacilli and bifidobacteria [9], [10]. Multiple in-vivo studies provide evidence that some probiotics can reduce diet-induced obesity in rodents[11]–[18], although there are reports of probiotics with no effect on body weight gain [19] or in some cases probiotics that actually cause weight-gain in rodents [20]. While many studies indicate probiotics intake causes functional changes, such as lower blood lipids in hyperlipidemic animals [21], evidence is lacking for the impact of probiotics containing individual or multiple bacterial species on gut microbiota diversity and composition of obese animals.

Importantly, different probiotic strains may have varying functional effects on the gut microbiota and obesity [22]. The apparent lack of microbiota changes in response to probiotics in some studies may be partly due to inter-individual variability in microbiota composition caused by genetic background, age, diet, or other environmental related factors. Some studies suggest a subset of microbial species appear to more widely spread colonizers of the human gastrointestinal tract, although no species appear to be universally present in all individuals [23], [24], while other studies suggest a common microbiome at the gene level may be shared between individuals [25], [26]. Pre-clinical models of diet-induced obesity in mice provide a useful way to assess physiologically relevant gut microbiota changes associated with both obesity and probiotic treatment, while controlling for the effects of genetic background, diet, age and other environmental factors on the gut microbiota.

The aim of this study was three fold as follows: to assess the functional effects of probiotic treatment on diet-induced obesity, to establish the effects of probiotic treatment on the gut microbiota of diet-induced obese mice and to assess the effects of probiotic treatment on the liver and adipose gene expression.

6.2 MATERIALS AND METHODS

6.2.1 ANIMALS, DIETS AND EXPERIMENTAL DESIGN

Male C57BL/6J mice (n = 36) aged 4 weeks were purchased from Jackson Laboratories (Bar Harbor, USA). All mice were individually housed at a constant temperature and humidity ($22\pm1°C$, 55 ± 10 percent) with a 12 h light/dark cycle. After 1 week allowing for adaptation, mice were fed a high-fat diet (n = 27, HFD; 20 percent fat and 1 percent cholesterol, w/w) to induce obesity or a normal diet (ND group, n = 9) for 8 weeks. Diet-induced obese mice were then randomly assigned to receive probiotics (HFD-probiotic group) or PBS (HFD-placebo group) for another 10 weeks, while the ND group was fed a normal diet. Yun et al. [27] tested the dose-dependent anti-diabetic effect of *Lactobacillus gasseri* ($2\times10^7 \sim 2\times10^{10}$ cfu/day), and observed that diabetic *db/db* mice receiving the bacteria exhibited dose-dependent improvement for several metabolic biomarkers. In our recent study, to maximize the interventional effects of two probiotics, *L. curvatus* HY7601 and *L. plantarum* KY1032, we also used a high-dose of bacteria, 5×10^9 cfu/day for each. *L. curvatus* HY7601 and *L. plantarum* KY1032 were isolated from Korean traditional fermented cabbage which is a rich source of *Lactobacillus* strains with potential probiotic properties [28]. *L. curvatus* HY7601 and *L. plantarum* KY1032 are reported to reduce adipogenesis in 3T3-L1 cells [29]. The probiotics were suspended in sterilized PBS and mixed with the diet immediately before being fed to the mice. Once the mice consumed the initial given amount of food, an additional amount of diet was added to the feed jar so that all the mice could consume all of the available food/probiotic mix every day. The composition of the diets was formulated based on the AIN-76 semi-synthetic diet (Table S1). A reference group (n = 9) was sacrificed to determine the accumulation of adipose tissue depots in diet induced obese mice after 8 weeks before probiotic treatment. Body weight was measured once a week. Before sacrifice, mice were fasted for 12 h and anesthetized with diethyl ether. Blood samples were taken from the inferior vena cava for plasma analysis. All adipose tissue depots were removed, rinsed with PBS and weighed. For real-time PCR analysis, the epididymal fat pad and liver tissue were frozen at −70°C right after removal. The experimental design was approved by the Ethics Committee at Korea Yakult Company Limited R&D center.

6.2.2 BACTERIAL 16S RRNA GENE AMPLIFICATION AND BARCODED PYROSEQUENCING

For analysis of the microbial content, metagenomic DNA was extracted from the fecal samples of all mice using the QIAamp DNA stool mini kit (Qiagen, Netherlands) according to the manufacturer's instruction. The extracted DNA was amplified using primers targeting the V1 to V3 hypervariable regions of the bacterial 16S rRNA gene (V1-9F: 5′-X-AC-GAGTTTGATCMTGGCTCAG-3′ and V3-541R: 5′-X-AC-WTTAC-CGCGGCTGCTGG-3′ where X denotes uniquely designed barcode for each mouse followed by a common linker AC). In this study, mixtures of barcodes with varied lengths (7 to 11 base pairs) were used. PCR reactions were carried out in a thermocycler (MJ Research, USA) under the following conditions: initial denaturation at 94°C for 5 min; followed by 20 cycles of denaturation at 94°C for 30 sec, annealing at 55°C for 45 sec, and elongation at 72°C for 1 min 30 sec. The amplified products were purified using resin columns, and 1 μg of PCR product for each mouse was mixed and subjected to pyrosequencing. The DNA sequencing was performed using the standard shotgun sequencing reagents and a 454 GS FLX Titanium Sequencing System (Roche, USA), according to the manufacturer's instructions by Chunlab Inc., Republic of Korea. The length of the fragment of the 16S rDNA pyrosequenced ranged from 118 to 526 base pairs and the average length was 472 base pairs. The pyrosequencing data are available in the EMBL SRA database under the accession number ERP000935.

6.2.3 ANALYSIS OF BACTERIAL 16S RRNA GENE SEQUENCES

Pre-processing and taxonomic assignment of sequencing reads were conducted using a JAVA based bioinformatic pipeline (Chunlab Inc., Republic of Korea) described in a previous study [30]. First, sequencing reads from the different samples were separated by unique barcodes. Then, the barcode, linker, and PCR primer sequences at both sides were removed from the original sequencing reads. Individual collections of sequences were depleted of non-16S rRNA sequences and chimaeras using HMMER 3.0 (http://hmmer.janelia.org) and BLAST. Sequences shorter than 300 nt, having one or more ambiguous base calls, an average quality below 25, or showing no match with the 16S rRNA EzTaxon-e database (http://eztaxon-e.ezbiocloud.net/) [31] were also excluded from the subsequent analyses.

The trimmed sequences were assigned taxonomically via alignment with the EzTaxon-e database which includes not only species within the formal nomenclatural system, but also phylotypes that represent both cultured and uncultured entries in the GenBank public database [31]. Sequences with identity scores >97% were resolved at the species level, between 97% and 94% at the genus level, between 94% and 90% at the family level, between 90% and 85% at the order level, between 85% and 80% at the class level and between 80% and 75% at the phylum level based on EzTaxon-e [31]. If the similarity was below the cutoff value, the read was assigned to an "unclassified" group.

The beta diversity measure was calculated in order to compare between pairs of taxonomic communities using the MOTHUR software. All taxa found in one or both samples were placed on a phylogenetic tree. The UniFrac algorithm calculated the distance between two samples as the ratio of the sum of branch lengths leading to taxa from both samples to the sum of all branch lengths leading to all taxa [32]. The Unweighted Pair Group Method with Arithmetic Mean (UPGMA) [33] was used to cluster the pairwise distances of the samples, which indicates samples sharing community structures shown in a dendrogram. Phylogenetic distances between samples were also visualized with principal coordinate analysis (PCoA) as previously described [34].

For calculation of alpha diversity measures, sequences were clustered and assigned to operational taxonomic units (OTUs) using the CD-HIT algorithm [35]. The OTUs were inputted into the MOTHUR software [36] to generate diversity indexes such as rarefaction curves [37] and ACE richness estimator [38]. Rarefaction curves showed the OTUs observed as a function of the sampling effort, showing that a steep slope represents a large portion of the species diversity not yet sampled. The ACE richness estimator predicts the species richness based on the number of rarely occurring OTUs.

EzTaxon-e derived taxonomic communities were used to calculate the relative abundance (%) of bacteria at the phylum taxa level and species taxa level in each sample, as well as the core microbiota present in all samples. The present/absence of all microbial species at the species-level across samples was visualized in a heatmap generated with the R software. There is no universal consensus on a core microbiota definition, so we calculated the core microbiota shared by each group population at multiple thresholds between 50–100% of the mice in each experimental group. A Venn diagram was used to show core microbiota species shared by >78% of the mice in each experimental group regardless of treatment.

6.2.4 HISTOLOGICAL ANALYSIS

Epididymal fat samples from each mouse were rinsed with sterilized PBS, fixed in 10 percent v/v formalin/PBS, and then embedded in paraffin for staining with hematoxylin and eosin (H&E). Images were obtained under a microscope (AxioObser Z1, Germany) at a magnification of ×200.

6.2.5 BLOOD ANALYSIS

Plasma, leptin, and insulin concentrations were determined using multiplex detection kits (Bio-Rad, USA) on the Bio-Plex Suspension array system (Bio-Rad, USA). The plasma total-cholesterol, triglyceride concentration, aspartate transaminase (AST) and alanine transaminase (ALT) activity were enzymatically determined using commercial kits (Asan Co., Republic of Korea). Plasma thiobarbituric acid-reacting substances (TBARS) were determined using a spectrophotometric method [31].

6.2.6 RT-QPCR

Total RNA was extracted from adipose (100 mg) and liver (15 mg) tissues using an RNAqueous kit (Ambion, USA). Total RNA (2 μg) was reverse-transcribed into cDNA with the high-capacity RNA-to-cDNA kit (Applied Biosystems Inc., USA). The cDNA was amplified on a 7500 Real Time PCR System (Applied Biosystems Inc., USA) using mouse-specific Taqman probe sets (Table S2) and normalized to GAPDH. The data are presented as the means ± SE.

6.2.7 STATISTICAL ANALYSIS

All data were presented as the means ± SE. For metabolic and gene expression data analysis, significant differences between groups (HFD+placebo versus ND, HFD+probiotic versus HFD+placebo) were determined using unpaired Student's t-test. For the relative abundance analysis of the gut microbiota, significant differences between groups (HFD+placebo versus ND, HFD+probiotic versus HFD+placebo) were determined using Kruskal–Wallis one-way analysis of variance with Bonferroni correction to control for multiple comparisons. All values were considered statistically significant when $p<0.05$.

6.3 RESULTS

6.3.1 EFFECTS OF PROBIOTIC TREATMENT ON BODY WEIGHT, FAT MASS AND ADIPOCYTES OF DIET-INDUCED OBESE MICE

Diet-induced obesity was induced for over 8 weeks (28.55±0.77 g versus 22.59±0.45 g, HFD+placebo and ND group respectively) (Figure

1A), but following probiotic treatment, HFD-induced body weight gain was 38 percent lower (p<0.01) in the probiotic group (8.53±0.20 g) than in the HFD+placebo group (13.75±1.07 g) (Figure 1B). Hence, after 10 weeks, the average body weight was 11 percent lower (p<0.05) in the HFD+probiotic group compared to the HFD+placebo group, although HFD+probiotic mice still gained more weight than those mice consuming the ND (Figure 1A).

Food intake in the probiotic group was not significantly different compared to the HFD+placebo mice, although mice receiving probiotics consumed 7~8% less food overall (Figure S1A). The food efficiency ratio (FER) represents total grams of body weight gained on a test food divided by the total grams of food consumed during an animal feeding study. In the HFD mice the FER was significantly increased compared to the ND-fed mice, reflecting greater efficiency of HFD on weight gain, conversely the FER was reduced by 29 percent (p<0.01) in the probiotic treatment group (Figure 1C) reflecting lower weight gain per grams of food consumed.

Liver toxicity biomarkers alanine transaminase (ALT) and aspartate transaminase (AST) were significantly elevated in the HFD compared to ND mice (Figure S1B and S1C). Conversely, plasma ALT was reduced by 70 percent (p<0.05) in the HFD+probiotic group, and plasma AST was non-significantly reduced by 20 percent compared to the HFD+placebo group.

White fat mass was significantly higher in the HFD+placebo group compared to the ND group after 18 weeks (p<0.001, Figure 1D). Fat accumulation was lower in the mice that received probiotic treatment since total white fat mass gain was 31 percent lower in the HFD+probiotic group (~5.69 g) than in the HFD+placebo group (~8.19 g). Hence, total white fat mass was reduced by 14 percent in the HFD+probiotic compared to the HFD+placebo group (p<0.05, Figure 1D). Analysis of adipose tissue depots revealed consistently higher mesenteric, intrascapular, subcutaneous, epididymal, retroperitoneal and perirenal fat in the HFD+placebo mice compared to the ND-fed mice. The mesenteric adipose tissue depot was reduced by 28 percent (p<0.05) in the HFD+probiotic mice compared to the HFD+placebo mice (Figure 1E). Furthermore, histological analysis of white (epididymal) adipose tissue showed the size of the

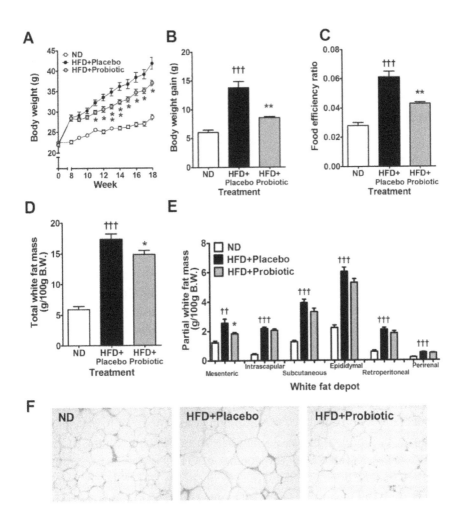

FIGURE 1: High-fat diet and probiotic effect on body weight, fat mass and adipocyte morphology. Effects of probiotic treatment on (A) body weight, (B) body weight gain, (C) food efficiency ratio, (D) total white fat mass, (E) partial white fat mass and (F) epididymal adipocyte morphology. Results are expressed as the means ± SE. Significant differences HFD-placebo versus ND are indicated as ††p<0.01 †††p<0.001. Significant differences between HFD-probiotic versus HFD-placebo are indicated as *p<0.05, **p<0.01. Epididymal adipose tissue morphology shown at ×200 magnification.

adipocytes was markedly increased in the HFD+placebo mice versus the ND mice but reduced in the mice receiving probiotic treatment (Figure 1F).

6.3.2 EFFECTS OF PROBIOTIC TREATMENT ON THE INDEXES OF GUT MICROBIAL DIVERSITY IN DIET-INDUCED OBESE MICE

To establish the gut microbiota changes caused by diet-induced obesity and the effect of probiotic treatment on the gut microbiota we performed fecal pyrosequencing. A total of 151,061 pyrosequencing reads for the fecal microbiota were analyzed with a mean of 6,564, 5,274 and 4,464 reads for the ND, HFD+placebo and HFD+probiotic groups, respectively (Table S3). The full pyrosequencing dataset is available in the EMBL SRA database, accession ERP000935. Beta diversity analysis using the hierarchical clustering algorithm UPGMA (Unweighted Pair-Group Method with Arithmetic mean) and dimensionality reduction using PCoA (Principal Coordinates Analysis) showed that the fecal samples were intermingled and did not form distinct non-overlapping clusters (Figure S2A and S2B).

To assess alpha diversity, pyrosequencing reads were assigned into operational taxonomic units (OTUs) with 97 percent sequence similarity and represented using rarefaction curves. Rarefaction analyses indicated individual rarefaction curves of the probiotic group appeared to plateau in the majority of samples (Figure 2A and S3), in agreement with the ACE richness estimator (Table S3). The number of OTUs observed and estimated showed that the diversity of gut microbiota of the HFD+placebo mice was lower ($p<0.001$) than that of the ND mice (Figure 2A, Table S3). The gut microbiota diversity was further lowered ($p<0.05$) in the HFD+probiotic compared to the HFD+placebo mice (Figure 2A, Table S3).

6.3.3 GUT MICROBIOTA SHARED BETWEEN MICE INDEPENDENT OF DIET AND TREATMENT

There is debate regarding whether a shared microbiota community exists between mammals, which is an important assumption in pre-clinical

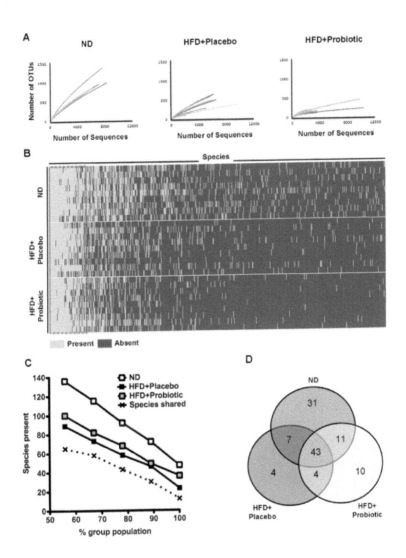

FIGURE 2: Shared microbiota and species diversity. (A) Rarefaction analysis of 151,061 pyrosequencing reads of 16S rRNA from feces using OTUs at a 97 percent sequence similarity cut-off value. (B) Microbiota species present or absent in ND, HFD+placebo and HFD+probiotic mice. Dark blue indicates species absent in the gut microbiota, light blue indicates species present in the gut microbiota. (C) Shared microbiota within and between groups varies depending on the percent group population cut-off used to define the shared microbiota. (D) Venn diagram of overlap in species shared by >78 percent of the mice from each group.

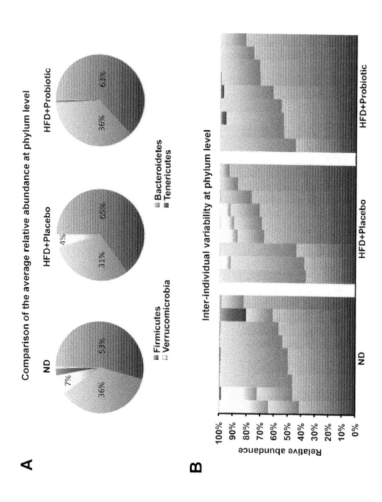

FIGURE 3: High-fat diet and probiotic effect on the gut microbiota composition at the phylum level. (A) The average relative abundance of the major microbial phyla in ND, HFD+placebo and HFD+probiotic mice. (B) Inter-individual variability in the relative abundance of the major microbial phyla in ND, HFD+placebo and HFD+probiotic mice. Values presented are percentage of relative abundance with respect to total bacterial sequences.

studies comparing gut microbiota between treatment groups; therefore, we determined the presence or absence of species across all samples and how many species were shared between samples. As shown in Figure 2B, there were 682 species detected overall (563, 355 and 265 species in the ND, HFD and HFD-probiotic group respectively), of which about a tenth of the microbial species (in the dotted red box) were present in over half of all the samples regardless of the treatment. Specifically, the number of bacterial species shared between the groups is dependent on how many mice in each group were used for the comparison between the groups (Figure 2C). For instance, when comparing 100% (9/9), 89% (8/9), 78% (7/9), 67% (6/9) and 56% (5/9) of the population in each group with one another, the number of species shared among all groups was 12, 30, 43, 58 and 65, respectively (Table S4). Figure 2D shows the number of shared species when the 78% criterion was applied; 43 species were shared among all three groups and many more species were shared between two groups or within each group.

6.3.4 EFFECTS OF PROBIOTIC TREATMENT ON THE GUT MICROBIOTA COMPOSITION OF DIET-INDUCED OBESE MICE

Gut microbial compositions for the most abundant two phyla *Firmicutes* and *Bacteroidetes* were not significantly different between the groups (Figure 3A, Table S5). Among the other phyla, the relative abundance of phylum *Tenericutes* was significantly lower in the HFD+placebo group compared to the ND group. In addition, the phylum *Verrucomicrobia* was absent and *Proteobacteria* was significantly lower in the probiotic treated group compared to the placebo treated HFD fed mice (Table S5). Inter-individual variability was also apparent at the phylum level within all groups (Figure 3B).

Next, we analyzed the differences in the gut microbiota composition at the species level. The relative abundance was determined for 682 gut bacterial species detectable in this study. We found that the relative abundance of 40 species was significantly ($p<0.05$) different in mice with diet-induced

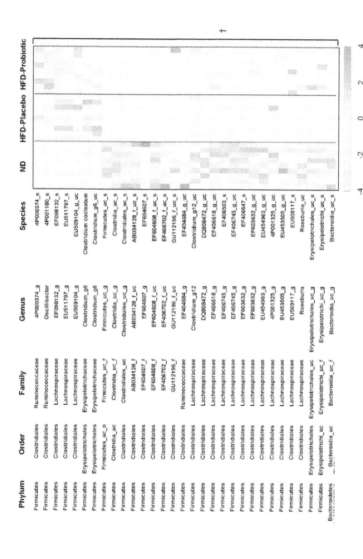

FIGURE 4: High-fat diet and probiotic effect on gut microbiota composition at the species level. Heatmap of the relative abundance of microbial species altered by diet-induced obesity or probiotic treatment. Data represents row scaled Z-scores. Significant differences between HFD-placebo versus ND are indicated as †$p < 0.05$. Significant differences between HFD+probiotic versus HFD+placebo are indicated as *$p < 0.05$.

FIGURE 4: *Cont.*

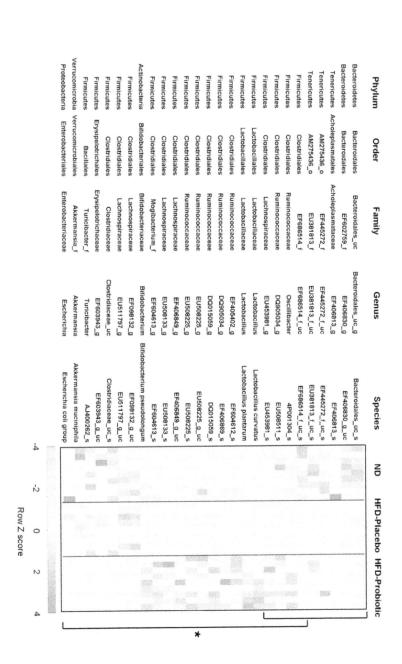

obesity, with an increase of 7 species (Figure 4, Table S6) and a decrease of 33 species (Figure 4, Table S7). The relative abundance of 4 species (EF686514_f_uc_s, 4P001304_s, EU508511_s and EU453981_s) belonging to the EF686514_f, *Ruminococcaceae* and *Lachnospiraceae* families of the order *Clostridiales* and phylum *Firmicutes*, which were decreased by HFD, were increased in mice receiving probiotic treatment (Figure 4, Table S7).

Gut microbial species not associated with changes caused by diet-induced obesity also appeared to be affected in mice receiving probiotic treatment. The relative abundance of 18 more species from diverse taxonomic orders including *Lactobacillales, Clostridiales, Bifidobacteriales, Erysipelotrichales, Bacillales, Verrucomicrobiales, Enterobacteriales* appeared to be different in the probiotic treated mice, with an increase of 11 species (Figure 4, Table S8) and a decrease of 7 species (Figure 4, Table S9). Following probiotic treatment *L. curvatus* and *L. plantarum* species were present at a relative abundance of 0.362±0.070 percent and 0.065±0.021 percent for all bacterial sequences in the HFD-probiotic group (Table S8). Furthermore, the relative abundance of endogenous *Bifidobacterium pseudolongum* was higher (p<0.01) in the HFD+probiotic mice compared to the HFD+placebo mice, although *B. pseudolongum* was not externally administered (Figure 4, Table S8).

6.3.5 EFFECTS OF PROBIOTIC TREATMENT ON BLOOD LIPID AND HORMONE LEVELS IN DIET-INDUCED OBESE MICE

We established a time-course of changes in plasma cholesterol and triglycerides in our pre-clinical model of diet-induced obesity. Cholesterol was consistently elevated in the HFD fed mice compared to the ND fed mice (Figure 5A), but plasma triglycerides were not significantly different (data not shown). Importantly, the time-course analysis revealed plasma cholesterol was significantly reduced by 17 percent (Figure 5A, p<0.05) after 10 weeks of treatment in the HFD+probiotic mice compared to the HFD+placebo mice.

Plasma leptin and insulin were both elevated in our experimental model of diet-induced obesity. Conversely, plasma leptin and insulin were lowered by 49 percent (p = 0.048) and 67 percent (p = 0.025), respectively, in the HFD+probiotic mice compared to the HFD+placebo mice (Figure 5B and 5C). Plasma TBARS, a measure of oxidative stress, was significantly elevated in the HFD mice compared to the ND mice (p<0.05); however, probiotic treatment caused a 30 percent decrease in TBARS compared to the placebo, but the difference was not significant (data not shown).

6.3.6 EFFECTS OF PROBIOTIC TREATMENT ON GENE EXPRESSION IN THE ADIPOSE TISSUE OF DIET-INDUCED OBESE MICE

Next, we measured gene expression in epididymal adipose tissue. HFD intake significantly increased the expression of epididymal adipose tissue genes controlling inflammation (TNFα, IL6, IL1β, MCP1) and fatty acid oxidation (CPT1, CPT2), as well as UCP2, LPL and SREBP1 (Figure 6). Conversely, HFD intake significantly decreased the expression of FAS and SCD1 genes. We found that TNFα (−42 percent), IL6 (−50 percent), IL1β (−33 percent), MCP1 (−41 percent), UCP2 (−43 percent) and LPL (−13 percent) gene expression in the epididymal fat were significantly lower in the HFD+probiotic mice compared to the HFD+placebo mice (Figure 6). Conversely, epididymal HSL (+28 percent) gene expression was significantly higher in the HFD+probiotic mice compared to the HFD+placebo mice.

6.3.7 EFFECTS OF PROBIOTIC TREATMENT ON LIPID AND CHOLESTEROL METABOLISM GENE EXPRESSION IN THE LIVER OF DIET-INDUCED OBESE MICE

We also examined the mRNA levels of genes related to lipid metabolism in the liver. As shown in Figure 7, HFD intake significantly decreased the expression of genes involved in fatty acid oxidation (PGC1α, CPT1) and increased the expression of genes involved in the regulation of adipogenesis (PPARγ, SREBP1, SCD1) and lipogenesis (LPL). Conversely, fatty acid oxidation related gene expression including PGC1α (+49 percent), CPT1 (+42 percent), CPT2 (+25 percent) and ACOX1 (+30

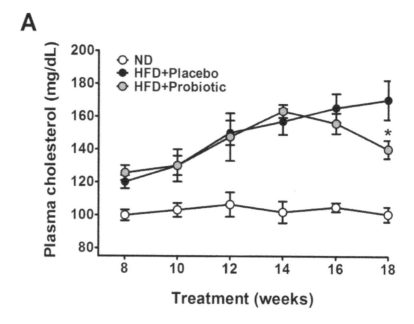

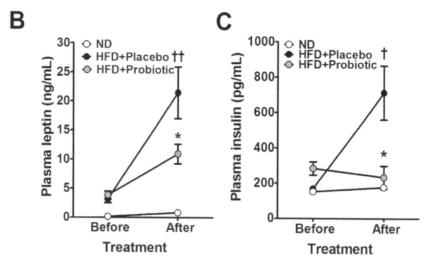

FIGURE 5: High-fat diet and probiotic effect on plasma cholesterol, leptin and insulin. Effects of probiotic treatment on (A) plasma cholesterol, (B) leptin and (C) insulin in diet-induced obese mice. Results are expressed as the means ± SE. Significant differences between HFD-placebo versus ND are indicated as †p<0.05, ††p<0.01. Significant differences between probiotic versus HFD are indicated as *p<0.05.

percent) was significantly higher in the HFD+probiotic mice compared to the HFD+placebo mice. In addition, LPL (−37 percent) and FAS (−41 percent) gene expression was significantly lower in the HFD+probiotic mice compared to the HFD+placebo mice. Additionally, the HSL mRNA level was significantly higher in the HFD mice compared to the ND mice and increased another 38 percent in mice receiving probiotic treatment (p<0.001). Finally, CYP7A1 and LDLR gene mRNA levels were significantly higher by 235 percent and 90 percent, respectively, in the probiotic treated mice compared to the placebo treated mice.

6.4 DISCUSSION

6.4.1 PROBIOTIC USE IS CORRELATED WITH A REDUCTION IN DIET-INDUCED OBESITY

The relationship between food intake and weight gain based on a given diet is very important in nutrition intervention studies. For this reason, the food efficiency ratio (FER) was used as an index for the efficiency of the given food. While mice treated with *L. curvatus* HY7601 and *L. plantarum* KY1032 showed 7~8% (~0.2 g) less food intake compared to the placebo-treated mice, probiotics-treated mice showed a greater reduction in body weight gain (~35% reduction) and total white fat mass gain (~31%) compared to the placebo-treated mice. These results indicate that the probiotics added diet does play a role in suppressing body weight gain compared to its control diet. Of note, fat accumulation was predominantly lower in the mesenteric adipose depot. There is some evidence to indicate other probiotics such as *L. gasseri* SBT2055 also reduce adipocyte size in the mesenteric fat depot of rats [39], which may be partly attributable to its close proximity to the gastrointestinal tract. A longer probiotic treatment duration may lead to greater changes in all visceral fat depots.

6.4.2 PROBIOTICS APPEAR TO MODULATE THE GUT MICROBIOTA OF DIET-INDUCED OBESE MICE

Probiotics may provide a way to alter the gut microbiota naturally and they partly explain the reduction in fat accumulation in response to

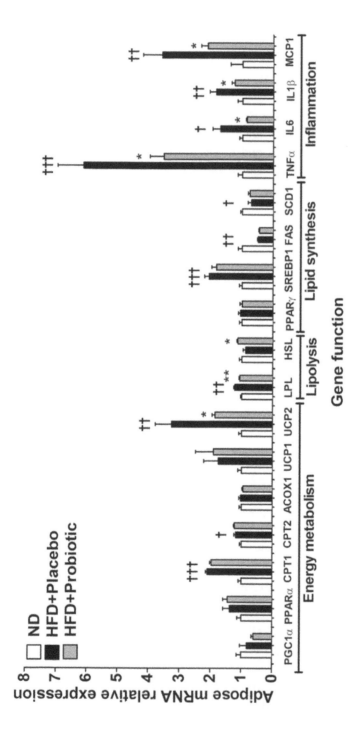

FIGURE 6: High-fat diet and probiotic effect on gene expression in epididymal fat. Results are expressed as the means ± SE. Significant differences between HFD-placebo versus ND are indicated as †p<0.05, ††p<0.01, †††p<0.001. Significant differences between HFD+probiotic versus HFD+placebo are indicated as *p<0.05, **p<0.01, ***p<0.001.

probiotic interventions. However, there was a recent report that *L. acidophilus* NCDC 13 supplementation has no detectable effect on obese animals [19]. Some of the discrepancies between findings may be due to the strain-specific effects of probiotics. Another contributing factor is inter-individual variability in the gut microbiota between individuals, which may be attributable to differences in genetic background, age and diet [40]. Therefore, it is essential when assessing the effect of probiotics on obesity and the gut microbiota that confounding factors such as genetic background, age, sex and diet are controlled. To minimize inter-individual variability in the gut microbiota, we used mice with the same genetic background, age and sex, and observed that about a tenth of all detected microbial species were shared by over half of the mice regardless of diet or treatment, which is an essential assumption for preclinical studies of probiotic interventions.

We tried to ensure the reliability of the species identity determined by pyrosequencing. We sequenced the 16 s rRNA gene region of *L. curvatus* HY7601 using the 16 s rRNA universal primers (27F, 1492R) and compared it to *L. curvatus* HY7601 pyrosequences. Both sequences were perfectly aligned. *L. plantarum* KY1032 also showed alignment between both sequences proving the reliability of the species identity carried out by pyrosequencing, in at least two species (Table S10).

At the phylum level, there is some evidence which indicates the ratio of *Bacteroidetes:Firmicutes* is decreased in diet-induced obese mice, ob/ob mice [41], obese humans [42], and conversely increased by weight-loss [42]. In contrast, other studies, particularly in humans, suggest the *Bacteroidetes:Firmicutes* ratio is not a factor in human obesity and the *Bacteroidetes:Firmicutes* ratio appears to be unrelated to diet [43]–[45]. In the present study, we did not find significant differences in the relative abundance of *Bacteroidetes* and *Firmicutes* among the experimental groups.

At the species level, we found significant differences between the groups. The relative abundance of 40 species was altered by diet-induced obesity, 4 of which were altered in mice receiving probiotic treatment. In addition, 18 species were different in mice with probiotic treatment independently of diet-induced obesity. Remarkably, the relative abundance of *Bifidobacterium pseudolongum* was about 10 times higher in the HFD-probiotic group than in the HFD-placebo group in present study, which appears to be correlated with the suppression of body weight gain or body fat reduction in diet-induced obese mice. Recent reports suggest that certain members of the genus *Bifidobacterium* have conferred health-promoting or probiotic effects [46], [47].

Alongside modulation of the gut microbiota at the species level, we found that mice in the probiotic treatment group also had lower gut microbiota diversity. Low gut microbiota diversity is usually a hallmark of intestinal dysbiosis. Our findings of reduced microbial diversity alongside reduced weight-gain are consistent with evidence from obese mice treated with antibiotics [48], [49] or wheat arabinoxylan [50]. In addition, germ-free mice which lack gut microbiota appear to be protected against diet-induced obesity [5], [7]. Some probiotic strains may reduce the diversity of the gut microbiota by either increased competition for nutrients or alternatively by production of antimicrobial peptides that reduce microbial growth [10]. Further study is required to establish whether probiotic strains commonly reduce the diversity of the gut microbiota and whether there are any long-term consequences of prolonged probiotic supplementation.

6.4.3 INFLAMMATION AND LIPID METABOLISM RELATED GENE EXPRESSION IN ADIPOSE AND LIVER TISSUE APPEARS TO BE ALTERED BY PROBIOTICS

Chronic low-grade inflammation is a characteristic of obesity [51]. Inflammatory cytokine related genes including TNFα, IL6, IL1β and MCP1, which were increased in parallel with plasma insulin levels in the diet-induced obese mice, were reduced in mice receiving probiotic treatment. Several potential mechanisms may explain the reduction of pro-inflammatory cytokine expression induced in mice receiving probiotic treatment. Pathogenic gut microbials are reported to stimulate LPS production and secretion from intestinal epithelial cells, which can then bind cytokine receptors on hepatocytes and adipocytes triggering pro-inflammatory cytokine release [52]. Intestinal barrier function is reported to be improved by some probiotic strains [53], hence reducing LPS release from the intestinal epithelial cells, leading to decreased pro-inflammatory cytokine

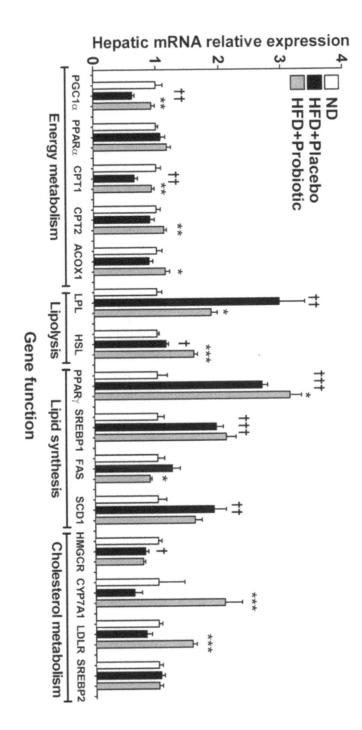

FIGURE 7: High-fat diet and probiotic effect on gene expression in liver. Results are expressed as the means ± SE. Significant differences between HFD-placebo versus ND are indicated as †p<0.05, ††p<0.01, †††p<0.001. Significant differences between HFD+probiotic versus HFD+placebo are indicated as *p<0.05, **p<0.01, ***p<0.001.

production in adipose tissue. It will be important in future studies to assess whether the probiotic strain we used herein leads to reduced inflammatory-related gene expression due to alteration in the intestinal barrier function or due to some other factors.

Energy metabolism related gene expression was increased in the liver of probiotic treated mice, including PGC1α, CPT1, CPT2 and ACOX1 which suggests some of the differences in fat accumulation may have been due to increased mitochondrial oxidation of long chain fatty acids [54] and increased fatty acid oxidation in the liver [55]. Although further studies are needed to determine whether probiotics exert any direct effect on energy metabolism genes or whether probiotic effects are predominantly mediated by changes in the gut microbiota.

Hepatic cholesterol uptake and bile synthesis related genes including LDLR and CYP7A1, were also higher in the probiotic treated mice, which was consistent with the lower cholesterol levels in the probiotic treated mice. Probiotic effects on cholesterol levels have been primarily attributable to lowered gastrointestinal cholesterol absorption or increased cholesterol excretion, mediated via bile metabolism [56]. In both adipose and liver tissues, lower LPL gene expression and higher HSL gene expression in the probiotic treated mice suggests that probiotic treatment may reduce fatty acid uptake and augment lipolysis [57], [58]. We acknowledge that the effects of the probiotic treatment on a relatively small panel of genes related to inflammation and metabolism were assessed. In future studies, it may be worthwhile to conduct global gene and proteomic profiling to further elucidate the underlying response of metabolic tissues to probiotic treatment.

6.5 CONCLUSIONS

Body weight gain was reduced in diet-induced obese mice treated with *L. curvatus* HY7601 and *L. plantarum* KY1032. The gut microbiota was also different in diet-induced obese mice receiving probiotic treatment. Furthermore, energy metabolism and inflammation related genes in liver and adipose tissue were also concomitantly different in mice receiving probiotic treatment. Taken together, these findings suggest *L. curvatus*

HY7601 and *L. plantarum* KY1032 supplementation might modulate the gut microbiota, at least in mice, and may provide a natural alternative to combat obesity. However, full scale trials in humans are required.

REFERENCES

1. DiBaise JK, Zhang H, Crowell MD, Krajmalnik-Brown R, Decker GA, et al. (2008) Gut microbiota and its possible relationship with obesity. Mayo Clin Proc 83: 460–469. doi: 10.4065/83.4.460
2. Turnbaugh PJ, Ley RE, Hamady M, Fraser-Liggett CM, Knight R, et al. (2007) The human microbiome project. Nature 449: 804–810. doi: 10.1038/nature06244
3. Abu-Shanab A, Quigley EMM (2010) The role of the gut microbiota in nonalcoholic fatty liver disease. Nat Rev Gastroenterol Hepatol 7: 691–701. doi: 10.1038/nrgastro.2010.172
4. Bäckhed F, Ding H, Wang T, Hooper LV, Koh GY, et al. (2004) The gut microbiota as an environmental factor that regulates fat storage. Proc Natl Acad Sci USA 101: 15718–15723. doi: 10.1073/pnas.0407076101
5. Bäckhed F, Manchester JK, Semenkovich CF, Gordon JI (2007) Mechanisms underlying the resistance to diet-induced obesity in germ-free mice. Proc Natl Acad Sci USA 104: 979–984. doi: 10.1073/pnas.0605374104
6. Fleissner CK, Huebel N, Abd El-Bary MM, Loh G, Klaus S, et al. (2010) Absence of intestinal microbiota does not protect mice from diet-induced obesity. Br J Nutr 104: 919–929. doi: 10.1017/S0007114510001303
7. Mestdagh R, Dumas M-E, Rezzi S, Kochhar S, Holmes E, et al. (2012) Gut microbiota modulate the metabolism of brown adipose tissue in mice. J Proteome Res 11: 620–630 doi:10.1021/pr200938v.
8. Turnbaugh PJ, Bäckhed F, Fulton L, Gordon JI (2008) Diet-induced obesity is linked to marked but reversible alterations in the mouse distal gut microbiome. Cell Host Microbe 3: 213–223. doi: 10.1016/j.chom.2008.02.015
9. Delzenne NM, Neyrinck AM, Bäckhed F, Cani PD (2011) Targeting gut microbiota in obesity: effects of prebiotics and probiotics. Nat Rev Endocrinol 7: 639–646. doi: 10.1038/nrendo.2011.126
10. Gerritsen J, Smidt H, Rijkers GT, de Vos WM (2011) Intestinal microbiota in human health and disease: the impact of probiotics. Genes Nutr 6: 209–240. doi: 10.1007/s12263-011-0229-7
11. Aronsson L, Huang Y, Parini P, Korach-André M, Håkansson J, et al. (2010) Decreased fat storage by *Lactobacillus* paracasei is associated with increased levels of angiopoietin-like 4 protein (ANGPTL4). PLoS ONE 5: e13087. doi: 10.1371/journal.pone.0013087
12. Chen JJ, Wang R, Li X, Wang R (2011) Bifidobacterium longum supplementation improved high-fat-fed-induced metabolic syndrome and promoted intestinal Reg I gene expression. Exp Biol Med 236: 823–831. doi: 10.1258/ebm.2011.010399

13. Kang J-H, Yun S-I, Park H-O (2010) Effects of *Lactobacillus gasseri* BNR17 on body weight and adipose tissue mass in diet-induced overweight rats. J Microbiol 48: 712–714 doi:10.1007/s12275-010-0363-8.

14. Kondo S, Xiao J-Z, Satoh T, Odamaki T, Takahashi S, et al. (2010) Antiobesity effects of Bifidobacterium breve strain B-3 supplementation in a mouse model with high-fat diet-induced obesity. Biosci Biotechnol Biochem 74: 1656–1661. doi: 10.1271/bbb.100267

15. Lee H-Y, Park J-H, Seok S-H, Baek M-W, Kim D-J, et al. (2006) Human originated bacteria, *Lactobacillus* rhamnosus PL60, produce conjugated linoleic acid and show anti-obesity effects in diet-induced obese mice. Biochim Biophys Acta 1761: 736–744. doi: 10.1016/j.bbalip.2006.05.007

16. Lee K, Paek K, Lee HY, Park JH, Lee Y (2007) Antiobesity effect of trans-10,cis-12-conjugated linoleic acid-producing *Lactobacillus* plantarum PL62 on diet-induced obese mice. J Appl Microbiol 103: 1140–1146. doi: 10.1111/j.1365-2672.2007.03336.x

17. Ma X, Hua J, Li Z (2008) Probiotics improve high fat diet-induced hepatic steatosis and insulin resistance by increasing hepatic NKT cells. J Hepatol 49: 821–830. doi: 10.1016/j.jhep.2008.05.025

18. An HM, Park SY, Lee DK, Kim JR, Cha MK, et al. (2011) Antiobesity and lipid-lowering effects of Bifidobacterium spp. in high fat diet-induced obese rats. Lipids Health Dis 10: 116. doi: 10.1186/1476-511X-10-116

19. Arora T, Anastasovska J, Gibson G, Tuohy K, Sharma RK, et al. (2012) Effect of *Lactobacillus* acidophilus NCDC 13 supplementation on the progression of obesity in diet-induced obese mice. Br J Nutr 108: 1382–1389. doi: 10.1017/S0007114511006957

20. Yin Y-N, Yu Q-F, Fu N, Liu X-W, Lu F-G (2010) Effects of four Bifidobacteria on obesity in high-fat diet induced rats. World J Gastroenterol 16: 3394–3401. doi: 10.3748/wjg.v16.i27.3394

21. Park D-Y, Ahn Y-T, Huh C-S, McGregor RA, Choi M-S (2013) Dual probiotic strains suppress high fructose-induced metabolic syndrome. World J Gastroenterol 19: 274–283. doi: 10.3748/wjg.v19.i2.274

22. McNulty NP, Yatsunenko T, Hsiao A, Faith JJ, Muegge BD, et al. (2011) The impact of a consortium of fermented milk strains on the gut microbiome of gnotobiotic mice and monozygotic twins. Sci Transl Med 3: 106ra106. doi: 10.1126/scitranslmed.3002701

23. Jalanka-Tuovinen J, Salonen A, Nikkilä J, Immonen O, Kekkonen R, et al. (2011) Intestinal microbiota in healthy adults: temporal analysis reveals individual and common core and relation to intestinal symptoms. PLoS ONE 6: e23035. doi: 10.1371/journal.pone.0023035

24. Qin J, Li R, Raes J, Arumugam M, Burgdorf KS, et al. (2010) A human gut microbial gene catalogue established by metagenomic sequencing. Nature 464: 59–65. doi: 10.1038/nature08821

25. Turnbaugh PJ, Hamady M, Yatsunenko T, Cantarel BL, Duncan A, et al. (2009) A core gut microbiome in obese and lean twins. Nature 457: 480–484. doi: 10.1038/nature07540

26. Kinross JM, Darzi AW, Nicholson JK (2011) Gut microbiome-host interactions in health and disease. Genome Med 3: 14. doi: 10.1186/gm228

27. Yun S-I, Park H-O, Kang J-H (2009) Effect of *Lactobacillus gasseri* BNR17 on blood glucose levels and body weight in a mouse model of type 2 diabetes. J Appl Microbiol 107: 1681–1686. doi: 10.1111/j.1365-2672.2009.04350.x

28. Chang J-H, Shim YY, Cha S-K, Chee KM (2010) Probiotic characteristics of lactic acid bacteria isolated from kimchi. J Appl Microbiol 109: 220–230 doi:10.1111/j.1365-2672.2009.04648.x.

29. Park D-Y, Ahn Y-T, Huh C-S, Jeon S-M, Choi M-S (2011) The inhibitory effect of *Lactobacillus* plantarum KY1032 cell extract on the adipogenesis of 3T3-L1 Cells. J Med Food 14: 670–675. doi: 10.1089/jmf.2010.1355

30. Chun J, Kim KY, Lee J-H, Choi Y (2010) The analysis of oral microbial communities of wild-type and toll-like receptor 2-deficient mice using a 454 GS FLX Titanium pyrosequencer. BMC Microbiology 10: 101 doi:10.1186/1471-2180-10-101.

31. Kim O-S, Cho Y-J, Lee K, Yoon S-H, Kim M, et al. (2012) Introducing EzTaxon-e: a prokaryotic 16S rRNA gene sequence database with phylotypes that represent uncultured species. Int J Syst Evol Microbiol 62: 716–721. doi: 10.1099/ijs.0.038075-0

32. Hamady M, Lozupone C, Knight R (2010) Fast UniFrac: facilitating high-throughput phylogenetic analyses of microbial communities including analysis of pyrosequencing and PhyloChip data. ISME J 4: 17–27. doi: 10.1038/ismej.2009.97

33. Felsenstein J (2004) Inferring phylogenies. Sunderland, Massachusetts: Sinauer Associates Inc.

34. Krzanowski WJ (2000) Principles of multivariate analysis. A user's perspective. Oxford, United Kingdom: Oxford University Press.

35. Li W, Godzik A (2006) Cd-hit: a fast program for clustering and comparing large sets of protein or nucleotide sequences. Bioinformatics 22: 1658–1659. doi: 10.1093/bioinformatics/btl158

36. Schloss PD, Westcott SL, Ryabin T, Hall JR, Hartmann M, et al. (2009) Introducing mothur: open-source, platform-independent, community-supported software for describing and comparing microbial communities. Appl Environ Microbiol 75: 7537–7541. doi: 10.1128/AEM.01541-09

37. Hurlbert S (1971) The nonconcept of species diversity: a critique and alternative parameters. Ecology 52: 577–586.

38. Chao A, Lee SM (1992) Estimating the number of classes via sample coverage. J Am Stat Assoc 87: 210–217.

39. Hamad EM, Sato M, Uzu K, Yoshida T, Higashi S, et al. (2009) Milk fermented by *Lactobacillus gasseri* SBT2055 influences adipocyte size via inhibition of dietary fat absorption in Zucker rats. Br J Nutr 101: 716–724. doi: 10.1017/S0007114508043808

40. Claesson MJ, Cusack S, O'Sullivan O, Greene-Diniz R, de Weerd H, et al. (2011) Composition, variability, and temporal stability of the intestinal microbiota of the elderly. Proc Natl Acad Sci USA 108 Suppl 14586–4591. doi: 10.1073/pnas.1000097107

41. Ley RE, Bäckhed F, Turnbaugh P, Lozupone CA, Knight RD, et al. (2005) Obesity alters gut microbial ecology. Proc Natl Acad Sci USA 102: 11070–11075. doi: 10.1073/pnas.0504978102

42. Ley RE, Turnbaugh PJ, Klein S, Gordon JI (2006) Microbial ecology: human gut microbes associated with obesity. Nature 444: 1022–1023. doi: 10.1038/4441022a

43. Schwiertz A, Taras D, Schäfer K, Beijer S, Bos NA, et al. (2010) Microbiota and SCFA in lean and overweight healthy subjects. Obesity 18: 190–195 doi:10.1038/oby.2009.167.

44. Mai V, McCrary QM, Sinha R, Glei M (2009) Associations between dietary habits and body mass index with gut microbiota composition and fecal water genotoxicity: an observational study in African American and Caucasian American volunteers. Nutr J 8: 49 doi:10.1186/1475-2891-8-49.

45. Duncan SH, Lobley GE, Holtrop G, Ince J, Johnstone AM, et al. (2008) Human colonic microbiota associated with diet, obesity and weight loss. Int J Obes 32: 1720–1724 doi:10.1038/ijo.2008.155.

46. Turroni F, Foroni E, Pizzetti P, Giubellini V, Ribbera A, et al. (2009) Exploring the diversity of the bifidobacterial population in the human intestinal tract. Appl Environ Microbiol 75: 1534–1545. doi: 10.1128/AEM.02216-08

47. Arvanitoyannis IS, Van Houwelingen-Koukaliaroglou M (2005) Functional foods: a survey of health claims, pros and cons, and current legislation. Crit Rev Food Sci Nutr 45: 385–404. doi: 10.1080/10408390590967667

48. Cani PD, Amar J, Iglesias MA, Poggi M, Knauf C, et al. (2007) Metabolic endotoxemia initiates obesity and insulin resistance. Diabetes 56: 1761–1772. doi: 10.2337/db06-1491

49. Membrez M, Blancher F, Jaquet M, Bibiloni R, Cani PD, et al. (2008) Gut microbiota modulation with norfloxacin and ampicillin enhances glucose tolerance in mice. FASEB J 22: 2416–2426. doi: 10.1096/fj.07-102723

50. Neyrinck AM, Possemiers S, Druart C, Van de Wiele T, De Backer F, et al. (2011) Prebiotic effects of wheat arabinoxylan related to the increase in bifidobacteria, Roseburia and Bacteroides/Prevotella in diet-induced obese mice. PLoS ONE 6: e20944 doi:10.1371/journal.pone.0020944.

51. Gregor MF, Hotamisligil GS (2011) Inflammatory mechanisms in obesity. Annu Rev Immunol 29: 415–445. doi: 10.1146/annurev-immunol-031210-101322

52. Musso G, Gambino R, Cassader M (2011) Interactions between gut microbiota and host metabolism predisposing to obesity and diabetes. Annu Rev Med 62: 361–380. doi: 10.1146/annurev-med-012510-175505

53. Ohland CL, Macnaughton WK (2010) Probiotic bacteria and intestinal epithelial barrier function. Am J Physiol Gastrointest Liver Physiol 298: G807–819 doi:10.1152/ajpgi.00243.2009.

54. Song S, Zhang Y, Ma K, Jackson-Hayes L, Lavrentyev EN, et al. (2004) Peroxisomal proliferator activated receptor gamma coactivator (PGC-1alpha) stimulates carnitine palmitoyltransferase I (CPT-Ialpha) through the first intron. Biochim Biophys Acta 1679: 164–173. doi: 10.1016/j.bbaexp.2004.06.006

55. Finck BN, Kelly DP (2007) Peroxisome proliferator-activated receptor gamma coactivator-1 (PGC-1) regulatory cascade in cardiac physiology and disease. Circulation 115: 2540–2548. doi: 10.1161/CIRCULATIONAHA.107.670588

56. Pereira DIA, Gibson GR (2002) Effects of consumption of probiotics and prebiotics on serum lipid levels in humans. Crit Rev Biochem Mol Biol 37: 259–281. doi: 10.1080/10409230290771519

57. Preiss-Landl K, Zimmermann R, Hämmerle G, Zechner R (2002) Lipoprotein lipase: the regulation of tissue specific expression and its role in lipid and energy metabolism. Curr Opin Lipidol 13: 471–481. doi: 10.1097/00041433-200210000-00002

58. Lafontan M, Langin D (2009) Lipolysis and lipid mobilization in human adipose tissue. Progress in Lipid Research 48: 275–297. doi: 10.1016/j.plipres.2009.05.001

There are several supplemental files that are not available in this version of the article. To view this additional information, please use the citation information cited on the first page of this chapter.

PART III

INFLAMMATION
AND INNATE IMMUNITY

CHAPTER 7

ANTIMICROBIAL PEPTIDES AND GUT MICROBIOTA IN HOMEOSTASIS AND PATHOLOGY

MAUREEN J. OSTAFF, EDUARD FRIEDRICH STANGE, AND JAN WEHKAMP

7.1 INTRODUCTION

We humans, like every other multi-cellular organism, are in a constant race to maintain, renew and replace our epithelial tissues. Mostly, this is not a fair fight as our cells are not only threatened by time itself but often challenged with environmental attacks, such as UV rays, oxidative stress or, of particular note, microbes. The latter not always explicitly classify as a threat since they can deliver beneficial properties to the host or leastwise bring no harm. Specific gut bacteria have for instance been associated with improvement of digestion, absorption, vitamin synthesis and the inhibition of pathogen growth (Saulnier et al, 2009), which classifies them as mutualistic inhabitants. But even when considered friendly, or at least commensal, their population needs to be tightly controlled to ensure it stays benevolent rather than taking advantage of a debilitated host (Eberl, 2010). Albeit every human epithelial interface has its own battles to fight,

This chapter was originally published under the Creative Commons Attribution License. Ostaff MJ, Stange EF, and Wehkamp J. Antimicrobial Peptides and Gut Microbiota in Homeostasis and Pathology. EMBO Molecular Medicine 5,10 (2013): pp. 1465–1483. doi: 10.1002/emmm.201201773.

the intestinal tract provides an exceptionally striking situation. Its epithelial renewal rate outruns every other tissue in our body (Gregorieff & Clevers, 2005), calling for an especially controlled and efficient regenerative balance. Along the way, it is constantly confronted with an immensely complex ecology of microorganisms, which again, demands a particularly well-balanced homeostasis. All together up to 10^{13} to 10^{14} microorganisms are harboured in the digestive tract of a typical person, corresponding to a mass of about 1–2 kg and by far more cells than the human body. Up to 1000 different species make up the community, which contains mainly bacteria but can also include some eucaryotes, viruses and archaea. The intestinal colonization starts immediately during birth and soon after, the intestinal lumen is hosting a diverse ecosystem. The microbial composition and distribution of the menagerie varies with age, state of health, residence and potentially diet (Lozupone et al, 2012). Present numbers and types also dramatically vary by intestinal region. Due to the bactericidal properties of the gastric and also bile acids, the stomach and proximal small intestine contain only few microorganisms. Patients with reduced gastric acid levels (achlorhydria or hypochlorhydria for example) may suffer from bacterial overgrowth and subsequent inflammatory or malignant complications (Friis-Hansen, 2006; Husebye, 2005; Naylor & Axon, 2003). With increasing distance from the stomach and less acidic pHs however, bacterial numbers are rising. The ileum for example contains a fairly large amount of aerobic and anaerobic bacteria such as *Enterobacter* and *Lactobacilli*. The most densely populated intestinal region is found in the colon with numbers of up to 10^{12} bacteria per gram of intestinal content and predominately anaerobic representatives such as *Bacteroides, Bifidobacteria, Fusobacteria, Clostridium* and *Peptostreptococci* (Sears, 2005). Most intestinal bacteria belong to the phyla *Bacteriodetes* or *Firmicutes* but their composition varies locally and is dependent on the present immune defense strategies as determined by the host's genetic make-up and environmental aspects, e.g. the individual nutritional life style.

Early on, gut microbes have been implicated in the development of the intestinal morphology and function (Thompson & Trexler, 1971) based on evidence from germ-free or gnotobiotic animal models. An influence of bacteria has also been studied in the development of Peyer's patches and other gut-associated lymphoid tissue as well as in epithelial cell renewal rates (Heitman et al, 1980; Sun et al, 2004; Yamanaka et al, 2003). It is therefore easily imaginable how the intestinal regenerative balance depends on the epithelium's homeostasis towards its microbiota. This relationship though is by far not restricted to a one-sided influence of the former on the latter, but rather dual. Epithelial innate antibiotic effector molecules, termed antimicrobial peptides (AMPs), can fend off ingested pathogens but also shape and control the composition of commensal inhabitants. In humans, AMPs are expressed both broadly and in specialized cells as well as inducible or constitutively. They represent an ancient or primitive defense mechanism found in virtually every multi-cellular organism. In non-vertebrates, where they often act as the major form of protection against microbes, AMPs have been intensively studied even though many questions still remain unanswered. In humans and other mammals, they also have gained acknowledgement as important immune system contributors and potential future drug candidates (Brogden & Brogden, 2011; Wiesner & Vilcinskas, 2010). Our antimicrobial defense system has undergone an extensive co-evolution with a diverse world of microorganisms. Such long-standing interactions established multiple mechanisms, which ensure a commensal or even better a mutualistic co-existence in the gut (Neish, 2009). Different protein families feature AMPs with the most prominent ones in the intestinal tract represented by defensins, cathelicidins (e.g. LL-37), C-type lectins (such as the regenerating islet-derived protein (REG) family), ribonucleases (RNases) and S100 proteins (e.g. calprotectin). All these families, as well their most important members have been extensively covered in many excellent reviews (Bevins, 2003; Gallo & Hooper, 2012; Harder et al, 2007; Lai & Gallo, 2009) and are therefore not further described in detail. We will nonetheless later on introduce the group of defensins as central AMPs of the gut, since their mechanisms of action, expression and functions are of particular importance for following discussions.

The recent advances in the field of intestinal AMPs continuously highlight their important role in regulating the gut microbial community while ensuring a beneficial homeostasis at the intestinal barrier (Salzman et al, 2010). One well established example in this context are the inflammation promoting consequences of reduced antimicrobial defenses, as they can be seen in chronic inflammatory bowel diseases (IBD) especially Crohn's disease (CD) (Wehkamp et al, 2008). A new ramification is additionally presented by gut bacterial translocation in liver cirrhosis, which could recently additionally be linked to reduced antimicrobial defense in a rodent model (Teltschik et al, 2011). In parallel, scientific advances in current mechanistic studies have revealed novel antimicrobial modes of actions that nicely illustrate their complex role in host protection. The newly identified defense strategies included a formation of bacteria trapping net structures (Chu et al, 2012), but also an environmental dependent activity activation (Schroeder et al, 2011b) as a newly discovered biological principle. Supplementary, major proceedings in our understanding of the checks and balance systems within epithelial proliferative gut networks provide new views on different intestinal disorders. Our group could, for instance, elucidate an involvement of disturbed Wnt signalling, which is crucial for epithelial proliferation but also Paneth cell antimicrobial function, in chronic small intestinal inflammation (Koslowski et al, 2012; Wehkamp et al, 2007). Moreover, we also reported an influence of gut bacteria regarding the expression of transcription factors controlling epithelial secretory lineage decision making as well as Goblet cell differentiation (Becker et al, 2013).

In this review, we therefore aim at discussing the importance of a well-balanced host microbe relationship in the context of intestinal epithelial homeostasis. We will feature several mechanisms that insure a beneficial interaction but nonetheless apologize in advance for not possibly being able to cover all the excellent papers in this very vast field. Due to the complex nature of the topic, we will mainly focus on the role of epithelial antimicrobial defenses, in particular defensins. In addition, we will highlight the influence of microbiota on homeostatic signalling and vice versa at the interface of intestinal epithelia.

7.2 MASTERING MICROBIOTA

Long-standing interactions during our evolution generated a homeostatic and mutualistic relationship between the host and its microbes. While the intestinal symbionts enjoy a more or less ideal habitat with a constant temperature and a continuous supply of nutrients, the human organism also receives considerable benefits, e.g. the synthesis of certain vitamins or the breakdown of otherwise indigestible nutritional components. The difference between this fairly peaceful homeostatic host–microbe coexistence and the harmful interactions with pathogens during infections, is however critically dependent on the fact that our intestinal mucosa can hold mutualistic inhabitants at bay. The famous saying "good fences make good neighbours" describes this scenario nicely, as commensal microbiota can also play an important or even central role in the emergence of illnesses which will be discussed in later chapters. The normally well-balanced host–microbe coexistence depends on a complex and multileveled intestinal barrier. The epithelium, as the outermost single cell layer holds an especially critical position. It forms the first line of defense and performs a variety of protective tasks to secure the homeostasis towards symbiotic inhabitants and to avoid invasion with potential pathogens. Intestinal epithelia employ different protective mechanisms that form an intricate innate immune strategy network. Intestinal epithelia probe the resident gut microbiota with pattern recognition receptors (PRR). Those receptors, unlike adaptive immune receptors, require no segmental gene rearrangement and recognize microbes by essential and highly conserved "pathogen-associated molecular patterns" (PAMPs) or "microbe-associated molecular patterns" (MAMPs) (Didierlaurent et al, 2002). The latter term has been proposed since the molecular PAMP motifs, which are recognized by PRRs can also be shared by commensal microorganisms. The M/PAMP-PRR involving way of monitoring gut microbiota has been proven to be crucial for a healthy intestinal barrier (Lee et al, 2006; Rakoff-Nahoum et al, 2004). When stimulated with their respective ligand, PRRs induce a rapid and continuous first line of defense. This includes the production and release of AMPs as well as coordinative signalling molecules and mucins (Cario, 2005; Lievin-Le & Servin, 2006) (Fig 1). Prominent intestinal PRR include the constitutively or inducibly expressed transmembranous surface "Toll like receptors" (TLR's) found on all gut cells, and the intracellular "Nucleotide-binding oligomerization domain containing molecules" (NODs), amongst others (reviewed in Lavelle et al, 2010). The cellular responses following PRR activation are mediated by different signalling molecules and cascades, e.g. "Myeloid differentiation primary response gene" (MyD)88, mitogen-activated protein kinases (MAPK) and "nuclear factor kappa-light-chain-enhancer of activated B cells" (NF-κB) signalling. The activated defense program aims at eliminating a potential hazard and can lead to subsequent chemokine-interceded recruitment of acute inflammatory cells and further fostering of NF-κB mediated responses (Santaolalla & Abreu, 2012). In recent years, studies on either the function of a specific PRR or the general intestinal innate recognition machinery have extended our understanding of barrier defense. The major responsibilities have thereby shifted from a short time battle scenario in case of pathogen challenges to a more complex picture with a focus on a sustainable homeostasis towards microbial symbionts. In this framework, it is clear that PRRs must allow a certain amount of tolerance towards the presence of commensal or mutualistic gut microbiota to avoid a constant over- activation. One strategy in promoting a low basal activity is to limit the expression of PRRs. For instance in the human colon, TLR3 (recognizing dsRNA associated with viral infection) and TLR5 (which senses bacterial flagellin) are abundantly expressed, whereas TLR2 (which can be stimulated by different lipopetide agonists (reviewed in Cario, 2008) and TLR4 (which recognises LPS) expression is low in a healthy gut but can be induced (Cario, 2010; Hausmann et al, 2002). An additional example for selective epithelial expression of PRRs is the intracellular, muramyldipeptide sensing 'Nucleotide-binding oligomerization domain containing molecule' (NOD)2, which is found in small intestinal epithelia not exclusively but predominantly in AMP producing Paneth cells (Lala et al, 2003). A second crucial factor in dampening PRR mediated inflammatory signalling, is the presence of a sophisticated mucus barrier. Small intestinal epithelia are covered by a single unattached layer of mucus, while the colonic situation exhibits two distinct mucus zones with the inner layer attached and the outer lower density zone remaining unattached (reviewed by Johansson et al, 2011). In the colon, the outer mucus layer constitutes a habitat for commensal bacteria, whereas the inner one functions as a rather sterile seal and is renewed continuously within 1 h (at least in mice) by surface goblet cells (Johansson, 2012). This mucus overlay is not only a physical shield; it retains epithelial produced antimicrobials and thereby provides a competent first line of defense against microbial attachment and invasion (Meyer-Hoffert et al, 2008). To a certain extent, the intestinal lining nonetheless has to come in contact with resident microbiota, as they are essential for different physiological processes. Using germ-free or gnotobiotic animal models as early as 1961, the presence of gut microbiota were already implicated in the development of a proper epithelial architecture (Gordon & Bruckner-Kardoss, 1961a,1961b; Heneghan, 1965). The importance of a somewhat continuous PRR signalling activity, even though it might be low, becomes evident in mice with an epithelial loss of MyD88. The intestinal tissue specific knock out (ko) of this important cytoplasmatic TLR signalling compound leads for example to impaired antimicrobial activity and diminished levels of mucin-2 (the major mucus component), cumulating in differences in gut microbial composition, a greater number of mucus-associated bacteria, translocation events and increased colitis susceptibility (Frantz et al, 2012). A previous study on the influence of MyD88 furthermore focused specifically on small intestinal Paneth cells. Therein, this PRR signalling compound proved to be essential in limiting bacterial penetration by triggering a complex antimicrobial program (Vaishnava et al, 2008). Recently the importance of a well-adjusted interplay between gut bacteria and host innate defenses has also gained awareness in obesity and obesity related metabolic disorders such as diet induced insulin resistance (reviewed in Harris et al, 2012). An especially intriguing example is provided by a study using TLR2 ko mice. Under germfree condition, the absence of this PRR receptor protects against obesity-induced insulin resistance. However, when housed under normal circumstances, the genetic benefit is lost; moreover it is reversed to an increased susceptibility. Loss of TLR2 in intestinal epithelia and subsequently diminished innate defenses preceded changes in the gut microbial composition and creating a menagerie which promoted diminished insulin sensitivity in the host, while overwriting the initial host genetic advantage in this setting (Caricilli et al, 2011).

Such in vivo models on epithelial innate immune signalling support a crucial role of basal PRR activation to maintain a beneficial homeostasis towards gut bacteria. They illustrate how a lack of continuous innate defense might promote a switch from a commensal and/or mutualistic relationship towards a pathobiontic character within the gut microbial community.

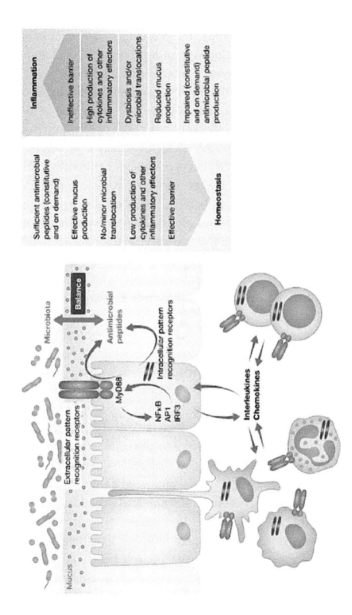

FIGURE 1: The relationship between resident microbiota and epithelial barrier functions is characterized by a delicate homeostasis Maturated epithelial cells provide not only a physical shield against the luminal content; they also generate potent biological effectors which help to control intestinal microbiota and keep the epithelial adjacent mucus barrier quite sterile. Among these, various AMPs sourced from all epithelia are crucial in maintaining a beneficial homeostasis in the gut. AMPs are in part constitutively expressed but can also be induced by PRR-activated signalling cascades after stimulation with microbial patterns.

6.3 GUT DEFENSINS

Intestinal epithelia generate specific and competent defensin weapon arsenals with activity against bacteria, viruses, protozoa and fungi reflecting the different threats and challenges, which are met at the mucosa. Members of both groups of gut defensins, α- and β-defensins, are at least in part dependent on innate immune PRRs either for their transcriptional induction or their secretion. In the small intestine, specialized Paneth cells, located at the bottom of crypts of Lieberkühn, store and secrete various antimicrobial effectors (e.g. lysozyme, phospholipase A2 group IIA (sPLA2, also known as PLA2G2A) or REGIIIα) (Clevers & Bevins, 2013; George et al, 2008) but their most abundant products are the α-defensins human defensin (HD)5 (gene name DEFA5) and HD6 (gene name DEFA6). HDs exhibit a 3–4 kDa small conserved amphipathic structure with cationic and hydrophobic residues. While HD6 so far only exhibited little bactericidal potential in vitro but employs additional defense strategies, which will be discussed in the next chapter, investigations on HD5 exposed an effective killing capacity against various bacteria (Ericksen et al, 2005). Mechanistic studies could also show that an artificial D-enantiomer version of HD5 shows significantly less activity than the native L-form isomer in killing *Staphylococcus aureus*, but equally bactericidal potential against *Escherichia coli* (Wei et al, 2009), revealing an unexpected functional complexity. Both Paneth cell α-defenins also seem to have antiviral activity (Doss et al, 2009; Klotman & Chang, 2006; Wang et al, 2013) but, depending on the setting, might also increase infectivity of certain viruses (Klotman et al, 2008). Furthermore, for HD5, anti-parasitic activity has been reported (Leitch & Ceballos, 2009). The expression of both Paneth cell α-defensins is controlled by different signalling pathways and may depend on an involvement of intracellular NOD2 (also known as CARD15) and the β-catenin dependent Wnt signalling cascade (Koslowski et al, 2009a). The small intestinal subgroup of CD (an IBD which will be discussed in detail below) is linked to major impairments in Paneth cell function and particularly low levels of both HD5 and HD6 (Wehkamp & Stange, 2010). This clinical relevance already indicates their decisive role in gut homeostasis and labels them as promising putative targets for future therapeutic interventions. A second defensin group found in gut epithelial cells, are β-defensins. Different from the Paneth cell restricted HD5 and HD6, with which they share their small size and cationic character, β-defensins are present in a variety of epithelial cells, including enterocytes. While the human β-defensin (HBD) 1 (also known by its gene name *DEFB101*) is constitutively expressed, others, like HBD2 (gene name *DEFB4*) show pathogen and/or inflammation dependent upregulation (Kubler et al, 2009; Ogushi et al, 2001a; Zilbauer et al, 2005, 2010) while also being inducible by probiotic bacteria (Schlee et al, 2007, 2008). Interestingly, HBDs are genetically clustered in a copy-number (CN) or gene dosage variable region with a diploid number of up to 12. CN divergence but also other sequence variations can be important for their level of gene expression (Groth et al, 2010). In a recent worldwide study, Hardwick et al could show how the respective cluster contains rapidly evolving noncoding regulatory sequences. These sites for example can influence the general transcriptional as well as cytokine responsiveness of *DEFB103* (also known as HBD3), an inducible AMP with important antibacterial and antiviral activity against many pathogens, which threaten epithelia. In East Asian individuals, variations resulting in a high HBD3 level were common and possibly linked to the geographically elevated and likely selection-driving incidence of influenza (Hardwick et al, 2011). Even though the work by Hardwick et al specifically focused on HBD3 in a distinct tissue setting, it is a striking example how the level of β-defensin inducibility can have important health related consequences. Another example is provided by colonic CD, which is associated with diminished on demand upregulation and secretion of HBD2 (Wehkamp et al, 2003a, 2008; Zilbauer et al, 2010). Data on β-defensin CN variations (CNV) are however ambiguous in this setting. Earlier evidence on low *DEFB4* copy numbers potentially underlying the impairment were not confirmed (Aldhous et al, 2009; Bentley et al, 2010; Fellermann et al, 2006). Different from the inducible β-defensins, HBD1 appears to be stable during infection or inflammation, but again shows general low mRNA in colonic CD. A single nucleotide polymorphism (SNP) variant in the *DEFB101* promoter however, was shown to act protective in this setting (Kocsis et al, 2008). In line with the widespread expression of HBD1 and therefore its seemingly grave importance in epithelial defense, the variant also holds relevance in additional clinical contexts, e.g. in HIV transmission (Braida et al, 2004; Milanese et al, 2006) and oral infections (Jurevic et al, 2003). The SNP is generally functionally linked to HBD1 mRNA level, and interestingly also involved in the transcriptional expression of HBD3, at least in keratinocytes (Kalus et al, 2009). In the gut, and potentially also other tissues, *DEFB101* is furthermore partly under the control of nuclear receptor peroxisome proliferator-activated receptor (PPAR)γ (Peyrin-Biroulet et al, 2010), an essential mediator for intestinal homeostasis in response to dietary signals, inflammation and microbiota (Desreumaux et al, 2001; Marion-Letellier et al, 2009; Pothoulakis, 2009; Wehkamp et al, 2003a). Intestinal HBD1 is moreover dependent on Hypoxia-inducible factor (Hif)-1α, which binds a specific response element in the gene's regulatory region (Kelly et al, 2013). Other tissue studies allowed the identification of yet other regulatory factors in *DEFB101* transcription. The oncogene PAX2 could be identified as a repressor for HBD1 in prostate cancer (Bose et al, 2009). Interestingly, high levels of glucose and activation of the insulin pathway have also been proposed to induce HBD1 in different in vitro experiments (Barnea et al, 2008; Malik & Al-Kafaji, 2007). The various reports on *DEFB101* expression provide a glimpse on how even a rather stably expressed AMP can be dependent on several distinctive regulatory mechanisms. Such multi-layered interconnections in the control of antimicrobial defense might not only complicate investigations on the genetic regulation of the respective factors but particularly also hamper mechanistic studies in disease settings.

6.4 AMPS IN MAINTAINING THE HOST–MICROBE-HOMEOSTASIS

Epithelial AMPs provide an important component within a complex barrier defense system and their production and secretion is an ongoing as well as an on demand process. From mice models we can get an idea about their essential functions in fencing of commensal but also pathogenic microbes. An induction of extensive Paneth cell degranulation (an excessive release of antimicrobials) via TLR9 stimulation for example, protects mice against *Salmonella typhimurium* infection (Rumio et al, 2004) but a lack of Paneth cell α-defensin (termed cryptdins in mice) activating enzyme conversely promotes a high susceptibility to orally administered pathogens (Wilson et al, 1999). A lack of the antimicrobial cathelecidin (mCRAMP in mice or LL-37 in humans), which is upregulated during ileitis or colitis dependent on the level of inflammation (Koon et al, 2011; Kubler et al, 2009; Schauber et al, 2006), leads to more severe symptoms and mucosal disruption in dextran sodium sulphate (DSS) chemically induced mouse colitis (Koon et al, 2011). Interestingly, the different abnormalities in this DSS challenged ko model, such as an increase in cytokine production and apoptotic cells, or impaired mucus production, can be reversed by intrarectal administration of or gene therapy with mCRAMP (Tai et al, 2013). Mice, which are transgenic for human defensin 5 and accordingly exhibit reshaped antimicrobial activity, are on the other hand protected against infections (Salzman et al,). Significant changes in the composition of gut microbiota when Paneth cell α-defensin defense is either doctored or diminished, also demonstrates its in vivo homeostatic role towards the symbionts (Salzman et al, 2010). Interestingly a person's nutritional status and lifestyle might play a crucial role in antimicrobial defense. Malnutrition for example, which is linked to diarrhea and inflammation, increased intestinal permeability and translocation of bacteria, has also been associated with differences in AMP expression and a dysbiosis of resident microbiota in the gut (Hashimoto et al, 2012; Hodin et al, 2011). Of special interest might be the fact that Paneth cells seem to be particularly affected by a lack of nutrition and show reduced AMP expression and granule abberations in a starvation mouse model (Hodin et al, 2011). This link between AMPs and intestinal barrier effectiveness did also become evident in a rat model of liver cirrhosis. Translocation of common intestinal microbiota could thereby be related to diminished epithelial α-defensins in the respective animals (Teltschik et al, 2011). Another study utilizing a mouse model of graft versus host disease (GVHD) also linked diminished Paneth cell antimicrobials to an increase of normally rare septicemia causing *E. coli* in expense of symbiotic diversity (Eriguchi et al, 2012). Of note, when comparing data from different mouse strains, one has to consider how a specific genetic background might differentially impact antimicrobial defense. C57BL/6 (B6) mice for example, exhibit 5 strain specific Paneth cell α-defensins, which have not been identified in other inbred mice (Shanahan et al, 2011). How this might be of general consequence in comparing results obtained in different models with otherwise seemingly comparable gene knockout approaches is easily imaginable. A study by Willing et al nicely employed how different mouse strains exhibit varying susceptibility to *Citrobacter rodentium* (a model of human pathogenic *E. coli* infections). They found that the different genetic background in investigated strains amass in variability in the architecture of the intestinal microbiotial community. The fact that transplantation of gut microbiota between strains promoted differentially activated innate defenses that could in turn partly abolish the symptom variability additionally nicely illustrates the reciprocity between host defense and symbiotic microbes (Willing et al, 2011). Such interplay might also be important in humans, for example in *Clostridium difficile* infections, where the transplantation of microbiota, or more precisely faecal transplants from healthy donors, have proven efficient in eradicating the pathogen and infection associated symptoms in patients (Borody & Khoruts, 2012). Faecal transplantation (FT) has also been introduced in other intestinal disorders, such as pseudomembranous colitis or irritable bowel syndrome amongst others, but large data sets on the different applications are still missing. Reports are often heterogeneous in the type of disease which was treated, what donors were used, as well as in their methodology and how they define a treatment response (Landy et al, 2011). Larger and randomized-controlled trials in addition to long-term follow-up studies are needed to gain evidence based insights on the procedure and its application before recommending faecal transplantation in a wider range of patients and disorders (Kassam et al, 2013; Khanna & Pardi, 2012). Effects of faecal transplantations on the microbiota compositions are yet also not fully clarified. Shifts from a disease related dysbiosis towards a healthier state in recipients have been reported but these often relate to quite small collectives, which are limited to *C. difficile* infected patients (Grehan et al, 2010; Khoruts et al, 2010). Recent works in this context reported high responding rates to FT, as well as a shift from a previous overabundance of Proteobacteria to a more normal composition of increased faecal bacterial diversity, similar to healthy donors, with an increase in *Bacteroidetes* (Shahinas et al, 2012; van et al, 2013). How long-standing such effects are and if and how FT affects the microbial ecology in the intestine of patients with other intestinal disorders is yet to be studied. Since the hosts genetic composition is also dramatically involved in shaping its microbiota, FT might be less effective in patients whose symptoms are not linked to a pathogenic catalyst but rather involve genetic susceptibility.

As mentioned, host AMPs for example exert a major influence on shaping microbial communities in the gut. It is therefore not surprising that the ability to evade them provided certain pathogenic strains with a selective evolutionary advantage (Gruenheid & Le, 2012; Koprivnjak & Peschel, 2011). This becomes clear in the case of *Helicobacter pylori*, which utilizes host cholesterol to gain resistance against cathelicidine (LL-37) (McGee et al, 2011). Furthermore, even though this gastritis promoting bacterium induces HBD2, it seems to selectively block another β-defensin, HBD3 (DEFB103) (Bauer et al, 2013). β-defensins share, like most AMPs, common characteristic biochemical properties like a positive charge and disulphide bonds that are important for their antimicrobial function (Boman, 2003). Even though these properties are quite similar between the respective HBDs, there can be vast differences in their effectiveness against different bacterial strains and in their modes of action. A striking example is provided by HBD1, for which earlier studies only reported weak antimicrobial function as compared to HBD2 or other defensins. The reason for this perceived lack of function became evident in work by Schroeder et al. The quite strong activity of HBD1 against various commensal bacteria and also a facultative pathogenic fungus depends on a biochemical activation in a reducing environment (Schroeder et al, 2011a,2011b). The "from zero to hero" story of HBD1 highlights how often artificial experiment settings might miss important conclusions on antimicrobial efficacy. It is thus likely that additional capacities of defensins and other antimicrobials have yet to be elucidated and that the experimental environment might become a determining factor in this context. Aside from HBD1, HD6 also represents an exception of the antimicrobial activity rule. As mentioned earlier, it likewise did not exhibit extensive anti-bacterial activity in original studies. Chu et al were recently able to demonstrate how this Paneth cell α-defensin nonetheless helps to keep the epithelium sterile. It is able to form structures, which do not directly kill microbes but can disable them in a trap like strategy. HD6 polymerizes and forms peptide nanonets around bacteria, which have the potential to prevent them from being translocating across the gut wall. This mechanism does not directly affect microbial viability but can have a huge impact on microbial infectivity. Chu et al also confirmed the inhibitory effect of HD6 on translocation events in a Salmonella infected HD6 transgenic mouse model. This model nicely displayed the nanonet formation in vivo and also underlines the critical importance that HD6 likely has in human intestinal barrier integrity (Chu et al, 2012).

6.5 CROHN'S DISEASE AND ULCERATIVE COLITIS: AMPS IN CHRONIC INFLAMMATION

In CD, a normally commensal or even mutualistic microbial community turns delinquent, leaving the host's immune system in a "with friends like these who needs enemies" situation that subsequently promotes an ongoing inflammatory response (Fig 2). Recurring and grave intestinal inflammations in such affected patients are characterized by frequent diarrhea, ulcerations and sometimes multiple fistula (Podolsky, 2002). It is well accepted that to a similar degree both, genetic but also environmental factors contribute to the development of the disease (Halfvarson et al, 2006; Schreiber et al, 2005) but the mechanisms underlying the disturbed homeostasis are still extensively discussed. Epithelia of CD patients display mucosal adherent bacteria, activated T cells, and antibodies aimed not at specific pathogens but rather towards regular gut microbiota (Duchmann et al, 1999; Sartor, 1997). Researchers and clinicians therefore started to favour the idea of an epithelial barrier defect to rationalize this breech in homeostasis (Wehkamp et al, 2005a, 2008). In 2001, with the identification of the PRR *NOD2* as the foremost genetic CD susceptibility factor (Hugot et al, 2001; Ogura et al, 2001) the importance of innate defenses and a crucial role of disturbed bacteria-host interactions became commonly acknowledged.

It is important to address that CD symptoms can be quite heterogeneously in different patients, which might support distinguishing the disorder as a collection of similar but slightly different sub diseases. The Montreal classification for example phenotypes patients according to the affected gastrointestinal location as either solely small intestinal, exclusive colonic (and/or rectal) disease, or as a presentation with both, small and

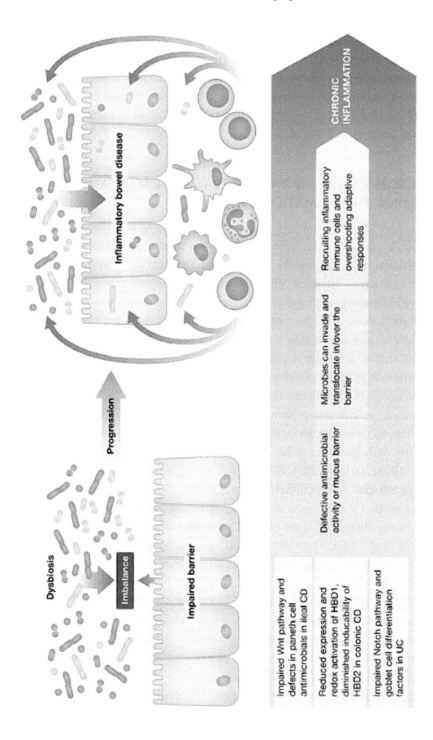

FIGURE 2: Proposed model for the pathogenesis of IBDs. IBD is characterized by mucosal adherent bacteria and the induction of continuous and overshooting immune responses against normally commensal gut microbiota. Different defects in the intestinal barrier integrity, which affect the innate immune system, are linked to specific subgroups of IBD. Small intestinal CD is associated with defects in Paneth cell antimicrobial defense, which includes reduced α-defensin expression and Impairments in the Wnt pathway. In the colon, Crohn's disease is characterized by reduced inducability of HBD2 as well as diminished constitutive expression of HBD1 and the HBD1 reducing, and thereby activating thioredoxin. UC on the other hand shows an impaired inflammation associated induction of factors, which are important for goblet cell differenciation, which affects the mucus layer effectiveness. Such defects in the first line of mucosal defense can result in mucosal adherent bacteria as well as microbial translocations, which then promote ongoing inflammatory and adaptive immune responses.

large intestine, involved. The patient's age of onset also plays an important part in subgrouping, as do the disease progression states which can range from a relatively weak "inflammatory," to a more severe stenotic (with intestinal strictures), or a penetrating course with internal fistulae. Whereas behavioural characteristics might change over time, location maintains a relatively stable entity throughout the disease course arguing for differing pathogenesis mechanisms in small intestinal and colonic CD subgroups (Gasche & Grundtner, 2005; Louis et al, 2001; Silverberg et al, 2005). In the last years, peculiar defects in epithelial antimicrobial defense were identified which might not only explain the location specificity, but additionally accommodate an involvement of host impairments and the microbial component in disease development (Wehkamp et al, 2005a, 2008). Colonic CD is associated with an attenuated production of β-defensins e.g. reduced inducibility of HBD2 but also low HBD1 level, as mentioned previously. Since HBD2 can be induced by pathogens but also probiotic bacteria, e.g. *E.coli* Nissle but also certain *Lactobacilli* via the activation of NF-κB and activator protein 1 (AP-1) (Mondel et al, 2008; Ogushi et al, 2001b; Schlee et al, 2007; Wehkamp et al, 2003c, 2004a), a specific defect in β-defensin inducibility and/or function might likely explain why probiotic treatment seems to have promising effects in pouchitis and maintenance of remission in ulcerative colitis (UC, another IBD), but no benefit in CD (Schultz & Lindstrom, 2008). Further investigations on intestinal β-defensins might one day help to thoroughly understand their involvement in colonic CD disease aetiology.

The molecular mechanisms underlying another colonic IBD, UC, are also still under fervent discussion. The impact of genetics on the disease risk is with 20% comparably smaller and poorly understood environmental issues predominate with an 80% involvement in UC pathogenesis. Nonetheless similar to CD, bacterial contamination of the colonic mucus (Swidsinski et al, 2002) suggests that a host barrier problem is likewise a key problem in the disorder. Especially during inflammation, UC is associated with a thinner and in part even absent mucus layer (Pullan et al, 1994; Strugala et al, 2008) while defensins are readily induced (Wehkamp et al, 2003b). As mentioned, the ability of the mucus to bind and retain AMPs is crucial in protecting intestinal epithelia from bacterial adhesion and invasion (Meyer-Hoffert et al, 2008). It might therefore be that even though defensins are upregulated, the antimicrobial barrier is nonetheless severely compromised in UC. A clinical relevance of impairments in the intestinal epithelia covering mucus layer has also been confirmed in various models, which exhibited spontaneous or more severe DSS-induced colitis (Heazlewood et al, 2008; Johansson et al, 2011; Petersson et al, 2011). Furthermore, an inflammation associated and likely protective increase of mucus promoting goblet cell differentiation factors is found in CD, but absent in UC (Gersemann et al, 2009). One of the key regulators in this context, human atonal 1 (Hath1) might even be completely missing in affected colonic UC tissue (Zheng et al, 2011). In addition to such goblet cell differentiation impairments, another mechanism discussed in the context of UC associated mucus depletion centres on mucolytic gut microbiota. These bacteria are more frequent in IBD and might directly and negatively influence mucus thickness and stability (Png et al, 2010).

In the small intestinal presentation of IBD, ileal CD, a prominent reduction of constitutively expressed Paneth cell α-defensins HD-5 and -6 furthermore endorses a disease concept of defective antimicrobial defense (Wehkamp & Stange, 2010). Expression levels of a total of eight other Paneth cell products show no such decrease and the specific effect can also be seen independent from current inflammation. Of interest in this context is the fact that the association of *NOD2* shows specificity for the small intestinal disease subgroup and that the PRR is prominently expressed in Paneth cells. In 2010, Biswas et al used a *NOD-2* deficient mouse model to study the effect on Paneth cell defensins. When inoculated with the opportunistic pathogen *Helicobacter hepaticus,* a strong inflammatory response could be rescued by transgenic expression of HD-5 in *NOD2* deficient mice but not by a wild-type bone marrow transplant (Biswas et al, 2010). An in vitro model using one of the disease associated *NOD2* variants, the frameshift mutation F3020insC, also underlined the PPRs important function in mediating antimicrobial defense (Begue et al, 2006). Whether disease relevant genetic variants of *NOD2* also precede even further reduced levels of Paneth cell α-defensins in humans, has been under ample discussion (Bevins et al, 2009; Simms et al, 2008; Wehkamp et al, 2004b, 2005b). A recent study in *NOD2* deficient mice on a BL6 background demonstrated only a reduced expression of cryptdin-related sequence 1C, but other Paneth cell antimicrobials were unchanged. The work by Shanahan et al also displayed how differences in faecal microbiota between the ko and wildtype mice were overwritten by cohousing the animals (Shanahan et al, 2013). If and how a change in mucosa adherent bacteria might still be present could be an interesting question in future research in this *NOD2* model. Not only the genetic background of laboratory mice influences epithelial antimicrobial defense (Gulati et al, 2012), but also their habitat exhorts a profound impact on gut microbiota (Ma et al, 2012). Since there are also profound differences between mice and humans regarding adaptive and innate immune functions in general (Mestas & Hughes, 2004; Seok et al, 2013), it is apparent how model systems might not always reflect the situation in patients who have defects in the studied genes. It is therefore essential for the study of NOD2 but also other factors in antimicrobial defense to follow-up on mechanistic studies in additional settings, e.g. primary, intestinal structure forming organoids from adult stem cells (Howell & Wells, 2011; McCracken et al, 2011).

Besides NOD2, also other CD pathogenesis involved factors and/ or associated genes are proposed in the context of Paneth cell antimicrobial defense (Table 1). Similar to *NOD2*, the genetic association of *"ATG16 autophagy related 16-like 1"* (*ATG16L1*) (Cadwell et al, 2008) shows an increased effect in the small intestinal subphenotype (Fowler et al, 2008; Hampe et al, 2007). The *ATG16L1* risk variant is accompanied by Paneth cell abnormalities in patients, which are correspondingly present in ATG16L1[HM] mice (Cadwell et al, 2008). The bona fide autophagy protein has essential functions in granule exocytosis pathways and thus in peptide export from secretory cells.

TABLE 1: Genetic associations in Crohn's disease with a relevance in the specialized antimicrobial producing Paneth cell

Factor	Full gene name	Core functions	Relevance in Paneth cell
Factors with a direct link to Paneth cell function			
NOD2/ CARD15*	Nucleotide-binding oligomerization domain-containing protein 2/cas-pase recruitment domain-containing protein 15	Intracellular PRR sensing bacterial muramyldipeptide	NOD2 is involved in the expression of Paneth cell defensins and the activation of innate antimicrobial defense strategies (Begue et al, 2006). Carriers of a frameshift risk variant have been reported to exhibit particularly low Paneth cell α-defensin levels (Bevins et al, 2009; Wehkamp et al, 2005b).
Atg16L1*	Autophagy related 16-like 1 (S. cere-visiae)	Part of a protein complex involved in autophagy, the major degradation system of cytoplasmatic components	ATG16L1 is involved in the granule exocytosis pathway and respectively the secretion of Paneth cell AMPs. Patients carrying the associated risk variants display Paneth cell abnormalities (Cadwell et al, 2008)
XBP1	X-box binding protein 1	Important transcription factor in the ER stress response as well as secretory cell development and maintenance	XBP1 deletion results in apoptotic Paneth cell loss and reduced antimicrobial activity. In addition to the association of common SNPs, the gene also exhibits rare hypomorphic non-synonymus variants in IBD patients (Kaser et al, 2008)
LRP6*	Low density lipoprotein related receptor 6	Wnt Co-receptor, R-Spondin receptor and LGR interaction partner with an important role in β-catenin dependent Wnt	LRP6 expression levels are linked to those of Paneth cell HD5 in vitro. The receptor's mRNA is furthermore reduced in small intestinal CD and an early onset associated non-synonymous risk variant precedes even further reduced levels of HDs (Koslowski et al, 2012)
TCF7L2*	Transcription factor 7-like 2 (T-cell specific, HMG-box), also known as TCF4	Transcription factor and interaction partner of β-catenin. Important regulator of Wnt target genes	TCF7L2 is reduced in and genetically associated with small intestinal CD. It binds the promoter region of HD5/6 and regulates the α-defensins transcriptional expression (Koslowski et al, 2009b; Wehkamp et al, 2007)

TABLE 1: *Cont.*

Factor	Full gene name	Core functions	Relevance in Paneth cell
Factors with a hypothesized role in diminished Paneth cell function in CD patients			
Lef1	Lymphoid enhancer-binding factor 1	Transcription factor and interaction partner of β-catenin. Important regulator of Wnt target genes and associated with CD (Dinu et al, 2012). It's role in canonical Wnt would support a potential involvement in Paneth cell function and in particular in the regulation of the α-defensins HD5 and HD6	A CDH1 CD risk haplotype precedes increased cytoplasmic E-cadherin likely due to a truncated form of the protein. This protein version also promotes impaired β-catenin localisation in vitro and might therefore be relevant for the canonical Wnt activity in Paneth cells (Muise et al, 2009)
CDH1	Cadherin-1 or epithelial cadherin (E-cadherin)	A calcium-dependent cell–cell adhesion glycoprotein involved in mechanisms regulating epithelial cell adhesion, mobility and proliferation	
KCNN4*	Potassium intermediate/ small conductance calcium-activated channel, subfamily N, member 4	Part of a voltage-independent potassium (K(+)) channel activated by intracellular calcium (Ca(2+))	The genetically associated KCNN4 encodes KCa3.1, which is found in Paneth cells. NOD2 risk variant carriers also exhibit reduced KCNN4 mRNA (Simms et al, 2010). In mice, a Ca(2+)-activated K(+) channel modulates Paneth cell secretion (Ayabe et al, 2002) which might allow to hypothesize a similar relevance of KCa3.1 in humans

*Associations are known to be stronger or specific to the small intestinal Crohn's disease subphenotype.

The maintenance of secretory cells as the AMP producing Paneth cell is also influenced by the CD associated *X-box binding protein 1* (*XBP1*) (Kaser et al, 2008), a key component of the endoplasmic reticulum (ER) stress response (Acosta-Alvear et al, 2007). Its deletion in mouse intestinal epithelia results in spontaneous enteritis and increased colitis susceptibility preceded by Paneth cell dysfunction amongst other epithelial impairments (Kaser et al, 2008). Another CD associated factor, the "*intermediate conductance calcium-activated potassium channel protein*" (*KCNN4*) encoded KCa3.1 protein has an important function in T cell Ca(2+) signalling and, like ATG16L1, a role in Paneth cell secretion. Besides its genetic association with the disease, *KCNN4* exhibits significantly reduced mRNA in *NOD2* mutated patients (Simms et al, 2010), highlighting a rather complex genetic interplay in the disease.

A new view on CD is based on an involvement of disturbed Wnt signalling in the small intestinal disease subgroup. The Wnt pathway is an important regulator of epithelial proliferation and interestingly also Paneth cell maturation (Crosnier et al, 2006). The β-catenin dependent Wnt cascade (also called "canonical"), depends on activation of Frizzled and 'low density lipoprotein receptor-related protein' (LRP) 5 or 6 receptors by Wnts and subsequent accumulation of cytoplasmatic β-catenin. In the absence of Wnt, β-catenin is associated with a complex containing adenomatous polyposis coli (APC), glycogen synthase kinase 3 β (GSK-3β) and axin amongst others (Aberle et al, 1997; Fagotto et al, 1999; Orford et al, 1997). This destruction complex mediates GSK3β- dependent phosphorylation and subsequent ubiquitination-dependent proteasomal degradation of β-catenin. Inhibition of the formation and/or activity of the destruction complex upon receptor ligand interaction promotes accumulation of β-catenin. The central pathway component can then enter the nucleus and activate target gene expression in cooperation with transcription factors of the "lymphoid enhancer-binding factor" (Lef)/'transcription factor (T-cell specific, high-mobility group (HMG)-box)' (TCF) family. Multiple studies could show a critical Paneth cell dependence on canonical Wnt (Andreu et al, 2005, 2008; van Es et al, 2005, 2012). In small intestinal CD, reduced expression (Perminow et al, 2010; Wehkamp et al, 2007; Zilbauer et al, 2011) and a genetic association (Koslowski et al, 2009b) of *TCF7L2* as well as an early onset associated coding variant in *LRP6* and generally low mRNA level of the Wnt co-receptor (Koslowski et al, 2012), support an important role of the pathway in disease aetiology. Furthermore, *E-cadherin* (*CDH1*) which has also been introduced in the context of CD susceptibility provides an additional bridge to disturbed canonical Wnt activity (Muise et al, 2009). Even though it has not directly been linked to Paneth cell function, its roles in β- catenin localization would support an influence on canonical signalling activity and subsequently the cell's maturation and gene program. Another indirect hit in the β-catenin dependent cascade was provided by a recent study using logic regression to reevaluate genetic data from a genome wide approach (Dinu et al, 2012). The used innovative statistical technique allows the selection of a model, which potentially involves multiple intersections and/or unions of SNPs within a certain gene, or any set of SNPs (e.g. various genes which are relevant in a specific pathway), that are associated with the phenotype of interest. In the analysis, the canonical Wnt signalling transcription factor *LEF1* was found to be amongst the genes with the strongest evidence for an association with the risk of CD. Impaired cell proliferation or differentiation as a novel pathogenesis concept might provide promising although complex opportunities for new and causal therapeutic intervention. In addition, studies on the interplay of the different Paneth cell affecting genetic hits and integrating the role of microbiota in this context could improve our understanding of symptomatic heterogeneity or disease severity and might one day assist in identifying critical risk patients.

6.6 THE EPITHELIAL REGENERATIVE HOMEOSTASIS

The human intestinal epithelial lining undergoes cell renewal at an extraordinary rate much faster than any other tissues in our body (Gregorieff & Clevers, 2005). All present cell types descend from multipotent stem cells located at the base of the crypts, right above and/or between the Paneth cells (Fig 3). They self-renew and generate an adjacent zone of rapidly cycling progenitors, which again increase their pool before differentiating into multiple lineages, creating up to 300 cells/cryp/day (Barker et al, 2008). The post-mitotic crypt necks and villus regions make up the biggest part of the intestinal epithelium (Crosnier et al, 2006) whereas Paneth

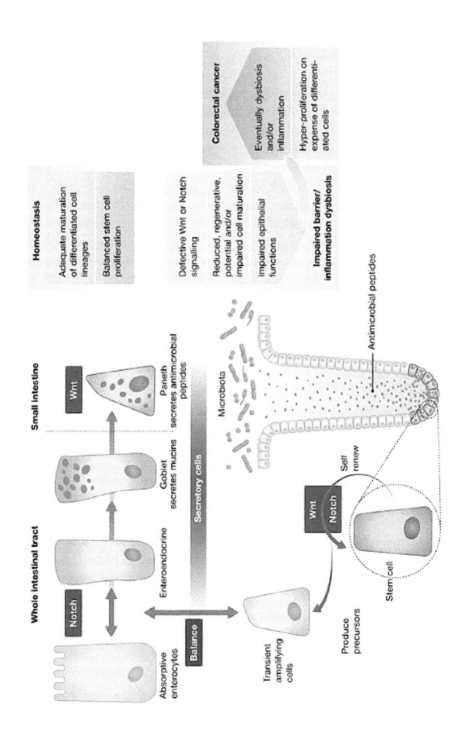

FIGURE 3: The gut is characterized by a delicately balanced regeneration. Intestinal epithelia underlie complex signalling networks, first and foremost the Notch and Wnt pathways, which control the symmetry of proliferation and differentiation. Notch furthermore directs the lineage decision between absorptive and secretory cells, while the β-catenin dependent Wnt cascade additionally regulates Paneth cell maturation and function. Different from all other secretory cell types (Enteroendocrine and Goblet cells), Paneth cells are normally confined to the bottom of small intestinal crypts of Lieberkühn but can under certain circumstances (e.g. inflammation) appear in other gastrointestinal epithelia. A disturbance of the epithelial cell homeostasis might have disastrous consequences promoting an either debilitated barrier or potentially tumour development. In both cases, effects of microbiota on the onset and/or progression of subsequent pathogenesis mechanisms are discussed. Bacteria have also been shown to influence epithelial differentiation factors in general, which highlights a circular symmetry of host microbe relationship in the gut.

Cells escape the upwards flow and reside at the crypt base for 3–6 weeks (Barker et al, 2008). As mentioned, proliferation is in large parts subject to the activity of Wnt (Korinek et al, 1998) but it is also dependent on Notch signalling (Fre et al, 2009). Both signals, Wnt and Notch are paradoxically also essential for the directed differentiation of specific cell types, Notch for the secretory lineage decision and Wnt for Paneth cell maturation (Jensen et al, 2000; van Es et al, 2005). In this context, the propable stem cell marker 'leucine-rich repeat G protein-coupled receptor' (LGR5) (Barker et al, 2007) also has important functions in Paneth cell maturation. It's deficiency results in premature Paneth cells but generates no major defects in other lineages, progenitor proliferation or cell migration in the small intestine (Garcia et al, 2009). Data on LGR4 show similar effects on gut homeostasis, it's disruption in mice leads to diminished Paneth cell numbers as well as increased DSS colitis severity (Liu et al, 2013). Recently two groups published almost simultaneously, how LGR5 and its homologues, like LGR4, can bind R-Spondins associate with Frizzled/LRP and potentiate Wnt-activity (Carmon et al, 2011; de et al, 2011) which nicely explains their importance for Paneth cell biology.

Even though intestinal proliferation pathway networks are quite complex, one needs to consider that they are also additionally subjected to various influences from innate immune and inflammatory signalling. The host–microbe homeostasis can hence be relevant for epithelial homeosta-

sis and vice versa since epithelia on their hand can, e.g. via AMP production, control the composition of gut microbiota. It was recently shown that
Lgr5+ putative intestinal stem cells express TLR4, which, when activated
via bacterial LPS, promotes apoptosis while reducing in vivo proliferation in mice (Neal et al, 2012). In the context of necrotizing enterocolitis
(NEC), the leading cause of death from gastrointestinal disease in preterm
infants, the role of TLR4 has furthermore been studied in mice models
and in vitro experiments. In both settings, TLR4 stimulation promoted
β-catenin inhibition via GSK3β activation cumulating in reduced cell proliferation rates (Sodhi et al, 2010). The same group also followed up with
functional studies on the effects of TLR4 in intestinal epithelia via deletion of the PRR in mice and cell culture. This deletion diminished Notch
pathway activity and increased goblet cell numbers in the small intestine
of mice and complementarily augmented goblet cell differentiation in cultured enterocytes (Sodhi et al, 2012). Another TLR4 mediated mechanism
with a role in NEC was recently identified in the context of epithelial autophagy. TLR4 activation induced autophagy in enterocytes, which was a
requirement for and not only a consequence of NEC development in the
studied mouse model (Neal et al, 2013). Different from the proliferation
inhibiting effects of TLR4, investigations on TLR2 and TLR5 implicated
them in promoting epithelial repair, growth and survival. The observed effects of those PRRs were not linked to the release of cytokines after TLR
stimulation, but rather to the activation of different receptor tyrosine kinases including members of the epidermal growth factor receptor (EGFR)
family (Shaykhiev et al, 2008). The setting of the respective work focused
on airway epithelial cells but since both receptors have also been implicated in hyper-proliferation of gastric epithelia (Song et al, 2011; Tye et
al, 2012), this mechanism might also be relevant in the gut. An influence
of TLR9 on gut epithelial homeostasis has also been investigated in ko
mice. Respective animals display increased numbers of proliferating cells
while levels of the Notch target gene hairy enhancer of split 1 (hes1), a differentiation factor directing cells towards the enterocyte fate, and vascular
endothelial growth factor (VEGF), which is important for epithelial cell
restitution, were reduced. TLR9-deficient mice were furthermore highly
susceptible to DSS induced inflammation and exhibited delayed wound
repair (Rose et al, 2012). Complementing this observation, an influence

of gut bacteria on the transcription of the Notch target Hes1 and other differentiation factors has also been proposed (Becker et al, 2013). The early
determination of secretory versus absorptive cell fate is regulated by an
antagonistic interplay of Hes1 and the basic helix–loop–helix transcription factor Hath1. Progenitor cells expressing Hes1 block Hath1, which
favours the absorptive lineage, while an inactive Notch/Hes1 signalling allows Hath1 transcription and a transit towards a secretory fate. Cells enter-
ing the secretory line require additional signals to mature into specific cell
types such as, for goblet cells, the zinc-finger transcription factor krüppel
like factor (KLF)4 or as mentioned for Paneth cells, active β-catenin. In
vitro expression of Hes1, Hath1, and to a minor degree also of KLF4, can
be reduced by a pathogenic or probiotic *E. coli*. Accommodatingly, germ
free mice also display diminished colonic expression of Hath1 and KLF4
in comparison to specific pathogen free or conventionalized counterparts,
even though a direct effect on goblet cell numbers cannot be observed
(Becker et al, 2013). Besides bacteria, other intestinal inhabitants can also
influence epithelial proliferation and differentiation. Mice infected with
Trichinella spiralis, a parasite that drives small intestinal inflammation,
show changes in mucosal architecture, e.g. an elevated amount of proliferative progenitors and Paneth cells (Walsh et al, 2009).

The relationship between microbes, innate immune and inflammatory
pathways, and cell proliferation seems to be quite complicated and complex but even more, it is also dual. β-catenin itself functions as a constitutive negative regulator of in vivo inflammation. Similar to the inhibitor
IkB, the central canonical Wnt pathway component can bind NF-κB and
can prevent its activity (Duan et al, 2007). In response to pathogenic (*Salmonella, Yersinia, Listeria* and enteropathogenic *E. coli* (EHEC)) but not
non-virulent bacteria, the physical interaction between the two signalling
components is compromised subsequent to GSK3β dependent β-catenin
degradation. Conversely, a study in colon and breast cancer cells could
demonstrate that GSK3β inhibition can also alter NF-κB activity through
β-catenin stabilization, which again links canonical Wnt with inflammatory signalling (Deng et al, 2004). Phosphorylation of GSK3β and β-catenin
stabilization seem to provide important control points in inflammatory
processes, suggesting that activated β-catenin may be a balancer of bacteria-induced inflammation in general and likely also in the gut. A failure of

the system could be fatal, shifting epithelial immune reactions towards a more inflammatory status. In monocytes such a pivotal role for GSK3β has been demonstrated in deciding inflammatory responses after TLR activation (Martin et al, 2005). In addition, it has also been reported that dendritic cells require β-catenin-dependent signalling to mediate gut tolerance to commensal microbes in mice. Ablation of β-catenin in dendritic cells reduced regulatory T cells and anti-inflammatory cytokines while increasing pro-inflammatory processes promoting an enhanced susceptibility to experimental colitis in this model (Manicassamy et al, 2010). For the epithelial setting it has furthermore been shown that levels of Wnt2, a ligand in the canonical cascade, are elevated after bacterial infection. An in vitro knock down of Wnt2 enhances bacteria induced epithelial IL8 expression, which is conversely less secreted in Wnt2 overexpressing cells (Liu et al, 2012). Upregulation of Wnt2 might hence be a host strategy to inhibit an overshooting inflammatory response during infection by activation of β-catenin.

Multiple crosstalks between proliferative, immunological and inflammatory pathways complicate the picture of epithelial homeostasis in the gut. This is especially tricky when considering tampering with specific pathways to test their therapeutic value. Blocking a signalling cascade might on the one hand dampen pro-inflammatory processes but might on the other hand impact epithelial differentiation. An example for this scenario is provided by TLR4. The PRR is upregulated during intestinal inflammation (Hausmann et al, 2002) and can induce autophagy in enterocytes (Neal et al, 2013). Blocking the PRRs with an antibody in fact ameliorates inflammation but unfortunately also delays mucosal healing in DSS treated mice (Ungaro et al, 2009).

6.7 COLORECTAL CANCER: A ROLE FOR MICROBES AND AMPS

Colorectal cancer (CRC) has recently been linked to a dysbiosis of gut microbiota (Sobhani et al, 2011). In their study, Sobhani et al identified 18 genera with an abundance of more than 1%. Thirteen of these genera (*Alistipes, Collinsella, Bacteroides, Lachnospira, Prevotella, Subdoligranulum, Dorea, Faecalibacterium, Roseburia, Coprococcus, Streptococcus,*

Bifidobacterium and *Ruminococcus*) corresponded to the previously de-scribed human intestinal microbiota phylogenetic core of which certain species were also specifically shown to be decreased in cancer patients: *Bifidobacterium longum*; BG; AY675246, *Clostridium clostridioforme*; 1-53; AY169422, *Ruminococcus sp.* DJF_VR66; EU728790, *Ruminococcus bromii*; L2-63; EU266549. Their analysis furthermore showed that more than 7% of the microbiota variability was impacted by the cancer status. This particular study could also connect variations in the distri-bution of bacterial genera in faecal samples with the disease status, and demonstrated a significantly elevated *Bacteroides/Prevotella* population, which correlated with an increase of IL-17 in mucosal samples of respec-tive patients. A more recent work by Ohigashi et al also consistently re-ported a divergence in faecal microbiota as well as a significant decrease of the concentrations of short chain fatty acids (SCFAs) in a similar setting and furthermore reported additional differences in the intestinal environ-ment, including an elevated pH (Ohigashi et al, 2013). Another study in six CRC patients did not focus on faecal microbiota but rather elucidated how tumour tissue directly seemed to harbour a specific microbiome which was strikingly different from adjacent non-malignant mucosa in five of the investigated CRC patients (Marchesi et al, 2011). The progression of colorectal cancer is coupled to deregulation of different signals and path-ways, amongst others, an augmentation of canonical Wnt, often mediated by deactivating mutations in APC (Goel & Boland, 2010; Saleh & Trinch-ieri, 2011; Vaiopoulos et al, 2012). Proinflammatory cytokines have been shown to enhance Wnt β-catenin/TCF transcriptional activity in this set-ting and patients with colonic IBD have been shown to bear an increased risk for CRC development in epidemiological studies (Saleh & Trinchieri, 2011). The cytokine IL-1β for example can promote GSK3β inactivation and subsequent β-catenin stabilization (Kaler et al, 2009). An impact of microbiota in this context has also been investigated. In azoxymethane (AOM), chemically induced inflammation of conventional, *Bacterioides vulgatus* mono-associated, and germfree IL-10$^{(-/-)}$ and Myd88$^{(-/-)}$ mice, it could be shown that the risk for colitis associated cancer seems to be TLR/MyD88 dependent and can be altered by manipulation of intestinal mi-crobes (Uronis et al, 2009). In a similar setting, Arthur et al could demon-strate that specific bacterial abilities can mediate cancer promoting effects and argued that colitis may foster the expansion of microbes with such deleterious capabilities (Arthur et al, 2012). In their study, commensal *E. coli NC101* promoted CRC in AOM treated IL-10-deficient mice while a deletion of the bacterium's polyketide synthase island decreased cancer multiplicity and invasion without affecting the inflammation in the model. CRC is not the only gastrointestinal malignancy with a connection to bacteria induced inflammation. Deregulation of NF-κB and canonical Wnt is also present in a majority of gastric cancers (Ooi et al, 2009) and induction of high nuclear β-catenin by *H. pylori*, a major cause of gastric malignancies, provides again, a link to bacteria. Besides the hosts genetic predisposition, *H. pylori*'s capacity to inhibit GSK3β activity is likely responsible for the outcome and persistence of intestinal metaplasia in gastritis (Hung et al, 2009). Intestinal colonization by another *Helicobacter* species, *H. hepaticus*, furthermore activates NF-κB-regulated networks both in the colon but also in liver and promotes hepatic cancer marked by canonical Wnt activation without bacterial translocation or hepatitis induction in mice (Fox et al, 2009).

Since AMPs are critical in controlling the enteric microbiota, they might well have a role in bacteria driven cancer development. Unfortunately this arc in the story of microbial influenced colonic cancer has not yet been investigated in detail. Other functions of AMPs however, have already been studied in this context. In addition to directly killing pathogens or regulating enteric symbionts, AMPs have a role in orchestrating adaptive immune responses. Some have chemotactic ability to recruit immune cells from monocytic and lymphocytic lineages (Lai & Gallo, 2009). HBDs have for instance been shown to recruit immune cells (e.g. monocytes, macrophages, and neutrophils but also T-cells) to the site of microbial invasion through interaction with the CC-chemokine receptor (CCR)6 and CCR2 (Rohrl et al, 2010a,2010b; Yang et al, 1999). CCR dependent mBD14 (the mouse ortholog of HBD3) recruitment of macrophages has been shown to indirectly promote tumourigenesis via the induction of proinflammatory cytokines (Rohrl et al, 2012a,2012b). Since in vitro results and data from mice models on the other hand also show anti-inflammatory influences of HBD3 on monocytes and macrophages (Semple et al, 2010, 2011), its role in inflammation promoted cancer could however be more complex. If and how the manipulation of AMP expression or a direct alteration of gut microbiota might be a preventative strategy in inflammation induced colon cancer, provides nonetheless interesting questions for supplementary future research.

6.8 CONCLUSIONS

As we highlighted in this review, the interconnections between AMPs, gut microbiota, innate immune signalling and epithelial proliferation pathways are quite complex. Disturbed antimicrobial function in the gut can provoke devastating consequences on barrier effectiveness and likely promotes a shift in the microbial community. In addition, an altered composition of gut microbiota can on its part influence and destabilize epithelial defenses. Such breeches of homeostasis on either the host or the microbiota side likely promote a vicious self-feeding cycle. A similar hostile chain of events could be enabled during the course of IBD or might even play a role in inflammation associated cancer risk. Further detailed investigations on the interplay of gut epithelial host–microbe interactions, inflammation and proliferation pathways are essential to complete our understanding in that matter. Such integral approaches are ambitious; nonetheless accepting this challenge holds promises for the development of new and causal therapeutic avenues in different intestinal disorders.

6.9 GLOSSARY

COMMENSALISM

A form of symbiosis when one organism profits from another without bringing any subsequent harm. In the gut, microorganisms, mainly bacteria, are commensal when they benefit from the host, e.g. by profiting from the available food sources, without negatively influencing it.

DYSBIOSIS

Defines a perturbation in the community of microbiota. This most often refers to a shift in the phyla composition of microbiota but can also relate to changes on the species level.

GNOTOBIOTIC ANIMAL MODELS

Model systems which house a defined microbiome. This technically also includes germ-free animals as the status of their microbiota is defined. It mostly refers to different mono-or multi-associated models. Gnotobiotic animals are normally reared sterile and then confronted with specific microbiota, single strands or defined communities, to study the relationship between the host and its potential symbionts or pathogens.

GUT MICROBIOME

The gut microbiome represents the millions of microbial genes of an ample and diverse co-evolved ecosystem of gut microbiota in our intestine.

GUT MICROBIOTA

A community of different microorganisms in the digestive tract. In humans it represents the largest reservoir of microorganisms and is made up by all together 10^{13} to 10^{14} microbial cells of which bacteria make up the largest part.

GUT PATHOBIONTS

Originally commensal or mutualistic gut inhabitants, which, due to a change in environment or any level within the host–microbiota relationship develop pathogenic potential and become pathobiontic.

HOMEOSTASIS

A status of relative stability where a system controls its internal properties and environment. In a living organism, regulatory mechanisms aim at maintaining different parameters at a constant level over potentially wide reaching variations, allowing it to function in a broad range of conditions.

MUTUALISM

Existence of a symbiotic relationship between different organisms in which both reciprocally profit from the situation. In the gut, microorganisms classify as mutualistic when they, in addition to being commensal, also have beneficial properties for the host, e.g. the ability to break down otherwise unavailable nutrients thereby improving digestion.

SYMBIONTS

Organisms living in a symbiotic relationship. In the human gut, this can refer to the different members within the gut microbiota.

REFERENCES

1. Aberle H, Bauer A, Stappert J, Kispert A, Kemler R (1997) Beta-catenin is a target for the ubiquitin-proteasome pathway. EMBO J 16: 3797-3804
2. Acosta-Alvear D, Zhou Y, Blais A, Tsikitis M, Lents NH, Arias C, Lennon CJ, Kluger Y, Dynlacht BD (2007) XBP1 controls diverse cell type- and condition-specific transcriptional regulatory networks. Mol. Cell 27: 53-66
3. Aldhous MC, Noble CL, Satsangi J (2009) Dysregulation of human beta-defensin-2 protein in inflammatory bowel disease. PLoS ONE 4: e6285
4. Andreu P, Colnot S, Godard C, Gad S, Chafey P, Niwa-Kawakita M, Laurent-Puig P, Kahn A, Robine S, Perret C, et al (2005) Crypt-restricted proliferation and commitment to the Paneth cell lineage following Apc loss in the mouse intestine. Development 132: 1443-1451
5. Andreu P, Peignon G, Slomianny C, Taketo MM, Colnot S, Robine S, Lamarque D, Laurent-Puig P, Perret C, Romagnolo B (2008) A genetic study of the role of the Wnt/beta-catenin signalling in Paneth cell differentiation. Dev Biol 324: 288-296

6.   Arthur JC, Perez-Chanona E, Muhlbauer M, Tomkovich S, Uronis JM, Fan TJ, Campbell BJ, Abujamel T, Dogan B, Rogers AB, et al (2012) Intestinal inflammation targets cancer-inducing activity of the microbiota. Science 338: 120-123

7.   Ayabe T, Wulff H, Darmoul D, Cahalan MD, Chandy KG, Ouellette AJ (2002) Modulation of mouse Paneth cell alpha-defensin secretion by mIKCa1, a Ca2+-activated, intermediate conductance potassium channel. J Biol Chem 277: 3793-3800

8.   Barker N, van Es JH, Kuipers J, Kujala P, van den BM, Cozijnsen M, Haegebarth A, Korving J, Begthel H, Peters PJ, et al (2007) Identification of stem cells in small intestine and colon by marker gene Lgr5. Nature 449: 1003-1007

9.   Barker N, van de WM, Clevers H (2008) The intestinal stem cell. Genes Dev 22: 1856-1864

10. Barnea M, Madar Z, Froy O (2008) Glucose and insulin are needed for optimal defensin expression in human cell lines. Biochem Biophys Res Commun 367: 452-456

11. Bauer B, Wex T, Kuester D, Meyer T, Malfertheiner P (2013) Differential expression of human beta defensin 2 and 3 in gastric mucosa of Helicobacter pylori-infected individuals. Helicobacter 18: 6-12

12. Becker S, Oelschlaeger TA, Wullaert A, Pasparakis M, Wehkamp J, Stange EF, Gersemann M (2013) Bacteria regulate intestinal epithelial cell differentiation factors both in vitro and in vivo. PLoS ONE 8: e55620

13. Begue B, Dumant C, Bambou JC, Beaulieu JF, Chamaillard M, Hugot JP, Goulet O, Schmitz J, Philpott DJ, Cerf-Bensussan N, et al (2006) Microbial induction of CARD15 expression in intestinal epithelial cells via toll-like receptor 5 triggers an antibacterial response loop. J Cell Physiol 209: 241-252

14. Bentley RW, Pearson J, Gearry RB, Barclay ML, McKinney C, Merriman TR, Roberts RL (2010) Association of higher DEFB4 genomic copy number with Crohn's disease. Am J Gastroenterol 105: 354-359

15. Bevins CL (2003) Antimicrobial peptides as effector molecules of mammalian host defense. Contrib Microbiol 10: 106-148

16. Bevins CL, Stange EF, Wehkamp J (2009) Decreased Paneth cell defensin expression in ileal Crohn's disease is independent of inflammation, but linked to the NOD2 1007fs genotype. Gut 58: 882-883

17. Biswas A, Liu YJ, Hao L, Mizoguchi A, Salzman NH, Bevins CL, Kobayashi KS (2010) Induction and rescue of Nod2-dependent Th1-driven granulomatous inflammation of the ileum. Proc Natl Acad Sci USA 107: 14739-14744

18. Boman HG (2003) Antibacterial peptides: basic facts and emerging concepts. J Intern Med 254: 197-215

19. Borody TJ, Khoruts A (2012) Fecal microbiota transplantation and emerging applications. Nat Rev Gastroenterol Hepatol 9: 88-96

20. Bose SK, Gibson W, Bullard RS, Donald CD (2009) PAX2 oncogene negatively regulates the expression of the host defense peptide human beta defensin-1 in prostate cancer. Mol Immunol 46: 1140-1148

21. Braida L, Boniotto M, Pontillo A, Tovo PA, Amoroso A, Crovella S (2004) A single-nucleotide polymorphism in the human beta-defensin 1 gene is associated with HIV-1 infection in Italian children. AIDS 18: 1598-1600

22. Brogden NK, Brogden KA (2011) Will new generations of modified antimicrobial peptides improve their potential as pharmaceuticals? Int J Antimicrob Agents 38: 217-225

23. Cadwell K, Liu JY, Brown SL, Miyoshi H, Loh J, Lennerz JK, Kishi C, Kc W, Carrero JA, Hunt S, et al (2008) A key role for autophagy and the autophagy gene Atg16l1 in mouse and human intestinal Paneth cells. Nature 456: 259-263

24. Caricilli AM, Picardi PK, de Abreu LL, Ueno M, Prada PO, Ropelle ER, Hirabara SM, Castoldi A, Vieira P, Camara NO, et al (2011) Gut microbiota is a key modulator of insulin resistance in TLR 2 knockout mice. PLoS Biol 9: e1001212

25. Cario E (2005) Bacterial interactions with cells of the intestinal mucosa: toll-like receptors and NOD2. Gut 54: 1182-1193

26. Cario E (2008) Barrier-protective function of intestinal epithelial Toll-like receptor 2. Mucosal Immunol S62-S66

27. Cario E (2010) Toll-like receptors in inflammatory bowel diseases: a decade later. Inflamm Bowel Dis 16: 1583-1597

28. Carmon KS, Gong X, Lin Q, Thomas A, Liu Q (2011) R-spondins function as ligands of the orphan receptors LGR4 and LGR5 to regulate Wnt/beta-catenin signaling. Proc Natl Acad Sci USA 108: 11452-11457

29. Chu H, Pazgier M, Jung G, Nuccio SP, Castillo PA, de Jong MF, Winter MG, Winter SE, Wehkamp J, Shen B, et al (2012) Human alpha-defensin 6 promotes mucosal innate immunity through self-assembled peptide nanonets. Science 337: 477-481

30. Clevers HC, Bevins CL (2013) Paneth cells: maestros of the small intestinal crypts. Annu Rev Physiol 75: 289-311

31. Crosnier C, Stamataki D, Lewis J (2006) Organizing cell renewal in the intestine: stem cells, signals and combinatorial control. Nat Rev Genet 7: 349-359

32. de Lau W, Barker N, Low TY, Koo BK, Li VS, Teunissen H, Kujala P, Haegebarth A, Peters PJ, van de Wetering M, et al (2011) Lgr5 homologues associate with Wnt receptors and mediate R-spondin signalling. Nature 476: 293-297

33. Deng J, Xia W, Miller SA, Wen Y, Wang HY, Hung MC (2004) Crossregulation of NF-kappaB by the APC/GSK-3beta/beta-catenin pathway. Mol Carcinog 39: 139-146

34. Desreumaux P, Dubuquoy L, Nutten S, Peuchmaur M, Englaro W, Schoonjans K, Derijard B, Desvergne B, Wahli W, Chambon P, et al (2001) Attenuation of colon inflammation through activators of the retinoid X receptor (RXR)/peroxisome proliferator-activated receptor gamma (PPARgamma) heterodimer. A basis for new therapeutic strategies. J Exp Med 193: 827-838

35. Didierlaurent A, Sirard JC, Kraehenbuhl JP, Neutra MR (2002) How the gut senses its content. Cell Microbiol 4: 61-72

36. Dinu I, Mahasirimongkol S, Liu Q, Yanai H, Sharaf EN, Kreiter E, Wu X, Jabbari S, Tokunaga K, Yasui Y (2012) SNP-SNP interactions discovered by logic regression explain Crohn's disease genetics. PLoS ONE 7: e43035

37. Doss M, White MR, Tecle T, Gantz D, Crouch EC, Jung G, Ruchala P, Waring AJ, Lehrer RI, Hartshorn KL (2009) Interactions of alpha-, beta-, and theta-defensins with influenza A virus and surfactant protein D. J Immunol 182: 7878-77887

38. Duan Y, Liao AP, Kuppireddi S, Ye Z, Ciancio MJ, Sun J (2007) beta-Catenin activity negatively regulates bacteria-induced inflammation. Lab Invest 87: 613-624

39. Duchmann R, May E, Heike M, Knolle P, Neurath M, Meyer zum Büschenfelde K.-H (1999) T cell specifity and cross reactivity towards enterobacteria, Bacteroides, Bifidobacterium, and antigens from resident intestinal flora in humans. Gut 44: 812-818

40. Eberl G (2010) A new vision of immunity: homeostasis of the superorganism. Mucosal Immunol 3: 450-460

41. Ericksen B, Wu Z, Lu W, Lehrer RI (2005) Antibacterial activity and specificity of the six human {alpha}-defensins. Antimicrob Agents Chemother 49: 269-275

42. Eriguchi Y, Takashima S, Oka H, Shimoji S, Nakamura K, Uryu H, Shimoda S, Iwasaki H, Shimono N, Ayabe T, et al (2012) Graft-versus-host disease disrupts intestinal microbial ecology by inhibiting Paneth cell production of alpha-defensins. Blood 120: 223-231

43. Fagotto F, Jho E, Zeng L, Kurth T, Joos T, Kaufmann C, Costantini F (1999) Domains of axin involved in protein-protein interactions, Wnt pathway inhibition, and intracellular localization. J Cell Biol 145: 741-756

44. Fellermann K, Stange DE, Schaeffeler E, Schmalzl H, Wehkamp J, Bevins CL, Reinisch W, Teml A, Schwab M, Lichter P, et al (2006) A chromosome 8 gene-cluster polymorphism with low human beta-defensin 2 gene copy number predisposes to Crohn disease of the colon. Am J Hum Genet 79: 439-448

45. Fowler EV, Doecke J, Simms LA, Zhao ZZ, Webb PM, Hayward NK, Whiteman DC, Florin TH, Montgomery GW, Cavanaugh JA, et al (2008) ATG16L1 T300A shows strong associations with disease subgroups in a large Australian IBD population: further support for significant disease heterogeneity. Am J Gastroenterol 103: 2519-2526

46. Fox JG, Feng Y, Theve EJ, Fry RC, Fiala JL, Doernte AL, Williams M, Raczynski AR, McFaline JL, Essigmann JM, et al (2009) Gut microbes define liver cancer risk in mice exposed to chemical and viral transgenic hepatocarcinogens. Gut 59: 88-97

47. Frantz AL, Rogier EW, Weber CR, Shen L, Cohen DA, Fenton LA, Bruno ME, Kaetzel CS (2012) Targeted deletion of MyD88 in intestinal epithelial cells results in compromised antibacterial immunity associated with downregulation of polymeric immunoglobulin receptor, mucin-2, and antibacterial peptides. Mucosal Immunol 5: 501-512

48. Fre S, Pallavi SK, Huyghe M, Laé M, Janssen KP, Robine S, Artavanis-Tsakonas S, Louvard D (2009) Notch and Wnt signals cooperatively control cell proliferation and tumorigenesis in the intestine. Proc Natl Acad Sci USA 106: 6309-6314

49. Friis-Hansen L (2006) Achlorhydria is associated with gastric microbial overgrowth and development of cancer: lessons learned from the gastrin knockout mouse. Scand J Clin Lab Invest 66: 607-621

50. Gallo RL, Hooper LV (2012) Epithelial antimicrobial defence of the skin and intestine. Nat Rev Immunol 12: 503-516

51. Garcia MI, Ghiani M, Lefort A, Libert F, Strollo S, Vassart G (2009) LGR5 deficiency deregulates Wnt signaling and leads to precocious Paneth cell differentiation in the fetal intestine. Dev Biol 331: 58-67

52. Gasche C, Grundtner P (2005) Genotypes and phenotypes in Crohn's disease: do they help in clinical management? Gut 54: 162-167

53. George MD, Wehkamp J, Kays RJ, Leutenegger CM, Sabir S, Grishina I, Dandekar S, Bevins CL (2008) In vivo gene expression profiling of human intestinal epithelial cells: analysis by laser microdissection of formalin fixed tissues. BMC Genomics 9: 209

54. Gersemann M, Becker S, Kubler I, Koslowski M, Wang G, Herrlinger KR, Griger J, Fritz P, Fellermann K, Schwab M, et al (2009) Differences in goblet cell differentiation between Crohn's disease and ulcerative colitis. Differentiation 77: 84-894

55. Goel A, Boland CR (2010) Recent insights into the pathogenesis of colorectal cancer. Curr Opin Gastroenterol 26: 47-52

56. Gordon HA, Bruckner-Kardoss E (1961a) Effect of normal microbial flora on intestinal surface area. Am J Physiol 201: 175-178

57. Gordon HA, Bruckner-Kardoss E (1961b) Effect of the normal microbial flora on various tissue elements of the small intestine. Acta Anat (Basel) 44: 210-225

58. Gregorieff A, Clevers H (2005) Wnt signaling in the intestinal epithelium: from endoderm to cancer. Genes Dev 19: 877-890

59. Grehan MJ, Borody TJ, Leis SM, Campbell J, Mitchell H, Wettstein A (2010) Durable alteration of the colonic microbiota by the administration of donor fecal flora. J Clin Gastroenterol 44: 551-561

60. Groth M, Wiegand C, Szafranski K, Huse K, Kramer M, Rosenstiel P, Schreiber S, Norgauer J, Platzer M (2010) Both copy number and sequence variations affect expression of human DEFB4. Genes Immun 11: 458-466

61. Gruenheid S, Le MH (2012) Resistance to antimicrobial peptides in Gram-negative bacteria. FEMS Microbiol Lett 330: 81-89

62. Gulati AS, Shanahan MT, Arthur JC, Grossniklaus E, von Furstenberg RJ, Kreuk L, Henning SJ, Jobin C, Sartor RB (2012) Mouse background strain profoundly influences Paneth cell function and intestinal microbial composition. PLoS ONE 7, e32403

63. Halfvarson J, Jess T, Magnuson A, Montgomery SM, Orholm M, Tysk C, Binder V, Jarnerot G (2006) Environmental factors in inflammatory bowel disease: a co-twin control study of a Swedish-Danish twin population. Inflamm Bowel Dis 12: 925-933

64. Hampe J, Franke A, Rosenstiel P, Till A, Teuber M, Huse K, Albrecht M, Mayr G, De La Vega FM, Briggs J, et al (2007) A genome-wide association scan of nonsynonymous SNPs identifies a susceptibility variant for Crohn disease in ATG16L1. Nat Genet 39: 207-211

65. Harder J, Glaser R, Schroder JM (2007) Human antimicrobial proteins effectors of innate immunity. J Endotoxin Res 13: 317-338

66. Hardwick RJ, Machado LR, Zuccherato LW, Antolinos S, Xue Y, Shawa N, Gilman RH, Cabrera L, Berg DE, Tyler-Smith C, et al (2011) A worldwide analysis of beta-defensin copy number variation suggests recent selection of a high-expressing DEFB103 gene copy in East Asia. Hum Mutat 32: 743-750

67. Harris K, Kassis A, Major G, Chou CJ (2012) Is the gut microbiota a new factor contributing to obesity and its metabolic disorders? J Obes 2012: 879151

68. Hashimoto T, Perlot T, Rehman A, Trichereau J, Ishiguro H, Paolino M, Sigl V, Hanada T, Hanada R, Lipinski S, et al (2012) ACE2 links amino acid malnutrition to microbial ecology and intestinal inflammation. Nature 487: 477-481

69. Hausmann M, Kiessling S, Mestermann S, Webb G, Spottl T, Andus T, Scholmerich J, Herfarth H, Ray K, Falk W, et al (2002) Toll-like receptors 2 and 4 are up-regulated during intestinal inflammation. Gastroenterology 122: 1987-2000

70. Heazlewood CK, Cook MC, Eri R, Price GR, Tauro SB, Taupin D, Thornton DJ, Png CW, Crockford TL, Cornall RJ, et al (2008) Aberrant mucin assembly in mice causes endoplasmic reticulum stress and spontaneous inflammation resembling ulcerative colitis. PLoS Med 5: e54

71. Heitman DW, Pool TB, Cameron IL (1980) Changes in proliferation and surface morphology in the rat ileum in response to total parenteral nutrition. J Anat 130: 603-615

72. Heneghan JB (1965) Imbalance of the normal microbial flora. The germ-free alimentary tract. Am J Dig Dis 10: 864-869

73. Hodin CM, Lenaerts K, Grootjans J, de Haan JJ, Hadfoune M, Verheyen FK, Kiyama H, Heineman E, Buurman WA (2011) Starvation compromises Paneth cells. Am J Pathol 179: 2885-2893

74. Howell JC, Wells JM (2011) Generating intestinal tissue from stem cells: potential for research and therapy. Regen Med 6: 743-755

75. Hugot J-P, Chamaillard C, Zouali H, Lesage S, Cezard J-P, Belaiche J, Almer S, Tysk C, O'Morain CA, Gassull M, et al (2001) Association of NOD2 leucine-rich repeat variants with susceptibility to Crohn's disease. Nature 411: 599-603

76. Hung KH, Wu JJ, Yang HB, Su LJ, Sheu BS (2009) Host Wnt/beta-catenin pathway triggered by Helicobacter pylori correlates with regression of gastric intestinal metaplasia after H. pylori eradication. J Med Microbiol 58: 567-576

77. Husebye E (2005) The pathogenesis of gastrointestinal bacterial overgrowth. Chemotherapy 51: 1-22

78. Jensen J, Pedersen EE, Galante P, Hald J, Heller RS, Ishibashi M, Kageyama R, Guillemot F, Serup P, Madsen OD (2000) Control of endodermal endocrine development by Hes-1. Nat Genet 24: 36-44

79. Johansson ME (2012) Fast renewal of the distal colonic mucus layers by the surface goblet cells as measured by in vivo labeling of mucin glycoproteins. PLoS ONE 7: e41009

80. Johansson ME, Larsson JM, Hansson GC (2011) The two mucus layers of colon are organized by the MUC2 mucin, whereas the outer layer is a legislator of host-microbial interactions. Proc Natl Acad Sci USA 108: 4659-44665

81. Jurevic RJ, Bai M, Chadwick RB, White TC, Dale BA (2003) Single-nucleotide polymorphisms (SNPs) in human beta-defensin 1: high-throughput SNP assays and association with Candida carriage in type I diabetics and nondiabetic controls. J Clin Microbiol 41: 90-96

82. Kaler P, Godasi BN, Augenlicht L, Klampfer L (2009) The NF-kappaB/AKT-dependent induction of Wnt signaling in colon cancer cells by macrophages and IL-1beta. Cancer Microenviron 2: 69-80

83. Kalus AA, Fredericks LP, Hacker BM, Dommisch H, Presland RB, Kimball JR, Dale BA (2009) Association of a genetic polymorphism (-44 C/G SNP) in the human DEFB1 gene with expression and inducibility of multiple beta-defensins in gingival keratinocytes. BMC Oral Health 9: 21

84. Kaser A, Lee AH, Franke A, Glickman JN, Zeissig S, Tilg H, Nieuwenhuis EE, Higgins DE, Schreiber S, Glimcher LH, et al (2008) XBP1 links ER stress to intestinal

inflammation and confers genetic risk for human inflammatory bowel disease. Cell 134: 743-756

85. Kassam Z, Lee CH, Yuan Y, Hunt RH (2013) Fecal microbiota transplantation for Clostridium difficile infection: systematic review and meta-analysis. Am J Gastroenterol 108: 500-508

86. Kelly CJ, Glover LE, Campbell EL, Kominsky DJ, Ehrentraut SF, Bowers BE, Bayless AJ, Saeedi BJ, Colgan SP (2013) Fundamental role for HIF-1alpha in constitutive expression of human beta defensin-1. Mucosal Immunol (Advance online publication), DOI: 10.1038/mi.2013.6

87. Khanna S, Pardi DS (2012) Clostridium difficile infection: new insights into management. Mayo Clin Proc 87: 1106-1117

88. Khoruts A, Dicksved J, Jansson JK, Sadowsky MJ (2010) Changes in the composition of the human fecal microbiome after bacteriotherapy for recurrent Clostridium difficile-associated diarrhea. J Clin Gastroenterol 44: 354-360

89. Klotman ME, Chang TL (2006) Defensins in innate antiviral immunity. Nat Rev Immunol 6: 447-456

90. Klotman ME, Rapista A, Teleshova N, Micsenyi A, Jarvis GA, Lu W, Porter E, Chang TL (2008) Neisseria gonorrhoeae-induced human defensins 5 and 6 increase HIV infectivity: role in enhanced transmission. J Immunol 180: 6176-6185

91. Kocsis AK, Lakatos PL, Somogyvari F, Fuszek P, Papp J, Fischer S, Szamosi T, Lakatos L, Kovacs A, Hofner P, et al (2008) Association of beta-defensin 1 single nucleotide polymorphisms with Crohn's disease. Scand J Gastroenterol 43: 299-307

92. Koon HW, Shih DQ, Chen J, Bakirtzi K, Hing TC, Law I, Ho S, Ichikawa R, Zhao D, Xu H, et al (2011) Cathelicidin signaling via the Toll-like receptor protects against colitis in mice. Gastroenterology 141: 1852-1863

93. Koprivnjak T, Peschel A (2011) Bacterial resistance mechanisms against host defense peptides. Cell Mol Life Sci 68: 2243-2254

94. Korinek V, Barker N, Moerer P, van DE, Huls G, Peters PJ, Clevers H (1998) Depletion of epithelial stem-cell compartments in the small intestine of mice lacking Tcf-4. Nat Genet 19: 379-383

95. Koslowski MJ, Beisner J, Stange EF, Wehkamp J (2009a) Innate antimicrobial host defense in small intestinal Crohn's disease. Int J Med Microbiol 300: 34-40

96. Koslowski MJ, Kubler I, Chamaillard M, Schaeffeler E, Reinisch W, Wang G, Beisner J, Teml A, Peyrin-Biroulet L, Winter S, et al (2009b) Genetic variants of Wnt transcription factor TCF-4 (TCF7L2) putative promoter region are associated with small intestinal Crohn's disease. PLoS ONE 4: e4496

97. Koslowski MJ, Teltschik Z, Beisner J, Schaeffeler E, Wang G, Kubler I, Gersemann M, Cooney R, Jewell D, Reinisch W, et al (2012) Association of a functional variant in the Wnt co-receptor LRP6 with early onset ileal Crohn's disease. PLoS Genet 8: e1002523

98. Kubler I, Koslowski MJ, Gersemann M, Fellermann K, Beisner J, Becker S, Rothfuss K, Herrlinger KR, Stange EF, Wehkamp J (2009) Influence of standard treatment on ileal and colonic antimicrobial defensin expression in active Crohn's disease. Aliment Pharmacol Ther 30: 621-633

99. Lai Y, Gallo RL (2009) AMPed up immunity: how antimicrobial peptides have multiple roles in immune defense. Trends Immunol 30: 131-141

100. Lala S, Ogura Y, Osborne C, Hor SY, Bromfield A, Davies S, Ogunbiyi O, Nunez G, Keshav S (2003) Crohn's disease and the NOD2 gene: a role for paneth cells. Gastroenterology 125: 47-57

101. Landy J, Al-Hassi HO, McLaughlin SD, Walker AW, Ciclitira PJ, Nicholls RJ, Clark SK, Hart AL (2011) Review article: faecal transplantation therapy for gastrointestinal disease. Aliment Pharmacol Ther 34: 409-415

102. Lavelle EC, Murphy C, O'Neill LA, Creagh EM (2010) The role of TLRs, NLRs, and RLRs in mucosal innate immunity and homeostasis. Mucosal Immunol 3: 17-28

103. Lee J, Mo JH, Katakura K, Alkalay I, Rucker AN, Liu YT, Lee HK, Shen C, Cojocaru G, Shenouda S, et al (2006) Maintenance of colonic homeostasis by distinctive apical TLR9 signalling in intestinal epithelial cells. Nat Cell Biol 8: 1327-1336

104. Leitch GJ, Ceballos C (2009) A role for antimicrobial peptides in intestinal microsporidiosis. Parasitology 136: 175-181

105. Lievin-Le MV, Servin AL (2006) The front line of enteric host defense against unwelcome intrusion of harmful microorganisms: mucins, antimicrobial peptides, and microbiota. Clin Microbiol Rev 19: 315-337

106. Liu X, Lu R, Wu S, Zhang YG, Xia Y, Sartor RB, Sun J (2012) Wnt2 inhibits enteric bacterial-induced inflammation in intestinal epithelial cells. Inflamm Bowel Dis 18: 418-429

107. Liu S, Qian Y, Li L, Wei G, Guan Y, Pan H, Guan X, Zhang L, Lu X, Zhao Y, et al (2013) Lgr4 deficiency increases susceptibility and severity of dextran sodium sulphate-induced inflammatory bowel disease in mice. J Biol Chem 288: 8794-8803

108. Louis E, Collard A, Oger AF, Degroote E, Aboul Nasr El Yafi FA, Belaiche J (2001) Behaviour of Crohn's disease according to the Vienna classification: changing pattern over the course of the disease. Gut 49: 777-782

109. Lozupone CA, Stombaugh JI, Gordon JI, Jansson JK, Knight R (2012) Diversity, stability and resilience of the human gut microbiota. Nature 489: 220-230

110. Ma BW, Bokulich NA, Castillo PA, Kananurak A, Underwood MA, Mills DA, Bevins CL (2012) Routine habitat change: a source of unrecognized transient alteration of intestinal microbiota in laboratory mice. PLoS ONE 7: e47416

111. Malik AN, Al-Kafaji G (2007) Glucose regulation of beta-defensin-1 mRNA in human renal cells. Biochem Biophys Res Commun 353: 318-323

112. Manicassamy S, Reizis B, Ravindran R, Nakaya H, Salazar-Gonzalez RM, Wang YC, Pulendran B (2010) Activation of beta-catenin in dendritic cells regulates immunity versus tolerance in the intestine. Science 329: 849-853

113. Marchesi JR, Dutilh BE, Hall N, Peters WH, Roelofs R, Boleij A, Tjalsma H (2011) Towards the human colorectal cancer microbiome. PLoS ONE 6: e20447

114. Marion-Letellier R, Dechelotte P, Iacucci M, Ghosh S (2009) Dietary modulation of peroxisome proliferator-activated receptor gamma. Gut 58: 586-593

115. Martin M, Rehani K, Jope RS, Michalek SM (2005) Toll-like receptor-mediated cytokine production is differentially regulated by glycogen synthase kinase 3. Nat Immunol 6: 777-784

116. McCracken KW, Howell JC, Wells JM, Spence JR (2011) Generating human intestinal tissue from pluripotent stem cells in vitro. Nat Protoc 6: 1920-1928

117. McGee DJ, George AE, Trainor EA, Horton KE, Hildebrandt E, Testerman TL (2011) Cholesterol enhances Helicobacter pylori resistance to antibiotics and LL-37. Antimicrob Agents Chemother 55: 2897-2904

118. Mestas J, Hughes CC (2004) Of mice and not men: differences between mouse and human immunology. J Immunol 172: 2731-2738

119. Meyer-Hoffert U, Hornef MW, Henriques-Normark B, Axelsson LG, Midtvedt T, Putsep K, Andersson M (2008) Secreted enteric antimicrobial activity localises to the mucus surface layer. Gut 57: 764-771

120. Milanese M, Segat L, Pontillo A, Arraes LC, de Lima Filho JL, Crovella S (2006) DEFB1 gene polymorphisms and increased risk of HIV-1 infection in Brazilian children. AIDS 20: 1673-1675

121. Mondel M, Schroeder BO, Zimmermann K, Huber H, Nuding S, Beisner J, Fellermann K, Stange EF, Wehkamp J (2008) Probiotic E. coli treatment mediates antimicrobial human beta-defensin synthesis and fecal excretion in humans. Mucosal Immunol 2: 166-172

122. Muise AM, Walters TD, Glowacka WK, Griffiths AM, Ngan BY, Lan H, Xu W, Silverberg MS, Rotin D (2009) Polymorphisms in E-cadherin (CDH1) result in a mis-localised cytoplasmic protein that is associated with Crohn's disease. Gut 58: 1121-1127

123. Naylor G, Axon A (2003) Role of bacterial overgrowth in the stomach as an additional risk factor for gastritis. Can J Gastroenterol 17: 13B-17B

124. Neal MD, Sodhi CP, Jia H, Dyer M, Egan CE, Yazji I, Good M, Afrazi A, Marino R, Slagle D, et al (2012) Toll-like receptor 4 is expressed on intestinal stem cells and regulates their proliferation and apoptosis via the p53 up-regulated modulator of apoptosis. J Biol Chem 287: 37296-37308

125. Neal MD, Sodhi CP, Dyer M, Craig BT, Good M, Jia H, Yazji I, Afrazi A, Richardson WM, Beer-Stolz D, et al (2013) A critical role for TLR4 induction of autophagy in the regulation of enterocyte migration and the pathogenesis of necrotizing enterocolitis. J Immunol 190: 3541-3551

126. Neish AS (2009) Microbes in gastrointestinal health and disease. Gastroenterology 136: 65-80

127. Ogura Y, Bonen DK, Inohara N, Nicolae DL, Chen FF, Ramos R, Britton H, Moran T, Karalluskas R, Duerr RH, et al (2001) A frameshift mutation in NOD2 associated with susceptibility to Crohn's diease. Nature 411: 603-606

128. Ogushi K, Wada A, Niidome T, Mori N, Oishi K, Nagatake T, Takahashi A, Asakura H, Makino S, Hojo H, et al (2001a) Salmonella enteritidis FliC (flagella filament protein) induces human beta-defensin-2 mRNA production by Caco-2 cells. J Biol Chem 276: 30521-30526

129. Ogushi K, Wada A, Niidome T, Mori N, Oishi K, Nagatake T, Takahashi A, Asakura H, Makino S, Hojo H, et al (2001b) Salmonella enteritidis FliC (flagella filament protein) induces human beta-defensin-2 mRNA production by Caco-2 cells. J Biol Chem 276: 30521-30526

130. Ohigashi S, Sudo K, Kobayashi D, Takahashi O, Takahashi T, Asahara T, Nomoto K, Onodera H (2013) Changes of the intestinal microbiota, short chain fatty acids, and fecal ph in patients with colorectal cancer. Dig Dis Sci 58: 1717-1726

131. Ooi CH, Ivanova T, Wu J, Lee M, Tan IB, Tao J, Ward L, Koo JH, Gopalakrishnan V, Zhu Y, et al (2009) Oncogenic pathway combinations predict clinical prognosis in gastric cancer. PLoS Genet 5: e1000676

132. Orford K, Crockett C, Jensen JP, Weissman AM, Byers SW (1997) Serine phosphorylation-regulated ubiquitination and degradation of beta-catenin. J Biol Chem 272: 24735-24738

133. Perminow G, Beisner J, Koslowski M, Lyckander LG, Stange E, Vatn MH, Wehkamp J (2010) Defective paneth cell-mediated host defense in pediatric ileal Crohn's disease. Am J Gastroenterol 105: 452-459

134. Petersson J, Schreiber O, Hansson GC, Gendler SJ, Velcich A, Lundberg JO, Roos S, Holm L, Phillipson M (2011) Importance and regulation of the colonic mucus barrier in a mouse model of colitis. Am J Physiol Gastrointest Liver Physiol 300: G327-G333

135. Peyrin-Biroulet L, Beisner J, Wang G, Nuding S, Oommen ST, Kelly D, Parmentier-Decrucq E, Dessein R, Merour E, Chavatte P, et al (2010) Peroxisome proliferator-activated receptor gamma activation is required for maintenance of innate antimicrobial immunity in the colon. Proc Natl Acad Sci USA 107: 8772-8777

136. Png CW, Linden SK, Gilshenan KS, Zoetendal EG, McSweeney CS, Sly LI, McGuckin MA, Florin TH (2010) Mucolytic bacteria with increased prevalence in IBD mucosa augment in vitro utilization of mucin by other bacteria. Am J Gastroenterol 105: 2420-2428

137. Podolsky DK (2002) Inflammatory bowel disease. N Engl J Med 347: 417-429

138. Pothoulakis C (2009) Review article: anti-inflammatory mechanisms of action of Saccharomyces boulardii. Aliment Pharmacol Ther 30: 826-833

139. Pullan RD, Thomas GA, Rhodes M, Newcombe RG, Williams GT, Allen A, Rhodes J (1994) Thickness of adherent mucus gel on colonic mucosa in humans and its relevance to colitis. Gut 35: 353-359

140. Rakoff-Nahoum S, Paglino J, Eslami-Varzaneh F, Edberg S, Medzhitov R (2004) Recognition of commensal microflora by toll-like receptors is required for intestinal homeostasis. Cell 118: 229-241

141. Rohrl J, Yang D, Oppenheim JJ, Hehlgans T (2010a) Human beta-defensin 2 and 3 and their mouse orthologs induce chemotaxis through interaction with CCR2. J Immunol 184: 6688-6694

142. Rohrl J, Yang D, Oppenheim JJ, Hehlgans T (2010b) Specific binding and chemotactic activity of mBD4 and its functional orthologue hBD2 to CCR6-expressing cells. J Biol Chem 285: 7028-7034

143. Rohrl J, Geissler EK, Hehlgans T (2012a) Friend or foe: a novel role of beta-defensins in tumor development. Oncoimmunology 1: 1159-1160

144. Rohrl J, Huber B, Koehl GE, Geissler EK, Hehlgans T (2012b) Mouse beta-defensin 14 (Defb14) promotes tumor growth by inducing angiogenesis in a CCR6-dependent manner. J Immunol 188: 4931-4939

145. Rose WA, Sakamoto K, Leifer CA (2012) TLR9 is important for protection against intestinal damage and for intestinal repair. Sci Rep 2: 574

146. Rumio C, Besusso D, Palazzo M, Selleri S, Sfondrini L, Dubini F, Menard S, Balsari A (2004) Degranulation of paneth cells via toll-like receptor 9. Am J Pathol 165: 373-381

147. Saleh M, Trinchieri G (2011) Innate immune mechanisms of colitis and colitis-associated colorectal cancer. Nat Rev Immunol 11: 9-20
148. Salzman NH, Gottsch JD, Huttner KM, Paterson Y, Bevins CL Protection against enteric salmonellosis in transgenic mice expressing a human intestinal defensin. Nature 422: 522-526
149. Salzman NH, Hung K, Haribhai D, Chu H, Karlsson-Sjoberg J, Amir E, Teggatz P, Barman M, Hayward M, Eastwood D, et al (2010) Enteric defensins are essential regulators of intestinal microbial ecology. Nat Immunol 11: 76-83
150. Santaolalla R, Abreu MT (2012) Innate immunity in the small intestine. Curr Opin Gastroenterol 28: 124-129
151. Sartor RB (1997) Review article: role of the enteric microflora in the pathogenesis of intestinal inflammation and arthritis. Aliment Pharmacol Ther 11: 17-22
152. Saulnier DM, Kolida S, Gibson GR (2009) Microbiology of the human intestinal tract and approaches for its dietary modulation. Curr Pharm Des 15: 1403-1414
153. Schauber J, Rieger D, Weiler F, Wehkamp J, Eck M, Fellermann K, Scheppach W, Gallo RL, Stange EF (2006) Heterogeneous expression of human cathelicidin hCAP18/LL-37 in inflammatory bowel diseases. Eur J Gastroenterol Hepatol 18: 615-621
154. Schlee M, Wehkamp J, Altenhoefer A, Oelschlaeger TA, Stange EF, Fellermann K (2007) The induction of human beta-defensin-2 by the probiotic Escherichia coli Nissle 1917 is mediated through flagellin. Infect Immun 75: 2399-2407
155. Schlee M, Harder J, Koten B, Stange EF, Wehkamp J, Fellermann K (2008) Probiotic lactobacilli and VSL#3 induce enterocyte beta-defensin 2. Clin Exp Immunol 151: 528-535
156. CrossRef | PubMed | CAS | Web of Science® Times Cited: 99 | Wiley Online Library
157. Schreiber S, Rosenstiel P, Albrecht M, Hampe J, Krawczak M (2005) Genetics of Crohn disease, an archetypal inflammatory barrier disease. Nat Rev Genet 6: 376-388
158. Schroeder BO, Stange EF, Wehkamp J (2011a) Waking the wimp: redox-modulation activates human beta-defensin 1. Gut Microbes 2: 262-266
159. Schroeder BO, Wu Z, Nuding S, Groscurth S, Marcinowski M, Beisner J, Buchner J, Schaller M, Stange EF, Wehkamp J (2011b) Reduction of disulphide bonds unmasks potent antimicrobial activity of human beta-defensin 1. Nature 469: 419-423
160. Schultz M, Lindstrom AL (2008) Rationale for probiotic treatment strategies in inflammatory bowel disease. Expert Rev Gastroenterol Hepatol 2: 337-355
161. Sears CL (2005) A dynamic partnership: celebrating our gut flora. Anaerobe 11: 247-251
162. Semple F, Webb S, Li HN, Patel HB, Perretti M, Jackson IJ, Gray M, Davidson DJ, Dorin JR (2010) Human beta-defensin 3 has immunosuppressive activity in vitro and in vivo. Eur J Immunol 40: 1073-1078
163. Semple F, MacPherson H, Webb S, Cox SL, Mallin LJ, Tyrrell C, Grimes GR, Semple CA, Nix MA, Millhauser GL, et al (2011) Human beta-defensin 3 affects the activity of pro-inflammatory pathways associated with MyD88 and TRIF. Eur J Immunol 41: 3291-3300
164. Seok J, Warren HS, Cuenca AG, Mindrinos MN, Baker HV, Xu W, Richards DR, Donald-Smith GP, Gao H, Hennessy L, et al (2013) Genomic responses in mouse

models poorly mimic human inflammatory diseases. Proc Natl Acad Sci USA 110: 3507-3512

165. Shahinas D, Silverman M, Sittler T, Chiu C, Kim P, len-Vercoe E, Weese S, Wong A, Low DE, Pillai DR (2012) Toward an understanding of changes in diversity associated with fecal microbiome transplantation based on 16S rRNA gene deep sequencing. MBio 3: DOI: 10.1128/mBio.00338-12

166. Shanahan MT, Tanabe H, Ouellette AJ (2011) Strain-specific polymorphisms in Paneth cell alpha-defensins of C57BL/6 mice and evidence of vestigial myeloid alpha-defensin pseudogenes. Infect Immun 79: 459-473

167. Shanahan MT, Carroll IM, Grossniklaus E, White A, von Furstenberg RJ, Barner R, Fodor AA, Henning SJ, Sartor RB, Gulati AS (2013) Mouse Paneth cell antimicrobial function is independent of Nod2. Gut (in press) DOI: 10.1136/gutjnl-2012-304190

168. Shaykhiev R, Behr J, Bals R (2008) Microbial patterns signaling via Toll-like receptors 2 and 5 contribute to epithelial repair, growth and survival. PLoS ONE 3: e1393

169. Silverberg MS, Satsangi J, Ahmad T, Arnott ID, Bernstein CN, Brant SR, Caprilli R, Colombel JF, Gasche C, Geboes K, et al (2005) Toward an integrated clinical, molecular and serological classification of inflammatory bowel disease: report of a working party of the 2005 Montreal World Congress of Gastroenterology. Can J Gastroenterol 19: 5-36

170. Simms LA, Doecke JD, Walsh MD, Huang N, Fowler EV, Radford-Smith GL (2008) Reduced alpha-defensin expression is associated with inflammation and not NOD2 mutation status in ileal Crohn's disease. Gut 57: 903-910

171. Simms LA, Doecke JD, Roberts RL, Fowler EV, Zhao ZZ, McGuckin MA, Huang N, Hayward NK, Webb PM, Whiteman DC, et al (2010) KCNN4 gene variant is associated with ileal Crohn's disease in the Australian and New Zealand population. Am J Gastroenterol 105: 2209-2217

172. Sobhani I, Tap J, Roudot-Thoraval F, Roperch JP, Letulle S, Langella P, Corthier G, Tran Van, NJ, Furet JP (2011) Microbial dysbiosis in colorectal cancer (CRC) patients. PLoS ONE 6: e16393

173. Sodhi CP, Shi XH, Richardson WM, Grant ZS, Shapiro RA, Prindle T, Jr, Branca M, Russo A, Gribar SC, Ma C, et al (2010) Toll-like receptor-4 inhibits enterocyte proliferation via impaired beta-catenin signaling in necrotizing enterocolitis. Gastroenterology 138: 185-196

174. Sodhi CP, Neal MD, Siggers R, Sho S, Ma C, Branca MF, Prindle T, Jr, Russo AM, Afrazi A, Good M, et al (2012) Intestinal epithelial Toll-like receptor 4 regulates goblet cell development and is required for necrotizing enterocolitis in mice. Gastroenterology 143: 708-718

175. Song EJ, Kang MJ, Kim YS, Kim SM, Lee SE, Kim CH, Kim DJ, Park JH (2011) Flagellin promotes the proliferation of gastric cancer cells via the Toll-like receptor 5. Int J Mol Med 28: 115-119

176. Strugala V, Dettmar PW, Pearson JP (2008) Thickness and continuity of the adherent colonic mucus barrier in active and quiescent ulcerative colitis and Crohn's disease. Int J Clin Pract 62: 762-769

177. Sun J, Hobert ME, Rao AS, Neish AS, Madara JL (2004) Bacterial activation of beta-catenin signaling in human epithelia. Am J Physiol Gastrointest Liver Physiol 287: G220-G227

178. Swidsinski A, Ladhoff A, Pernthaler A, Swidsinski S, Loening-Baucke V, Ortner M, Weber J, Hoffmann U, Schreiber S, Dietel M, et al (2002) Mucosal flora in inflammatory bowel disease. Gastroenterology 122: 44-54

179. Tai EK, Wu WK, Wang XJ, Wong HP, Yu L, Li ZJ, Lee CW, Wong CC, Yu J, Sung JJ, et al (2013) Intrarectal administration of mCRAMP-encoding plasmid reverses exacerbated colitis in Cnlp($^{-/-}$) mice. Gene Ther 20: 187-193

180. Teltschik Z, Wiest R, Beisner J, Nuding S, Hofmann C, Schoelmerich J, Bevins CL, Stange EF, Wehkamp J (2011) Intestinal bacterial translocation in rats with cirrhosis is related to compromised paneth cell antimicrobial host defense. Hepatology 55: 1154-1163

181. Thompson GR, Trexler PC (1971) Gastrointestinal structure and function in germ-free or gnotobiotic animals. Gut 12: 230-235

182. Tye H, Kennedy CL, Najdovska M, McLeod L, McCormack W, Hughes N, Dev A, Sievert W, Ooi CH, Ishikawa TO, et al (2012) STAT3-driven upregulation of TLR2 promotes gastric tumorigenesis independent of tumor inflammation. Cancer Cell 22: 466-478

183. Ungaro R, Fukata M, Hsu D, Hernandez Y, Breglio K, Chen A, Xu R, Sotolongo J, Espana C, Zaias J, et al (2009) A novel Toll-like receptor 4 antagonist antibody ameliorates inflammation but impairs mucosal healing in murine colitis. Am J Physiol Gastrointest Liver Physiol 296: G1167-G1179

184. Uronis JM, Mühlbauer M, Herfarth HH, Rubinas TC, Jones GS, Jobin C (2009) Modulation of the intestinal microbiota alters colitis-associated colorectal cancer susceptibility. PLoS ONE 4: e6026

185. Vaiopoulos AG, Kostakis ID, Koutsilieris M, Papavassiliou AG (2012) Colorectal cancer stem cells. Stem Cells 30: 363-371

186. Vaishnava S, Behrendt CL, Ismail AS, Eckmann L, Hooper LV (2008) Paneth cells directly sense gut commensals and maintain homeostasis at the intestinal host-microbial interface. Proc Natl Acad Sci USA 105: 20858-20863

187. van Es JH, Jay P, Gregorieff A, van Gijn ME, Jonkheer S, Hatzis P, Thiele A, van den BM, Begthel H, Brabletz T, et al (2005) Wnt signalling induces maturation of Paneth cells in intestinal crypts. Nat Cell Biol 7: 381-386

188. van Es JH, Haegebarth A, Kujala P, Itzkovitz S, Koo BK, Boj SF, Korving J, van den BM, van OA, Robine S, et al (2012) A critical role for the wnt effector tcf4 in adult intestinal homeostatic self-renewal. Mol Cell Biol 32: 1918-1927

189. van Nood E, Vrieze A, Nieuwdorp M, Fuentes S, Zoetendal EG, de Vos WM, Visser CE, Kuijper EJ, Bartelsman JF, Tijssen JG, et al (2013) Duodenal infusion of donor feces for recurrent Clostridium difficile. N Engl J Med 368: 407-415

190. Walsh R, Seth R, Behnke J, Potten CS, Mahida YR (2009) Epithelial stem cell-related alterations in Trichinella spiralis-infected small intestine. Cell Prolif 42: 394-403

191. Wang A, Chen F, Wang Y, Shen M, Xu Y, Hu J, Wang S, Geng F, Wang C, Ran X, et al (2013) Enhancement of antiviral activity of human alpha-defensin 5 against herpes simplex virus 2 by arginine mutagenesis at adaptive evolution sites. J Virol 87: 2835-2845

192. Wehkamp J, Stange EF (2010) Paneth's disease. J Crohn's Colitis 4: 523-531

193. Wehkamp J, Harder J, Weichenthal M, Mueller O, Herrlinger KR, Fellermann K, Schroeder JM, Stange EF (2003a) Inducible and constitutive beta-defensins are

differentially expressed in Crohn's disease and ulcerative colitis. Inflamm Bowel Dis 9: 215-223

194. Wehkamp J, Harder J, Weichenthal M, Mueller O, Herrlinger KR, Fellermann K, Schroeder JM, Stange EF (2003b) Inducible and constitutive beta-defensins are differentially expressed in Crohn's disease and ulcerative colitis. Inflamm Bowel Dis 9: 215-223

195. Wehkamp J, Schmidt K, Herrlinger KR, Baxmann S, Behling S, Wohlschlager C, Feller AC, Stange EF, Fellermann K (2003c) Defensin pattern in chronic gastritis: HBD-2 is differentially expressed with respect to Helicobacter pylori status. J Clin Pathol 56: 352-357

196. Wehkamp J, Harder J, Wehkamp K, Wehkamp-von Meissner B, Schlee M, Enders C, Sonnenborn U, Nuding S, Bengmark S, Fellermann K, et al (2004a) NF-kappaB- and AP-1-mediated induction of human beta defensin-2 in intestinal epithelial cells by Escherichia coli Nissle 1917: a novel effect of a probiotic bacterium. Infect Immun 72: 5750-5758

197. Wehkamp J, Harder J, Weichenthal M, Schwab M, Schaffeler E, Schlee M, Herrlinger KR, Stallmach A, Noack F, Fritz P, et al (2004b) NOD2 (CARD15) mutations in Crohn's disease are associated with diminished mucosal alpha-defensin expression. Gut 53: 1658-1664

198. Wehkamp J, Fellermann K, Herrlinger KR, Bevins CL, Stange EF (2005a) Mechanisms of disease: defensins in gastrointestinal diseases. Nat Clin Pract Gastroenterol Hepatol 2: 406-415

199. Wehkamp J, Salzman NH, Porter E, Nuding S, Weichenthal M, Petras RE, Shen B, Schaeffeler E, Schwab M, Linzmeier R, et al (2005b) Reduced Paneth cell alpha-defensins in ileal Crohn's disease. Proc Natl Acad Sci USA 102: 18129-18134

200. Wehkamp J, Wang G, Kubler I, Nuding S, Gregorieff A, Schnabel A, Kays RJ, Fellermann K, Burk O, Schwab M, et al (2007) The Paneth cell alpha-defensin deficiency of ileal Crohn's disease is linked to Wnt/Tcf-4. J Immunol 179: 3109-3118

201. Wehkamp J, Koslowski M, Wang G, Stange EF (2008) Barrier dysfunction due to distinct defensin deficiencies in small intestinal and colonic Crohn's disease. Mucosal Immunol 1: S67-S74

202. Wei G, de LE, Pazgier M, Yuan W, Zou G, Wang J, Ericksen B, Lu WY, Lehrer RI, Lu W (2009) Through the looking glass, mechanistic insights from enantiomeric human defensins. J Biol Chem 284: 29180-29192

203. Wiesner J, Vilcinskas A (2010) Antimicrobial peptides: the ancient arm of the human immune system. Virulence 1: 440-464

204. Willing BP, Vacharaksa A, Croxen M, Thanachayanont T, Finlay BB (2011) Altering host resistance to infections through microbial transplantation. PLoS ONE 6: e26988

205. Wilson CL, Ouellette AJ, Satchell DP, Ayabe T, Lopez-Boado YS, Stratman JL, Hultgren SJ, Matrisian LM, Parks WC (1999) Regulation of intestinal alpha-defensin activation by the metalloproteinase matrilysin in innate host defense. Science 286: 113-117

206. Yamanaka T, Helgeland L, Farstad IN, Fukushima H, Midtvedt T, Brandtzaeg P (2003) Microbial colonization drives lymphocyte accumulation and differentiation in the follicle-associated epithelium of Peyer's patches. J Immunol 170: 816-822

207. Yang D, Chertov O, Bykovskaia SN, Chen Q, Buffo MJ, Shogan J, Anderson M, Schröder JM, Wang JM, Howard OMZ, et al (1999) β-defensins: linking innate and adaptive immunity through dendritic and T cell CCR6. Science 286: 525-528

208. Zheng X, Tsuchiya K, Okamoto R, Iwasaki M, Kano Y, Sakamoto N, Nakamura T, Watanabe M (2011) Suppression of hath1 gene expression directly regulated by hes1 via notch signaling is associated with goblet cell depletion in ulcerative colitis. Inflamm Bowel Dis 17: 2251-2260

209. Zilbauer M, Dorrell N, Boughan PK, Harris A, Wren BW, Klein NJ, Bajaj-Elliott M (2005) Intestinal innate immunity to Campylobacter jejuni results in induction of bactericidal human beta-defensins 2 and 3. Infect Immun 73: 7281-7289

210. Zilbauer M, Jenke A, Wenzel G, Postberg J, Heusch A, Phillips AD, Noble-Jamieson G, Torrente F, Salvestrini C, Heuschkel R, et al (2010) Expression of human beta-defensins in children with chronic inflammatory bowel disease. PLoS ONE 5: e15389

211. Zilbauer M, Jenke A, Wenzel G, Goedde D, Postberg J, Phillips AD, Lucas M, Noble-Jamieson G, Torrente F, Salvestrini C, et al (2011) Intestinal alpha-defensin expression in pediatric inflammatory bowel disease. Inflamm Bowel Dis 17: 2076-2086.

CHAPTER 8

MATRIX METALLOPROTEINASE 13 MODULATES INTESTINAL EPITHELIAL BARRIER INTEGRITY IN INFLAMMATORY DISEASES BY ACTIVATING TNF

ROOSMARIJN E. VANDENBROUCKE, ELINE DEJONCKHEERE, FILIP VAN HAUWERMEIREN, SOFIE LODENS, RIET DE RYCKE, ELIEN VAN WONTERGHEM, AN STAES, KRIS GEVAERT, CARLOS LÓPEZ-OTIN, AND CLAUDE LIBERT

8.1 INTRODUCTION

Matrix metalloproteinases (MMPs) are important mediators during the process of inflammation and are consequently involved in several pathological processes, such as cancer (Decock et al, 2011; Overall & Lopez-Otin, 2002), sepsis (Vandenbroucke et al, 2011a, 2012; Vanlaere & Libert, 2009), lung diseases (Vandenbroucke et al, 2011b), ischaemia/reperfusion (Dejonckheere et al, 2011) and arthritis (Burrage et al, 2006). They constitute a group of structurally and functionally related zinc-dependent endopeptidases responsible for cleaving and rebuilding connective tissue com-

This chapter was originally published under the Creative Commons Attribution License. Vandenbroucke RE, Dejonckheere E, Van Hauwermeiren F, Lodens S, De Rycke R, Van Wonterghem E, Staes A, Gevaert K, López-Otin C, and Libert C. Matrix Metalloproteinase 13 Modulates Intestinal Epithelial Barrier Integrity In Inflammatory Diseases by Activating TNF. EMBO Molecular Medicine 5,7 (2013): pp. 1000–1016. doi:10.1002/emmm.201202100.

ponents such as collagen, elastin, gelatin and casein (Zitka et al, 2010). Moreover, several extracellular and intracellular non-matrix substrates of MMPs have been identified, including chemokines, cytokines, growth factors, junction proteins, molecular chaperones and cytoskeletal proteins (Cauwe & Opdenakker, 2010; Cauwe et al, 2007).

MMP13 (collagenase-3) belongs to the family of collagenases together with MMP1 and MMP8. Matrix substrates of MMP13 include native collagen, gelatin and aggrecan and non-matrix substrates include MCP-3 and pro-MMP9. MMP13 activity in chondrocytes and synovial cells appears to be critical in cartilage formation and in joint diseases (Takaishi et al, 2008). MMP13 has also been implicated in tumour invasion and metastasis (Fukuda et al, 2011; Wu et al, 2012), lung diseases (Shukla et al, 2006), and periodontal disease (de Aquino et al, 2009). Additionally, some reports suggest that MMP13 is important in IBD, an umbrella term that includes Crohn's disease and ulcerative colitis (UC), two chronic relapsing inflammatory disorders of the gut. Significantly increased levels of MMP13 mRNA were found in IBD biopsy specimens (Rath et al, 2006). Moreover, a positive correlation was found between MMP13 expression and the histological inflammation scores in mucosal samples from IBD patients (Vizoso et al, 2006). Recently, both endothelial cells and infiltrating leucocytes were identified as the major sources of MMP13 in UC (Rath et al, 2010).

IBD, as well as other pathological events such as sepsis, are associated with impairment of the intestinal epithelial barrier (John et al, 2011; Turner, 2009). Consequently, intestinal lumen components (i.e., bacteria, PAMPs and alarmins) leak into the bloodstream, inducing a systemic inflammatory response syndrome (SIRS), which can result in lethal multi-organ failure (Balzan et al, 2007). Tight junctions play an important role in the formation and maintenance of the intestinal epithelial barrier, as they tightly seal adjacent intestinal epithelial cells (IECs) at the apical site (Farquhar & Palade, 1963). Tight junctions transmembrane proteins such as occludin and claudins mediate adhesion by linkage to the underlying plaque proteins, which in turn associate with the cytoskeleton. Examples of plaque proteins are zona occludens (ZO) 1, −2 and −3 (Niessen, 2007). Several papers have reported that MMPs play a direct or indirect role in increasing epithelial barrier permeability (Ailenberg & Sefton, 2009; Huet et al, 2011; Vandenbroucke et al, 2012).

In this study, we investigated whether MMP13 plays a role in epithelial barrier disruption during pathological events such as sepsis and IBD, by using endotoxemia and DSS-induced colitis models, respectively. We found that MMP13 contributes to intestinal permeability by causing TNF shedding, which increases the levels of soluble, bioactive TNF. Consequently, TNF induces endoplasmic reticulum (ER) stress mediated mucus depletion in the gut, increased intestinal inflammation, reduced functionality of the tight junctions, and increased intestinal permeability. These changes lead to leakage of luminal components into the periphery, systemic inflammation, organ damage and eventually death. In conclusion, our results suggest that MMP13 is a potential therapeutic target for treatment of inflammatory disorders associated with TNF-dependent dysfunction of the intestinal barrier, such as sepsis and IBD.

8.2 RESULTS

8.2.1 MMP13 DEFICIENCY PROTECTS MICE FROM LPS-INDUCED SYSTEMIC INFLAMMATION AND LETHALITY

To investigate whether MMP13 contributes to the lethal effects of sepsis, we compared the response of wild type (MMP13$^{+/+}$) and MMP13-deficient (MMP13$^{-/-}$) mice in the endotoxemia model, i.e., i.p. injection of LPS, a model of human sepsis (Cantaluppi et al, 2008; Cruz et al, 2007, 2009). Early after endotoxemia induction, we observed strong up-regulation of MMP13 in all tested organs (Fig 1A–D). MMP13$^{-/-}$ mice were significantly protected against LPS-induced hypothermia (Fig 1E) and death (Fig 1F). We also subjected MMP13$^{+/+}$ and MMP13$^{-/-}$ mice to caecal ligation and puncture (CLP), the gold standard model for human sepsis (Dejager et al, 2011), and this revealed that MMP13$^{-/-}$ mice are also significantly protected against CLP-induced death (Fig 1G). Next, we studied the cyto- and chemokine levels in sera of LPS-injected mice. We observed substantial differences in the absolute concentrations, time courses and clearance of the tested cyto- and chemokines. Most inflammatory mediators reached their maximum around 6–12 h, with the exception of TNF, which reached a peak after 1 h, followed by a rapid decline (Fig 1H–K and Supporting Information Fig S1). We observed that 12 h after LPS injection, all cytokines (IL1β, IL6, IL10, IL12p40, IL12p70, IL17 and IFN-γ) and chemokines (G-CSF, GM-CSF, KC, MCP1 and Rantes) were lower in MMP13$^{-/-}$ mice than in MMP13$^{+/+}$ mice. Moreover, serum levels of IL1β (Fig 1G), TNF (Fig 1H), IL17 (Fig 1I) and MCP1 (Fig 1J) were lower even at the earlier time points after challenge in MMP13$^{-/-}$ mice. These results indicate that MMP13 plays a detrimental role in sepsis-induced systemic inflammation and lethality.

8.2.2 MMP13 DEFICIENCY PROTECTS MICE FROM LPS-INDUCED INTESTINAL PERMEABILITY, MUCUS DEPLETION AND ER STRESS

The "gut as motor of sepsis" hypothesis has been postulated based on the importance of the intestinal epithelium as a physical barrier between the intestinal lumen and the immune cells in the lamina propria (Carrico et al, 1986; Deitch & Berg, 1987). Indeed, in critically ill sepsis patients, intestinal permeability is correlated with bacterial translocation and subsequent multi-organ failure (Faries et al, 1998; Swank & Deitch, 1996).

We first addressed which cell type in the ileum is responsible for MMP13 expression. Immunostaining revealed MMP13 expression both in epithelial and inflammatory cells (Fig 2A). Four hours of LPS stimulation resulted in decreased MMP13 staining in the epithelial cells at the top of the villi, which suggests LPS-induced MMP13 secretion, while MMP13 expression in the inflammatory cells in the lamina propria increased further after LPS injection (Fig 2B). To exclude compensation by other MMPs in the ileum of MMP13$^{-/-}$ mice, we analysed MMP expression in ileum lysates. None of the tested MMPs were up-regulated, except MMP3 which displayed a two-fold down-regulation in MMP13$^{-/-}$ lysates when compared to MMP13$^{+/+}$ mice (Supporting Information Fig S2).

To study intestinal leakage in MMP13$^{+/+}$ and MMP13$^{-/-}$ mice after LPS challenge, fluorescently labeled FITC-dextran was administered orally

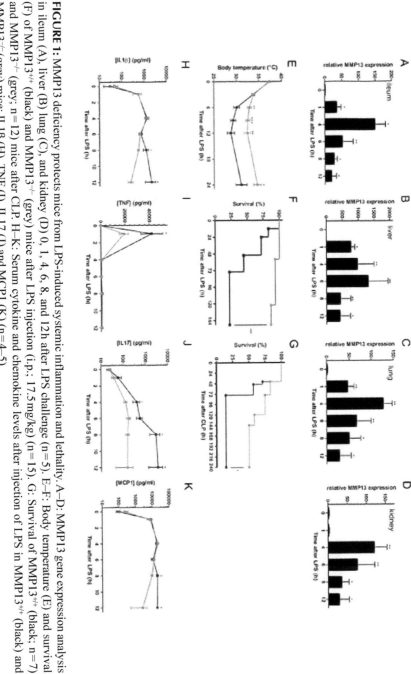

FIGURE 1: MMP13 deficiency protects mice from LPS-induced systemic inflammation and lethality. A–D: MMP13 gene expression analysis in ileum (A), liver (B) lung (C), and kidney (D) 0, 1, 4, 6, 8, and 12h after LPS challenge (n=5). E–F: Body temperature (E) and survival (F) of MMP13^{++} (black) and MMP13$^{-/-}$ (grey) mice after LPS injection (i.p.; 17.5 mg/kg) (n=15). G: Survival of MMP13^{++} (black; n=7) and MMP13$^{-/-}$ (grey; n=12) mice after CLP. H–K: Serum cytokine and chemokine levels after injection of LPS in MMP13^{++} (black) and MMP13$^{-/-}$ (grey) mice: IL1β (H), TNF (I), IL17 (J) and MCP1 (K) (n=4–5).

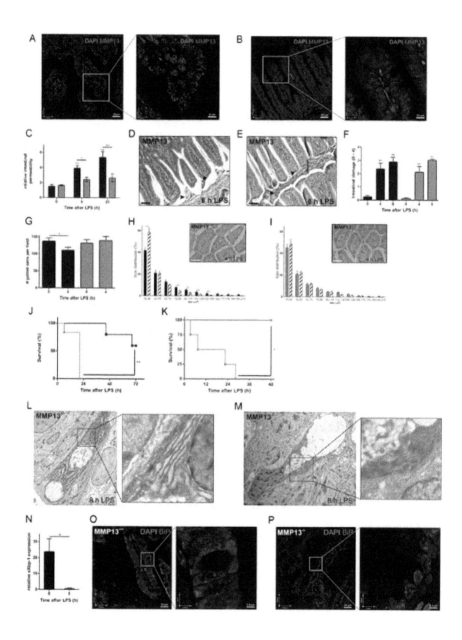

FIGURE 2: MMP13 deficiency protects mice from LPS-induced intestinal permeability, mucus depletion and ER stress. A,B: Representative confocal images of MMP13 (red) and DAPI (blue) immunostaining of unstimulated (A) and LPS-stimulated (B) (4 h) ileum sections. C: Intestinal permeability in MMP13$^{+/+}$ (black) and MMP13$^{-/-}$ (grey) mice 0, 8 and 20 h after LPS injection. Fluorescently labeled FITC-dextran was administered orally to the mice and 5 h later plasma was collected and fluorescence was measured. D,E: Representative hematoxylin and eosin stained sections of the ileum of MMP13$^{+/+}$ (D) and MMP13$^{-/-}$ (E) 8 h after LPS injection. Bar=50 μm. The presence of epithelial cells and cell debris in the lumen is indicated with an arrow. F: Quantification of intestinal tissue damage in MMP13$^{+/+}$ (black) and MMP13$^{-/-}$ (grey) mice: four neutral observers evaluated ileal sections stained with hematoxylin and eosin (n=5) in a blinded setup. LPS-induced intestinal damage is characterized by decreased villus height, disappearance of the mucus layer and goblet cells along the villus, cell death at the villus top, and cell debris in the lumen. G–I: Goblet cell amount (G) and size distribution (H-I) in MMP13$^{+/+}$ (black; H) and MMP13$^{-/-}$ (grey; I) mice 0 (blank) and 4 h (hatched) after LPS injection. The insert displays a representative image of Alcian blue stained ileal sections of MMP13$^{+/+}$ (H) and MMP13$^{-/-}$ (I) mice. Bar=50 μm. J: Survival of MMP13$^{+/+}$ mice (black) and MMP13$^{+/+}$ mice pretreated with the mucus depleting agent pilocarpine (grey) after LPS injection (i.p.; 6 mg/kg; LD50 in MMP13$^{+/+}$) (n=5). K: Survival of LPS-injected (i.p.; 17.5 mg/kg; LD0 in MMP13$^{-/-}$ mice) untreated (square; n=4) and pilocarpine treated (circle; n=3) MMP13$^{-/-}$ mice (grey). L,M: Representative morphological TEM images of MMP13$^{+/+}$ (L) and MMP13$^{-/-}$ (M) mice 8 h after LPS injection. The insert is a close-up of the ER. N: mRNA expression analysis of spliced Xbp-1 (sXbp-1) in ileum lysates of MMP13$^{+/+}$ (black) and MMP13$^{-/-}$ (grey) 8 h after LPS injection (n=5). O,P: Representative confocal images of BiP (red) and DAPI (blue) immunostaining of MMP13$^{+/+}$ (O) and MMP13$^{-/-}$ (P) ileum sections 8 h after LPS injection.

to the mice. We observed an increase of fluorescence in plasma of LPS-treated MMP13$^{+/+}$ mice, which is a measure of leakage from the intestinal lumen into the peripheral blood (Fig 2C). In contrast, MMP13$^{-/-}$ mice did not suffer from increased intestinal permeability. Despite the difference in intestinal permeability, morphological analysis revealed similar intestinal damage in MMP13$^{+/+}$ and MMP13$^{-/-}$ mice after LPS challenge (Fig 2D–F). Similarly, TUNEL staining showed equal levels of apoptosis induction in MMP13$^{+/+}$ and MMP13$^{-/-}$ mice (Supporting Information Fig S3). However, detailed analysis of the goblet cells by Alcian blue and MUC2 staining did reveal important differences both in the amount and size of Alcian blue positive goblet cells early after LPS challenge. Fig 2G shows that LPS reduces the amount of Alcian blue positive goblet cells in MMP13$^{+/+}$ mice, but not in MMP13$^{-/-}$ mice. Additionally, size distribution analysis shows that the percentage of goblet cells with reduced mucus content increases substantially in MMP13$^{+/+}$ mice 4 h after LPS challenge, whereas size distribution was unaffected in MMP13$^{-/-}$ mice (Fig 2H–I). Those observations were further confirmed by MUC2 immunostaining, both at 4 and 24 h (Supporting Information Fig S4). Treatment with pilocarpine, a mucus depleting agent (Albanese et al, 1994), sensitized both MMP13$^{+/+}$ (Fig 2J) and MMP13$^{-/-}$ (Fig 2K) mice to endotoxemia, pointing towards a crucial role of mucus in the protection against sepsis. More detailed analysis of goblet cell morphology by transmission electron microscopy (TEM) revealed that the ER of wild type goblet cells was dilated after LPS challenge (Fig 2L). This was not the case in MMP13$^{-/-}$ mice (Fig 2M). Additionally, two markers for ER stress, namely spliced Xbp1 (sXbp1) mRNA (Fig 2N) and BiP protein (Fig 2O–P) were higher in LPS-stimulated MMP13$^{+/+}$ compared to MMP13$^{-/-}$ mice. These results show that MMP13 deficiency protects from LPS-induced intestinal permeability, mucus depletion and goblet cell ER stress after systemic LPS injection.

8.2.3 MMP13 CONTRIBUTES TO TIGHT JUNCTION DESTABILIZATION

Intercellular junctions, such as tight junctions, play a crucial role in the formation and maintenance of the intestinal epithelial barrier. Consequently, intestinal permeability is often linked to tight junction malfunctioning (John et al, 2011). Several MMPs have been shown to cleave the components of tight junctions, thereby influencing their functionality. For example, it has been reported that hypoxia-induced MMP13 results in disorganization and fragmentation of the intracellular tight junction scaffolding protein ZO-1 (zona occludens), which results in hyperpermeablility of the blood–brain barrier (Lu et al, 2009). Western blot analysis of intestinal mucosal scrapings showed that LPS did not induce a decrease in the amount of full length ZO-1 protein (Fig 3A). Similar results were obtained for occludin (Fig 3B) and claudin-1 (Fig 3C). However, IEM analysis did reveal severe differences in the amount of immunogold-labeled ZO-1 located at the apical tight junctions: after LPS challenge, much more tight junction-localized ZO-1 could be detected in the IECs of MMP13$^{-/-}$ mice compared to MMP13$^{+/+}$ mice (Fig 3D–E). This observation was confirmed by immunofluorescent ZO-1 staining (Supporting Information Fig S5). Apparently, although total ZO-1 protein levels were equal in MMP13$^{+/+}$ and MMP13$^{-/-}$ mice, there was a profound difference in localization after LPS challenge.

Tight junctions are part of specialized lipid raft-like membrane microdomains (Nusrat et al, 2000). It was recently shown that sepsis causes redistribution of tight junctions in membrane microdomains and that this redistribution is responsible for increased permeability (Li et al, 2009). Mucosal scrapings from the ileum were homogenized and separated by ultracentrifugation. As shown in Fig 3F, after ultracentrifugation, the upper fractions contain the lipid rafts and the lower fractions the non-lipid rafts. Comparison of mucosal scrapings from the ilea of challenged MMP13$^{+/+}$ and MMP13$^{-/-}$ mice revealed that caveolin-1, an essential molecule in lipid raft microdomains, was present in different fractions. In LPS-treated MMP13$^{-/-}$ mice, caveolin-1 was in the lipid raft fraction, but it shifted almost completely to the non-lipid-raft fraction in the LPS-treated MMP13$^{+/+}$ mice (Fig 3G). This indicates that MMP13 deficiency protects from LPS-induced tight junction redistribution and therefrom resulting increased intestinal permeability.

8.2.4 MMP13 CLEAVES PROTNF, RESULTING IN THE FORMATION OF MATURE, BIOACTIVE TNF

Marchiando et al. recently showed that TNF induces caveolin-1-dependent endocytosis of tight junction proteins, which results in increased intestinal permeability (Marchiando et al, 2010). TNF is translated as a 26-kDa transmembrane precursor protein (tmTNF) that is proteolytically cleaved to release the soluble and biologically active 17-kDa C-terminal part (soluble TNF; sTNF). sTNF is known to induce a concentration- and time-dependent increase in epithelial permeability both in vitro and in vivo

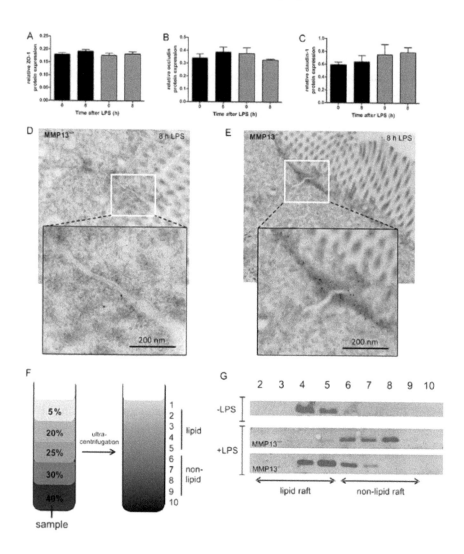

FIGURE 3: MMP13 contributes to tight junction destabilization. Source data is available for this figure in the Supporting Information. A–C: Western blot quantification of the protein expression levels of ZO-1 (A), occludin (B) and claudin (C) in mucosal scrapings of ilea from MMP13[+/+] (black) and MMP13[−/−] (grey) mice 0 and 8 h after LPS injection (n=3–4). D,E: Representative ZO-1 immunogold-labeled TEM images of MMP13[+/+] (D) and MMP13[−/−] (E) mice 8 h after LPS injection. F: Schematic overview of the separation of the lipid raft and non-lipid-raft fractions by ultracentrifugation. G: Caveolin-1 western blot analysis of fractions obtained after ultracentrifugation of mucosal scrapings from MMP13[+/+] and MMP13[−/−] mice 0 and 8 h after LPS challenge.

(Gitter et al, 2000; He et al, 2012; Ma et al, 2004, 2005; Marchiando et al, 2010; Schmitz et al, 1999). Although the major sheddase responsible for proTNF cleavage is TACE (tumour necrosis factor-α-converting enzyme; Adam17), Adam10 (Le Gall et al, 2009) and MMP-mediated shedding of TNF might also be important (Overall & Blobel, 2007). Several MMPs were shown to be able to cleave proTNF in vitro: MMP1, −2, −3, −7, −9, −12, −14 and −15 (Chandler et al, 1996; d'Ortho et al, 1997; Gearing et al, 1995; Tam et al, 2004).

To study whether MMP13 can cleave proTNF, the two proteins were co-incubated in vitro. As shown in Fig 4A and B, MMP13 can cleave proTNF in vitro to generate different N-terminal TNF fragments (~17, ~15, ~13 and ~11 kDa). Comparison of the TNF bioactivity revealed that 10 min co-incubation of proTNF with TACE or activated MMP13 (1:1 ratio) results in 218 and 227 U/mg bioactive TNF, respectively. By LC-MS/MS analysis, we could identify three different MMP13 cleavage sites, namely S68, A90 and A111 (Fig 4C). To determine if shedding of TNF is also dependent on MMP13 in vivo, we analysed TNF bioactivity in ileal lysates from MMP13$^{+/+}$ and MMP13$^{-/-}$ mice obtained 1 h after LPS challenge. Fig 4D shows that TNF bioactivity was significantly higher in ileum of MMP13$^{+/+}$ mice, which suggests that MMP13 can also cleave proTNF into soluble, bioactive TNF in vivo.

MMP13-dependent TNF cleavage was further confirmed both in vitro and ex vivo. Primary mouse macrophages from MMP13$^{+/+}$ mice were isolated by peritoneal lavage and stimulated in vitro with LPS in the absence or presence of MMP13 inhibitor. As shown in Fig 4E, MMP13 inhibition results in a decrease in TNF release into the supernatant. Similarly, ileum explants of LPS injected MMP13$^{+/+}$ mice were incubated ex vivo with different concentrations of MMP13 inhibitor. This resulted in a dose dependent decrease in TNF (Fig 4F).

If the LPS resistance of the MMP13$^{-/-}$ mice can be attributed to TNF, one would expect that MMP13$^{-/-}$ mice are as sensitive to systemic TNF injection as MMP13$^{+/+}$ mice. Indeed, no significant difference in response of MMP13$^{+/+}$ and MMP13$^{-/-}$ mice upon TNF injection could be detected (Fig 4G).

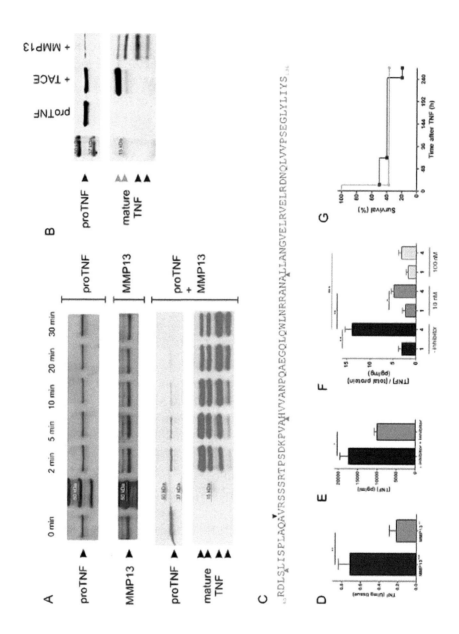

FIGURE 4: MMP13 cleaves proTNF to generate mature, bioactive TNF. Source data is available for this figure in the Supporting Information. A: Silver staining of proTNF (47 kDa) and MMP13 (52 kDa) samples incubated at 37°C for 0, 2, 5, 10, 20 and 30 min followed by SDS-PAGE. Anti-TNF western blot analysis of co-incubated proTNF (47 kDa) and MMP13 (52 kDa) samples at 37°C for 0, 2, 5, 10, 20 and 30 min with formation of mature TNF. B: Anti-TNF western blot analysis of proTNF (47 kDa), incubated at 37°C for 10 min with TACE and MMP13. Cleavage of proTNF by TACE results in two mature TNF fragments (~17 and ~15 kDa; grey). Cleavage of proTNF by MMP13 results in four cleavage fragments (~17, ~15, ~13 and ~11 kDa). C: Identified proTNF cleavage sites of MMP13 by LC-MS/MS (red arrow) and known TACE cleavage site (black arrow). D: TNF bioactivity of ileal lysates of MMP13$^{+/+}$ (black) and MMP13$^{-/-}$ (grey) mice 1 h after LPS injection (n=5). E: TNF levels of in vitro LPS-stimulated MMP13$^{+/+}$ macrophages incubated in the absence or presence of MMP13 inhibitor. F: TNF levels of ileum explants from in vivo LPS stimulated MMP13$^{+/+}$ mice incubated ex vivo with and without MMP13 inhibitor. G: Survival of MMP13$^{+/+}$ (black) and MMP13$^{-/-}$ (grey) mice injected with TNF (25 µg/20 g) (n=8).

8.2.5 MMP13-DEPENDENT INTESTINAL TNF ACTIVATION RESULTS IN MUCUS DEPLETION AND INCREASED INTESTINAL INFLAMMATION

TNF has been shown to induce mucus secretion (McElroy et al, 2011), so the depletion of mucus observed in MMP13$^{+/+}$ mice might be a direct effect of increased TNF levels. Indeed, incubation with TNF in vitro resulted in goblet cell Muc2 gene expression up-regulation (Fig 5A) and TNF injection in vivo resulted in a reduction of total goblet cell mucus (Fig 5B). The latter was confirmed by immunofluorescent staining of intestinal MUC2 before (Fig 5C) and after (Fig 5D) TNF injection. In the absence of a proper mucus layer, intestinal bacteria can interact with the underlying IECs (McGuckin et al, 2011). To address the importance of intestinal bacteria in LPS-induced shock, we first treated wild type mice with antibiotics to remove all bacteria from the gut. Next, we injected sterile and non-sterile MMP13$^{+/+}$ mice with LPS and analysed the effect on LPS lethality and IL-6 levels. Fig 5E shows that sterile mice were protected against the lethal effects of LPS. To address the importance of TNF in the endotoxemia model, we treated mice with Etanercept that acts as a TNF inhibitor (Kerensky et al, 2012). TNF inhibition resulted in protection of the mice in terms of survival rate (Fig 5F), intestinal permeability (Fig 5G) and amount of mucus containing goblet cells (Fig 5H and I). Additionally, mice deficient in the TNF receptor TNFR1, which is implicated in TNF-induced acute toxicity (Van Hauwermeiren et al, 2011), were protected against LPS-induced lethality (Supporting Information Fig S6).

The absence of mucus can lead to increased interaction of bacteria with the IECs (McGuckin et al, 2011). This, together with elevated TNF levels, could induce epithelial cell inflammation. Indeed, we observed more intestinal inflammation in MMP13$^{+/+}$ mice than in MMP13$^{-/-}$ mice. LPS injection resulted in strong up-regulation of IL-6 (Fig 5J) and iNOS (Fig 5K) in the ileum of MMP13$^{+/+}$ mice. This up-regulation was significantly lower in MMP13$^{-/-}$ mice. Moreover, we observed increased Paneth cell activation in MMP13$^{+/+}$ mice. This was reflected in increased MMP7 (Fig 5L) and RegIIIγ (Fig 5M) gene expression levels after LPS challenge in MMP13$^{+/+}$ mice, while no induction of Paneth-specific genes was observed in MMP13$^{-/-}$ mice.

8.2.6 MMP13-DEPENDENT INTESTINAL LEAKAGE RESULTS IN SYSTEMIC INFLAMMATION AND MULTI-ORGAN FAILURE

After LPS challenge, MMP13$^{+/+}$ mice, in contrast to MMP13$^{-/-}$ mice, displayed an increase in intestinal permeability (Fig 2C). This increased permeability can result in leakage of intestinal lumen components into the periphery. Indeed, serum analysis of LPS-injected mice showed high ileal fatty acid-binding protein (IL-FABP) levels in MMP13$^{+/+}$ mice (Fig 5N), a non-invasive marker for intestinal mucosal damage (Lieberman et al, 1997). IL-FABP levels were significantly lower in MMP13$^{-/-}$ mice. Leakage of intestinal content into the periphery can induce a further increase in systemic inflammation, which eventually results in multi-organ failure. Serum levels of lactate dehydrogenase (LDH), a marker for general tissue damage, were below detection limit in unchallenged mice (data not shown). However, LDH levels were higher in MMP13$^{+/+}$ than in MMP13$^{-/-}$ mice 8 h after LPS challenge (Fig 5O), which suggests multi-organ failure in MMP13$^{+/+}$, but not in MMP13$^{-/-}$ mice.

8.2.7 MMP13 DEFICIENCY RESULTS IN REDUCED SIGNS OF CLINICAL COLITIS AFTER DSS TREATMENT

Both TNF and MUC2 play a major role in the development of DSS-induced colitis via their involvement in epithelial barrier function, and they are altered before epithelial cell damage occurs (Dharmani et al, 2011). On the basis of our findings, we hypothesized that the absence of MMP13 could be protective in this colitis model. When MMP13$^{+/+}$ and MMP13$^{-/-}$ mice were given 2% DSS in the drinking water for 5 days, the knockout mice showed milder disease in terms of weight loss, stool consistency and rectal bleeding (Fig 6A). In agreement with this, we observed a significant increase in MMP13 gene expression after DSS treatment (Fig 6B). The DSS-induced model of colitis is associated with a significant decrease in colon length, and evaluation of colon length is believed to be the least variable parameter. Measurement of colon length in MMP13$^{+/+}$ and MMP13$^{-/-}$ mice 6 days after the start of DSS treatment revealed that MMP13 deficiency reduces the effect of DSS-induced colitis on the length of the colon (Fig 6C). Again, this was associated with reduced TNF bioactivity in colon lysate (Fig 6D).

8.3 DISCUSSION

The intestinal epithelium separates the intestinal lumen from the underlying lamina propria and thereby provides an important physical barrier against entry of luminal microbiota. Apical tight junctions are multifunctional structures that form a seal between adjacent epithelial cells and prevent paracellular diffusion of luminal material across the epithelium (Farquhar & Palade, 1963). Consequently, inflammation-induced disruption of tight junctions can contribute to leakage of luminal components into the periphery (John et al, 2011). Intestinal epithelial dysfunction is believed to be a common final pathway contributing to organ dysfunction and mortality in sepsis (Fink, 2003). In line with this, we observed a huge increase in intestinal permeability and IL-FABP serum levels, a marker for intestinal damage, in MMP13$^{+/+}$ mice after LPS challenge. This was associated with

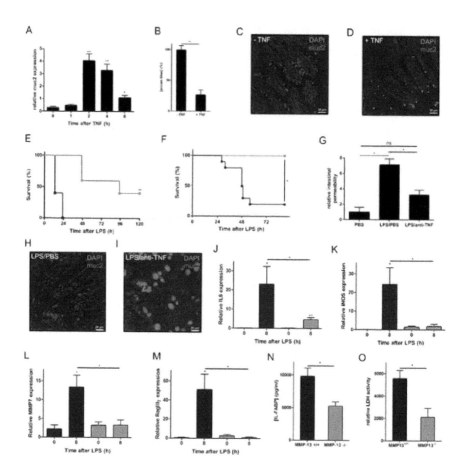

FIGURE 5: MMP13-dependent intestinal TNF activation results in mucus depletion, increased intestinal inflammation, systemic inflammation and organ damage. A: TNF (2000 U/ml) induces upregulation of Muc2 gene expression in goblet cells in vitro (n=6). B: Quantification of total goblet cell mucus before and 8h after TNF injection in vivo by Alcian blue staining of isolated ileum samples, followed by laxative treatment and absorbance measurement of the supernatant (n=8). C,D: Representative images of MUC2 (red) and DAPI (blue) immunostainings of ileal sections in the absence of TNF (C) and 8h after TNF injection (D). E: Survival curve of non-sterile (black) and sterile, antibiotics treated (grey) mice after LPS injection (i.v.; 250 µg/20 g) (n=12). F,G: Survival curve (F) and intestinal permeability (G) of LPS-injected MMP13$^{+/+}$ mice pretreated with PBS (black; n=10) or anti-TNF (grey; n=3) (i.p.; 17.5 mg/kg). H,I: Representative mucin-2 (red) confocal images of ileal sections of LPS-injected mice pretreated with PBS (H) and anti-TNF (I). J,K: Gene expression analysis of IL6 and iNOS in ileum lysates of MMP13$^{+/+}$

(black) and MMP13$^{-/-}$ (grey) mice 0 and 8 h after LPS injection (n=4–5). L,M: Gene expression analysis of the Paneth-cell-specific genes MMP7 (H) and RegIIIγ (I) in ileum lysates of MMP13$^{+/+}$ (black) and MMP13$^{-/-}$ (grey) mice 0 and 8 h after LPS injection (n=4–5). N: IL-FABP levels in serum of MMP13$^{+/+}$ (black) and MMP13$^{-/-}$ (grey) mice 8 h after LPS injection (n=5–7). O: Relative serum LDH activity 8 h after LPS injection in MMP13$^{+/+}$ (black) and MMP13$^{-/-}$ (grey) mice (n=6–14).

high serum levels of cytokines, chemokines and LDH, the latter being an indicator of general tissue damage. In contrast, LPS-injected MMP13$^{-/-}$ mice maintained a functional epithelial barrier and exhibited less severe systemic inflammation and organ damage. Eventually, this results in survival of the MMP13$^{-/-}$ mice, while almost all MMP13$^{+/+}$ mice succumbed. Similar protection was observed in the mouse model that is considered as the 'gold standard' for sepsis research, namely CLP (Dejager et al, 2011).

Both in vivo and in vitro studies have demonstrated that TNF is one of the crucial factors involved in the pathogenesis of intestinal permeability and that tight junction destabilization is implicated in this process (Gitter et al, 2000; He et al, 2012; Ma et al, 2004, 2005; Marchiando et al, 2010; Schmitz et al, 1999). ProTNF is a transmembrane protein that is cleaved into soluble, biological active TNF. Although TACE is the main sheddase involved in this process, it is likely that TACE and MMPs have complementary roles in the rapid shedding and activation of proTNF in response to different stimuli (Overall & Blobel, 2007). This idea is strengthened by the fact that TACE$^{-/-}$ cells still secrete 10–20% sTNF compared to TACE$^{+/+}$ cells (Killar et al, 1999). Noncleavable transmembrane TNF transgenic mice were fully protected from endotoxic shock, pointing towards the importance of TNF cleavage in the endotoxemia model (Mueller et al, 1999). Here, we clearly show that MMP13 can cleave and activate proTNF in vitro and we could identify three cleavage sites, one upstream and two downstream of the TACE cleavage site, resulting in similar bioactivity. However, substrate specificity of MMPs is partly regulated by their cellular localization, which makes it dangerous to directly interpret substrates identified in vitro as in vivo substrates. We detected MMP13 expression in epithelial and inflammatory cells in the ileum and confirmed via several approaches that TNF is a direct substrate of MMP13.

In vivo, bioactive, soluble TNF levels were higher in the inflamed tissue of MMP13$^{+/+}$ compared to MMP13$^{-/-}$ mice in LPS-induced shock. Moreover, LPS stimulation of both primary mouse macrophages and ileum explants incubated with MMP13 inhibitor resulted in reduced TNF levels. Additionally, MMP13$^{+/+}$ and MMP13$^{-/-}$ mice showed a similar response upon systemic TNF injection. The latter indicates that the resistance of the MMP13$^{-/-}$ mice to LPS challenge can at least partially be attributed to the MMP13-dependent cleavage of TNF. To exclude the involvement of other proteases that have been described to cleave and activate TNF, we measured Adam17 and -10 as well as MMP1, -2, -3, -7, -9, -12, -14 and -15 expression (Chandler et al, 1996; d'Ortho et al, 1997; Gearing et al, 1995; Tam et al, 2004). Only MMP7 was significant higher expressed in LPS-stimulated MMP13$^{+/+}$ mice compared to MMP13$^{-/-}$ mice. Consequently, it is possible that MMP7 contributes to the observed difference in TNF activation in MMP13$^{+/+}$ mice. However, the fact that MMP13 inhibition results in lower TNF levels, argues against this. Rather, this difference in MMP7 expression is likely a reflection of the increased Paneth cell activation, which is observed in the MMP13$^{+/+}$ mice, which is a consequence of the observed LPS-induced mucus loss.

It was recently shown that TNF can affect tight junctions via the induction caveolin-dependent endocytosis of tight junction proteins (Marchiando et al, 2010). In agreement with this, we observed that caveolin-1 translocated from the lipid raft to the non-lipid-raft fraction after LPS challenge in MMP13$^{+/+}$, but not in MMP13$^{-/-}$ mice. In addition, by IEM and immunofluorescence, we observed severe effects of LPS on the subcellular localization of ZO-1, which is crucial for clustering of claudins with the actin cytoskeleton, again only in the MMP13$^{+/+}$ mice. It is believed that ZO-1 forms a direct link between actin and the transmembrane tight junction proteins. Consequently, translocation of ZO-1 and thereby the associated contraction of cytoskeletal actin is thought to play an important role in the regulation of epithelial barrier function (Umeda et al, 2006). We did not observe LPS-dependent effects on the total protein level of different tight junction proteins, such as ZO-1, occludin and claudin-1, but it is known that it is mainly not the expression level but the expression pattern of tight junction proteins that determines epithelial permeability (Iwaya et al, 2012).

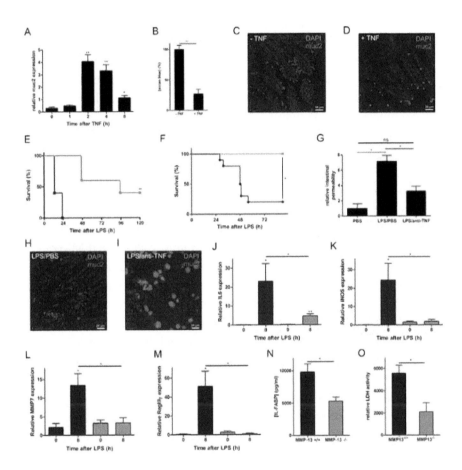

FIGURE 6: MMP13 deficiency results in reduced clinical signs of DSS-induced colitis. A: Clinical score of MMP13$^{+/+}$ (black) and MMP13$^{-/-}$ (grey) mice after 5 days of treatment with 2% DSS (n=12–14). Clinical scores are a composite of body weight loss, rectal bleeding and stool consistency scores. B: MMP13 gene expression before and 6 days after 2% DSS treatment. C: Colon length of MMP13$^{+/+}$ (black) and MMP13$^{-/-}$ (grey) mice on day 6 after the start of the DSS treatment (n=4). D: TNF bioactivity of colon lysates of MMP13$^{+/+}$ (black) and MMP13$^{-/-}$ (grey) mice 6 days after 2% DSS treatment (n=4; one-tailed t-test).

Not only the epithelial cell layer itself, but also the overlying mucus barrier, which consists of large glycoproteins called mucins, is extremely important for the intestinal barrier function. This is underlined by the observation that mice deficient in Muc2, the most abundant mucin in the small intestine, develop spontaneous intestinal inflammation (Van der Sluis et al, 2006). In vitro, we observed a TNF-dependent up-regulation of Muc2 gene expression in goblet cells, which is in agreement with literature where it was described that incubation of goblet cells with TNF induces mucin secretion within the first 24 h (Smirnova et al, 2001). Additionally, TNF injection in vivo resulted in a loss of goblet cells containing mucus, determined by quantification of total mucus and MUC2 immuno-fluorescence. This shows that TNF induces not only expression of mucus but also its secretion, finally resulting in the depletion of mucus. Indeed, we observed an LPS-induced decrease in mucus in MMP13$^{+/+}$ but not in MMP13$^{-/-}$ mice. The depletion of mucus by pilocarpine treatment resulted in sensitization for LPS-induced shock both in MMP13$^{+/+}$ and MMP13$^{-/-}$ mice, which further strengthens the notion of the important role of the mucus layer in endotoxemia. Recently, it was reported that spontaneous mucus depletion in *Winnie* and *Eeyore* mice, created by random mutagenesis of the Muc2 gene, was associated with ER stress (Heazlewood et al, 2008). In agreement with this, we observed, but only in MMP13$^{+/+}$ mice, LPS-induced evidence of ER stress in goblet cells (by TEM) and altered intestinal expression of spliced Xbp1 and BiP, both of which are involved in ER stress (Kaser et al, 2011). Disappearance of the mucus layer in MMP13$^{+/+}$ mice allows the intestinal bacteria to interact with IECs and Paneth cells, resulting in increased local inflammation and activation of Paneth cells. In LPS-injected MMP13$^{+/+}$ mice this was reflected in up-regulation of inflammatory genes, such as IL6 and iNOS, and Paneth-cell specific genes, such as RegIIIg and MMP7. RegIIIγ is an antibacterial agent present in the Paneth cells induced by the commensal microbes (Wlodarska & Finlay, 2010). The importance of the intestinal bacteria was further strengthened by the observation that sterile MMP13$^{+/+}$ mice were more resistant than non-sterile MMP13$^{+/+}$ mice to LPS-induced shock.

Both TNF and mucin might be selectively altered before epithelial cell damage in DSS-induced colitis (Dharmani et al, 2011), one of the most comprehensively tested models of colitis that mimics the clinical and histological features of human UC (Yan et al, 2009). The absence or inhibition of TNF activity ameliorates disease progression in different experimental IBD models and in human patients. Treatment with a TNF neutralizing antibody, a locally active TNF inhibitor, antisense oligonucleotides and siRNA molecules specific for TNF were shown to be effective in the DSS-induced colitis model (Dharmani et al, 2011; Murthy et al, 2002; Myers et al, 2003; Ocampo et al, 2012). As expected, we observed that MMP13$^{-/-}$ mice were less sensitive to DSS-induced colitis than MMP13$^{+/+}$ mice and that this was correlated with reduced bioactive TNF levels. However, the protection was moderate, especially since treatment with a TNF-neutralizing antibody markedly reduces the DSS-induced clinical score (Dharmani et al, 2011). This can be due to the fact that MMP13 is not the only important TNF sheddase in this model or because other processes are also involved. Indeed, the chemical DSS model is of great value for a better understanding of acute inflammatory disease processes in IBD, but during the recovery phase, also other processes such as wound healing play an important role. Wound healing is known to be delayed in MMP13$^{-/-}$ mice (Hartenstein et al, 2006). It has been suggested that altered sensitivity of genetically modified mice to DSS must be viewed in the context of epithelial cell injury and repair and should not be interpreted as a function of disrupted tight junction permeability alone (Brown & Mayer, 2007; Williams et al, 2001).

Although we do not exclude that also other MMP13 substrates play a role in the observed LPS resistance, we proved that the observed phenotype is highly dependent on TNF activity. Indeed, anti-TNF treatment of endotoxemic mice resulted in reduction of mortality, intestinal permeability and mucus containing goblet cell loss and TNFR1$^{-/-}$ mice were protected against LPS-induced lethality.

In conclusion (Fig 7), LPS-induced shock and DSS-induced colitis induce MMP13 up-regulation in the gut. This results in MMP13-mediated shedding of transmembrane-bound TNF and release of bioactive, soluble TNF. Subsequently, sTNF induces mucin expression and secretion by goblet cells, and eventually ER-stress, which results in mucus depletion and increased interaction of bacteria with IECs and Paneth cells. Additionally, TNF induces caveolin-dependent endocytosis, which destabilizes tight junctions. This causes loss of tight junction functionality and increased intestinal permeability. Consequent leakage of intestinal components increases systemic inflammation, which leads to organ damage and eventually to death.

Our results suggest that MMP13 is a potential therapeutic target for treatment of inflammatory disorders associated with TNF-dependent dysfunction of the intestinal barrier, such as sepsis and IBD. Unfortunately, the clinical use of pharmacologic MMP inhibitors has been hampered by their lack of specificity (Dorman et al, 2010). A major goal should be to identify compounds targeting MMP13 without interfering with other MMPs, not only for the previously suggested treatment of joint diseases (Takaishi et al, 2008), but as shown by our data also for the treatment of pathologies such as sepsis and IBD.

8.4 MATERIALS AND METHODS

8.4.1 ANIMALS

C57BL/6J MMP13$^{-/-}$ mice (Inada et al, 2004) were housed in an SPF animal facility with ad libitum access to food and water. We used both male and female mice (8–12 weeks old). All experiments were approved by the ethics committee of the Faculty of Science of Ghent University.

8.4.2 ENDOTOXEMIA MODEL AND TNF, PILOCARPINE AND ANTI-TNF INJECTIONS

Mice were injected intraperitoneally (i.p.) with LPS from *Salmonella enterica* serotype *abortus equi* (Sigma; LD100 in MMP13$^{+/+}$ mice: 17.5 mg/kg body weight) or with recombinant mouse TNF (LD100 in MMP13$^{+/+}$ mice: 1.25 mg/kg body weight) produced in *Escherichia coli* and endotoxin-free purified in our lab. In the experiments on antibiotic-treated mice, the mice were injected with 12.5 mg/kg LPS intravenously (i.v.) instead of i.p. to avoid injection into the swollen caecum. In the pilocarpine experiments, MMP13$^{+/+}$ mice were injected with 200 mg/kg pilocarpine 45 min prior to a sublethal LPS injection (i.p.; 6 mg/kg body weight). For MMP13$^{-/-}$ mice,

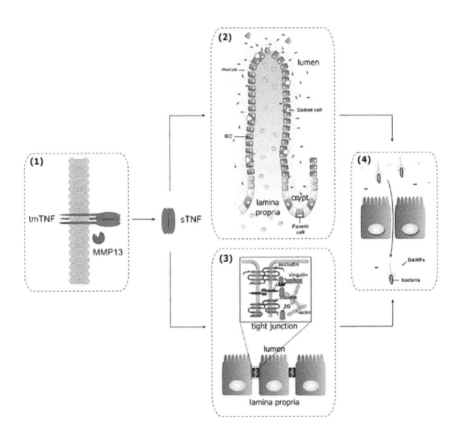

FIGURE 7: Effect of MMP13 on intestinal barrier dysfunction. LPS-induced shock and DSS-induced colitis result in MMP13 up-regulation in the gut. This leads to MMP13-mediated shedding of transmembrane-bound TNF and release of bioactive, soluble TNF (1). Subsequently, sTNF induces goblet cell mucin expression and secretion and eventually results in ER-stress, which leads to mucus depletion and increased interaction of bacteria with IECs and Paneth cells (2). Additionally, TNF induces caveolin-dependent endocytosis, resulting in destabilization of tight junctions. This is associated with loss of tight junction functionality and increased intestinal permeability (3). Consequent leakage of intestinal components increases systemic inflammation, which leads to organ damage and eventually to death (4).

17.5 mg/kg body weight LPS (i.p.) was used. Control animals received injections of PBS. Rectal bodytemperature was measured at different times after challenge. Mice were bled by heart puncture, and serum or EDTA plasma was prepared and stored at −20°C. Anti-TNF (etanercept; 400 μg) was administered to the mice 30 min prior to LPS injection.

8.4.3 DSS MODEL

Acute colitis was induced by addition of 2% DSS (dextran sulfate sodium; 36–50 kD; MP Biomedicals) to the drinking water for 5 days. Body weight, occult or gross blood lost per rectum, and stool consistency were determined daily. Faecal blood was determined using Hemoccult SENSA (Beckman Coulter) analysis. The baseline clinical score was determined on day 0. No weight loss was scored as 0, weight loss of 1–5% below baseline as 1, 5–10% as 2, 10–20% as 3, and >20% as 4. For bleeding, a score of 0 was assigned for no blood, 2 for positive Hemoccult, and 4 for gross bleeding. For stool consistency, a score of 0 was assigned for well-formed pellets, 2 for pasty stool, and 4 for liquid stool. These scores were combined and divided by three, resulting in a total clinical score ranging from 0 (healthy) to 4 (maximal colitis). To eliminate any diagnostic bias, mice were scored blindly. Postmortem, the entire colon was removed from caecum to anus, its length was measured as an indicator inflammation, and colon samples were taken for RNA isolation, protein analysis and for preparing PFA-fixed, paraffin-embedded sections.

8.4.4 MMP13 INHIBITOR EXPERIMENTS

Four days after 4 ml of 3% thioglycollate injection, macrophages were isolated by peritoneal lavage and two million cells were plated in six-well plates. Four hours later culture medium was refreshed and cells were stimulated with LPS (100 ng/ml) in the absence or presence of MMP13 inhibitor (1 nM; Calbiochem) and medium was collected after different time points. For the explant experiments, mice were injected with LPS

(17.5 mg/kg) and ileum was harvested 15 min later. Flushed ileum pieces of 1.5 cm were incubated ex vivo in the presence or absence of different concentrations MMP13 inhibitor (10 nM and 100 nM; Calbiochem).

8.4.5 CAECAL LIGATION AND PUNCTURE MODEL

Severe sepsis was induced in isoflurane anesthetized mice by ligation of the cecum, followed by twice puncturing with a 21-gauge needle as described earlier (Rittirsch et al, 2009). All animals received two doses of antibiotic therapy i.p. (ceftriaxone 25 mg/kg and metronidazole 12.5 mg/kg) at 9 and 24 h after CLP.

8.4.6 DEPLETION OF COMMENSAL INTESTINAL BACTERIA

For antibiotic-mediated depletion of commensal bacteria, the drinking water was supplemented with 200 mg/L ciprofloxacin (Sigma–Aldrich), 1 g/L ampicillin (Sigma–Aldrich), 1 g/L metronidazole (Sigma–Aldrich) and 500 mg/L vancomycin (Labconsult). After 2 weeks, the presence of colonic microflora was determined by culturing faecal samples in brain heart infusion (BD Biosciences) and in thioglycollate medium (Sigma–Aldrich).

8.4.7 REAL TIME QPCR

Organs were stored in RNALater (Ambion) and RNA was isolated by using the RNeasy Mini Kit (Qiagen). cDNA was synthesized by the iScript cDNA Synthesis Kit (BioRad). Real time PCR was performed on the Light Cycler 480 system (Roche) using the LightCycler 480 SYBR Green I Master (Roche). Expression levels were normalized to the expression of the two most stable housekeeping genes, which were determined for each organ using the geNorm Housekeeping Gene Selection Software (Vandesompele et al, 2002).

8.4.8 CYTOKINE/CHEMOKINE MEASUREMENTS

Quantification of cytokines and chemokines (in pg/ml) in serum was performed using the Bio-Plex cytokine assays (Bio-Rad), according to the manufacturer's instructions. TNF bioactivity (in U/mg tissue) was determined by using the L929 bioassay system.

8.4.9 INTESTINAL PERMEABILITY

FITC-labeled dextran (4 kDa, Sigma) was administered to mice by gavage at 150 mg/kg body weight. Five hours later, blood obtained by heart puncture was collected in EDTA-coated tubes (Sarstedt) and plasma was prepared. Leakage of FITC-labeled dextran into the circulation was determined by measurement of the plasma fluorescence ($\lambda ex/\lambda em = 488/520$ nm). Values were normalized to the lowest value.

8.4.10 HISTOPATHOLOGY OF SMALL INTESTINE

Tissues were fixed with 4% PFA, embedded in paraffin, sectioned at 4 µm, dewaxed and stained. After hematoxylin (Fluka) and eosin (Merck) staining, sections were mounted and the degree of damage was evaluated on entire organ sections by four neutral observers in a blinded fashion. Intestinal damage is characterized by decreased villus height, epithelial cell death at the villus top, and loss of mucus layer and goblet cells. Taking into account all histological features, a damage score ranging from 0 (normal) to 4 (abnormal) was given to each mouse. Alcian blue staining was performed by incubating the ileum sections for 30 min in 0.1% Alcian blue, followed by two washing steps and counterstaining with nuclear fast red for 5 min. Finally, sections were rehydrated and mounted. The amount and size distribution of Alcian blue positive goblet cells was measured automatically by using the Volocity software (Perkin–Elmer).

8.4.11 IMMUNOSTAINING

Tissues were fixed with 4% PFA, embedded in paraffin, sectioned at 4 μm, dewaxed and stained. For immunofluorescent labelling, sections were boiled in 10 mM sodium citrate buffer for antigen retrieval, incubated for 1 h in blocking buffer (10 mM Tris–HCl pH 7.4, 0.1 M $MgCl_2$, 0.5% Tween20, 1% BSA and 5% serum), and incubated overnight with anti-BiP (1/40; C50B12, Cell signaling) or anti-MUC2 antibody (1/200; sc-15334, Santa Cruz). After rinsing with TBS/0.1% Tween-20, sections were incubated with fluorescently labeled secondary antibody DAR555 (1/400; Invitrogen). After another washing step, sections were counterstained with DAPI and mounted. Fluorescent images were taken by a laser scanning confocal microscope (Leica TCS SP5).

8.4.12 TRANSMISSION ELECTRON MICROSCOPY (TEM)

The excised ileum was fixed in a solution of glutaraldehyde and formaldehyde (0.3%/2.5% for morphological EM analysis and 2.5%/4% immune-EM (IEM)) dissolved in 0.1 M sodium cacodylate buffer containing 20 mg/100 ml $CaCl^2$. Fixed specimens were dehydrated through a graded ethanol series and embedded in Spurr's resin for morphological EM analysis or in LR White's resin for IEM. Ultrathin sections of a gold interference colour were cut using an ultramicrotome (Leica EM UC6) and sections were collected on formvar-coated copper slot grids. For IEM, grids were incubated with blocking solution (5% BSA, 1% FSG in PBS) for 20 min, followed by thorough washing with PBS/1% BSA. Next, sections were incubated for 2 h with anti-ZO-1 (1/5; 617300, Life Technologies) diluted in PBS/1% BSA. After another washing step, grids were incubated for 30 min with protein A-10-nm gold (PAG10nm; Cell Biology Department, Utrecht University) and with PBS/0.1% BSA, PBS, and double-distilled water. Control experiments consisted of treating sections with PAG10nm alone. Finally, sections were post-stained with uranyl acetate for 40 min and lead citrate for 7 min in a Leica EM AC20 and viewed with a transmission electron microscope (JEOL 1010; JEOL, Tokyo, Japan).

8.4.13 TIGHT JUNCTION PROTEIN ANALYSIS

The excised ileum was washed with ice-cold PBS, cut open longitudinally, and mucosal samples were obtained by scraping to enrich for villi. Mucosal scrapings were homogenized in lysis buffer (50 mM Tris, 25 mM KCl, 5 mM $MgCl_2.6H_2O$, 2 mM EDTA, 40 mM NaF, 4 mM Na_3VO_4, pH 7.4) containing 1% Triton X-100 and a protease inhibitor mixture solution. For total protein analysis, samples were centrifuged for 15 min at maximal speed and supernatant was collected. Tight junction membrane microdomains were isolated according to a previously described method (Li et al, 2008). The homogenized samples were mixed with an equal volume of 80% sucrose in lysis buffer and loaded at the bottom of an ultracentrifuge tube. A discontinuous sucrose gradient was layered on top of the sample by layering 30, 25, 20 and 5% sucrose (2 ml each). The gradients were ultracentrifuged (250,000 g, 18 h at 4°C) in a Ti90 rotor in an Optima L-80XP ultracentrifuge (Beckman). Ten 1-ml fractions were collected from the top of each tube. Protein concentration was determined by BCA assay (Pierce) and samples were analysed by Western blot analysis. Blots were incubated overnight with anti-actin (1/10,000; 691002, MP Biomedicals), anti-claudin-1 (1/5000; 519000, Life Technologies), anti-occludin (1/250; 422400, Life Technologies), anti-ZO-1 (1/1000; 617300, Life Technologies) or anti-caveolin (1/500; ab2910, AbCam) antibody overnight at 4°C, followed by 1 h incubation with IRDye antibody (1/10,000; Westburg) at room temperature. Immunoreactive proteins were visualized and quantified using the Odyssey™ Infrared Imaging System and Odyssey software as described by the manufacturer (Li-Cor).

8.4.14 CELL CULTURE

HT29-MTX goblet cells were a kind gift from Dr. Thécla Lesuffleur (INSERM UMR S 938, Paris, France) (Lesuffleur et al, 1993) and were grown in DMEM supplemented with 25 mM glucose and 10% FBS. Cells were seeded in six-well plates and 21 days later, 2000 U/ml recombinant human TNF was added and samples were collected at different times, followed by RNA isolation. Recombinant human TNF was produced in *E. coli* and endotoxin-free purified.

8.4.15 QUANTIFICATION OF TOTAL GOBLET CELL MUCUS

(Kitagawa et al, 1986). The excised ileum was soaked for 2 h in 2 ml of 0.1% Alcian blue, dissolved in 0.16 M sucrose buffered with 0.05 M sodium acetate (pH 5.8). Uncomplexed dye was removed by two successive washes in 2 ml of 0.25 M sucrose for 15 and 45 min. Next, the mucus-complexed dye was extracted by treatment with laxative (30% disodium octyl sulfosuccinate) for 2 h. After centrifugation (3000 rpm for 10 min), the optical density of the extracted solution was read at 620 nm and the concentration of the extracted Alcian blue was calculated in comparison with a calibration curve obtained from known concentrations of Alcian blue solutions.

8.4.16 IL-FABP ELISA

Concentrations of ileal fatty acid binding protein in plasma were determined by a standard enzyme-linked immunosorbent assay (ELISA) for mouse IL-FABP according to manufacturer's instructions (Hycult Biotechnology).

8.4.17 LDH ACTIVITY

LDH activity in plasma was measured by the CytoTox 96 Assay (Promega), according the manufacturer's instructions.

8.4.18 PROTNF CLEAVAGE ASSAY

Recombinant MMP13 (511-MM-010, R&D) was diluted to 100 μg/ml in assay buffer (50 mM Tris, 10 mM $CaCl_2$, 150 mM NaCl, 0.05% Brij-35, pH 7.5) and activated by incubation for 2 h at 37°C in the presence of 1 mM APMA. Recombinant proTNF fusion protein (1012-PS-010, R&D systems) was diluted in 50 mM Tris pH 8 at a concentration of 200 μg/ml. ProTNF was incubated with activated MMP13 at 37°C in a 1:1 ratio (w:w) and samples were taken at different times points. Reaction was stopped by addition of loading buffer followed by snap freezing. As a control for self-cleavage, proTNF and activated MMP13 samples were treated similarly, but without co-incubation. Equal amounts of sample were loaded on a 15% SDS–PAGE. Control samples (proTNF and MMP13 alone) were visualized by silver staining. Samples of co-incubated proTNF and MMP13 were analysed by western blot. Blots were incubated overnight with anti-TNF antibody (1/1000; SAB4502982, Sigma–Aldrich) followed by 1 h incubation with IRDye 800CW goat anti-rabbit IgG antibody (1/10,000) at room temperature. Immunoreactive proteins were visualized using the Odyssey™ Infrared Imaging System and Odyssey software as described by the manufacturer (Li-Cor).

8.4.19 IN-GEL STABLE-ISOTOPE LABELLING AND LC-MS/MS ANALYSIS

(Asara et al, 2006). The gel bands containing full length and possible TNF fragments upon cleavage by MMP13 were excised from the coommassie-stained SDS–PAGE and washed consecutively with water (Milli-Q purified, Millipore), water/acetonitrile (1/1, with acetonitrile HPLC grad; Biosolve) and acetonitrile, each for 15 min. After these washing steps, the gel bands were vacuum dried. Each gel band was then re-swollen in 1 mg NHS-trideutero-acetate (synthesized in-house according to (Staes et al, 2011)) dissolved in 100 μl 50 mM triethylammonium bicarbonate (Sigma–Aldrich) pH 8. Trideutero-acetylation of primary amines, i.e., ε-amines of lysines and α-amines of free (neo)N-termini, was allowed for 1 h at 30°C, followed by washing the gel bands again with water followed by acetonitrile, each for 15 min and vacuum dried. These trideutero-acetylation and washing steps were once repeated in order to reach maximal trideutero-acetylation. Subsequent washing the gel bands with 50 mM ammonium bicarbonate (Sigma–Aldrich) quenches any remaining NHS-ester, after which the gel bands were vacuum dried. Hydroxylamine (2 μl, 50 wt%; Sigma–Aldrich) in 100 μl 50 mM ammonium bicarbonate was added to each gel band for 20 min at 30°C in order to reverse possible O-trideutero-acetylation of Ser, Thr and Tyr. Samples were washed consecutively for

15 min with 50 mM ammonium bicarbonate and acetonitrile and vacuum dried. Each gel band was re-swollen with 10 μl 50 ng sequence grade trypsin (Promega Corporation). Gel bands were completely immersed in 50 mM ammonium bicarbonate and trypsin digestion was allowed overnight at 37°C. Two microliters of 100% formic acid was added to deactivate trypsin, the peptide mixtures were vacuum dried and re-dissolved in 20 μl of 0.1% trifluoroacetic acid (Biosolve) in 2% acetonitrile.

The peptide mixtures were then introduced into an LC-MS/MS system, the Ultimate 3000 RSLC nano (Dionex) in-line connected to an LTQ Orbitrap Velos (Thermo Fisher Scientific) for peptide identification. Sample mixture (2.5 μl) was loaded on a trapping column (made in-house, 100 μm internal diameter (I.D.) × 20 mm length, 5 μm C18 Reprosil-HD beads; Dr. Maisch). After flushing from the trapping column, the sample was loaded on a reverse-phase column (made in-house, 75 μm ID × 150 mm, 5 μm C18 Reprosil-HD beads; Dr. Maisch). Peptides were separated with a 30 min linear gradient from 2% solvent A (0.1% formic acid) to 50% solvent B (0.1% formic acid in 80% acetonitrile) at a flow rate of 300 nl/min followed by a wash with solvent B.

The mass spectrometer was operated in data-dependent mode, automatically switching between MS and MS/MS acquisition for the 10 most abundant peaks in a MS spectrum. Full scan MS spectra were acquired in the Orbitrap at a target value of 1E6 with a resolution of 60,000. The 10 most intense ions were isolated for fragmentation in the linear ion trap, with a dynamic exclusion of 20 s and fragmented after filling the ion trap at a target value of 1E4 ion counts. From the MS/MS data in each LC run, Mascot Generic Files were created using the Distiller software (version 2.4.2.0, Matrix Science, www.matrixscience.com/Distiller). These peak lists were then searched with the Mascot search engine (Matrix Science) using the Mascot Daemon interface (version 2.3, Matrix Science). Spectra were searched against the Swiss-Prot database (version 2012_05 of the UniProtKB/Swiss-Prot protein database) restricted to human proteins concatenated with the TNFα part of the fusion protein. Variable modifications were set to methionine oxidation, pyro-glutamate formation of N-terminal glutamine, S-propionamide formation of cysteines, acetylation of the peptide N-terminus and tri-deuteroacetylation of the peptide N-terminus. Fixed modifications were set to tri-deuteroacetylation on lysine. Mass tolerance on peptide ions was set to 10 ppm (with Mascot's C13 option set to 1), and to 0.5 Da for peptide fragment ions. The peptide charge was set to 1+, 2+, 3+ and instrument setting was put on ESI-TRAP. Enzyme was set to semi-ArgC/P, allowing for 1 missed cleavage, and cleavage was also allowed when arginine is followed by proline. Only peptides that were ranked one and scored above the threshold score, set at 99% confidence, were withheld. All further data management was done by ms_lims (Helsens et al, 2010).

8.4.20 STATISTICAL ANALYSIS

Data are presented as means $\pm$ SEM. Data were analysed with an unpaired Mann–Whitney U-test, unless mentioned differently. Survival curves were compared using a log-rank test. Significances were calculated for differences from the corresponding 0 h time point and/or between MMP13$^{+/+}$ and MMP13$^{-/-}$ mice, as indicated (*, $0.01 \leq p < 0.05$; **, $0.001 \leq p < 0.01$; ***, $p < 0.001$).

REFERENCES

1.   Ailenberg M, Sefton MV (2009) Effect of a matrix metalloproteinase sequestering biomaterial on Caco-2 epithelial cell barrier integrity in vitro. Acta Biomater 5: 1898-1904
2.   Albanese CT, Cardona M, Smith SD, Watkins S, Kurkchubasche AG, Ulman I, Simmons RL, Rowe MI (1994) Role of intestinal mucus in transepithelial passage of bacteria across the intact ileum in vitro. Surgery 116: 76-82
3.   Asara JM, Zhang X, Zheng B, Christofk HH, Wu N, Cantley LC (2006) In-gel stable-isotope labeling (ISIL): a strategy for mass spectrometry-based relative quantification. J Proteome Res 5: 155-163
4.   Balzan S, de Almeida Quadros C, de Cleva R, Zilberstein B, Cecconello I (2007) Bacterial translocation: overview of mechanisms and clinical impact. J Gastroenterol Hepatol 22: 464-471
5.   Brown SJ, Mayer L (2007) The immune response in inflammatory bowel disease. Am J Gastroenterol 102: 2058-2069
6.   Burrage PS, Mix KS, Brinckerhoff CE (2006) Matrix metalloproteinases: role in arthritis. Front Biosci 11: 529-543

7. Cantaluppi V, Assenzio B, Pasero D, Romanazzi GM, Pacitti A, Lanfranco G, Puntorieri V, Martin EL, Mascia L, Monti G, et al (2008) Polymyxin-B hemoperfusion inactivates circulating proapoptotic factors. Intensive Care Med 34: 1638-1645

8. Carrico CJ, Meakins JL, Marshall JC, Fry D, Maier RV (1986) Multiple-organ-failure syndrome. Arch Surg 121: 196-208

9. Cauwe B, Opdenakker G (2010) Intracellular substrate cleavage: a novel dimension in the biochemistry, biology and pathology of matrix metalloproteinases. Crit Rev Biochem Mol Biol 45: 351-423

10. Cauwe B, Van den Steen PE, Opdenakker G (2007) The biochemical, biological, and pathological kaleidoscope of cell surface substrates processed by matrix metalloproteinases. Crit Rev Biochem Mol Biol 42: 113-185

11. Chandler S, Cossins J, Lury J, Wells G (1996) Macrophage metalloelastase degrades matrix and myelin proteins and processes a tumour necrosis factor-alpha fusion protein. Biochem Biophys Res Commun 228: 421-429

12. Cruz DN, Perazella MA, Bellomo R, de Cal M, Polanco N, Corradi V, Lentini P, Nalesso F, Ueno T, Ranieri VM, et al (2007) Effectiveness of polymyxin B-immobilized fiber column in sepsis: a systematic review. Crit Care 11: R47

13. Cruz DN, Antonelli M, Fumagalli R, Foltran F, Brienza N, Donati A, Malcangi V, Petrini F, Volta G, Bobbio Pallavicini FM, et al (2009) Early use of polymyxin B hemoperfusion in abdominal septic shock: the EUPHAS randomized controlled trial. JAMA 301: 2445-2452

14. de Aquino SG, Guimaraes MR, Stach-Machado DR, da Silva JA, Spolidorio LC, Rossa C Jr (2009) Differential regulation of MMP-13 expression in two models of experimentally induced periodontal disease in rats. Arch Oral Biol 54: 609-617

15. Decock J, Thirkettle S, Wagstaff L, Edwards DR (2011) Matrix metalloproteinases: protective roles in cancer. J Cell Mol Med 15: 1254-1265

16. Deitch EA, Berg R (1987) Bacterial translocation from the gut: a mechanism of infection. J Burn Care Rehabil 8: 475-482

17. Dejager L, Pinheiro I, Dejonckheere E, Libert C (2011) Cecal ligation and puncture: the gold standard model for polymicrobial sepsis? Trends Microbiol 19: 198-208

18. Dejonckheere E, Vandenbroucke RE, Libert C (2011) Matrix metalloproteinase8 has a central role in inflammatory disorders and cancer progression. Cytokine Growth Factor Rev 22: 73-81

19. Dharmani P, Leung P, Chadee K (2011) Tumor necrosis factor-alpha and Muc2 mucin play major roles in disease onset and progression in dextran sodium sulphate-induced colitis. PLoS ONE 6: e25058

20. Dorman G, Cseh S, Hajdu I, Barna L, Konya D, Kupai K, Kovacs L, Ferdinandy P (2010) Matrix metalloproteinase inhibitors: a critical appraisal of design principles and proposed therapeutic utility. Drugs 70: 949-964

21. d'Ortho MP, Will H, Atkinson S, Butler G, Messent A, Gavrilovic J, Smith B, Timpl R, Zardi L, Murphy G (1997) Membrane-type matrix metalloproteinases 1 and 2 exhibit broad-spectrum proteolytic capacities comparable to many matrix metalloproteinases. Eur J Biochem 250: 751-757

22. Faries PL, Simon RJ, Martella AT, Lee MJ, Machiedo GW (1998) Intestinal permeability correlates with severity of injury in trauma patients. J Trauma 44: 1031-1035 (discussion 1035–1036)

23. Farquhar MG, Palade GE (1963) Junctional complexes in various epithelia. J Cell Biol 17: 375-412

24. Fink MP (2003) Intestinal epithelial hyperpermeability: update on the pathogenesis of gut mucosal barrier dysfunction in critical illness. Curr Opin Crit Care 9: 143-151

25. Fukuda H, Mochizuki S, Abe H, Okano HJ, Hara-Miyauchi C, Okano H, Yamaguchi N, Nakayama M, D'Armiento J, Okada Y (2011) Host-derived MMP-13 exhibits a protective role in lung metastasis of melanoma cells by local endostatin production. Br J Cancer 105: 1615-1624

26. Gearing AJ, Beckett P, Christodoulou M, Churchill M, Clements JM, Crimmin M, Davidson AH, Drummond AH, Galloway WA, Gilbert R, et al (1995) Matrix metal-loproteinases and processing of pro-TNF-alpha. J Leukoc Biol 57: 774-777

27. Gitter AH, Bendfeldt K, Schmitz H, Schulzke JD, Bentzel CJ, Fromm M (2000) Epithelial barrier defects in HT-29/B6 colonic cell monolayers induced by tumor necrosis factor-alpha. Ann N Y Acad Sci 915: 193-203

28. Hartenstein B, Dittrich BT, Stickens D, Heyer B, Vu TH, Teurich S, Schorpp-Kistner M, Werb Z, Angel P (2006) Epidermal development and wound healing in matrix metalloproteinase 13-deficient mice. J Invest Dermatol 126: 486-496

29. He F, Peng J, Deng XL, Yang LF, Camara AD, Omran A, Wang GL, Wu LW, Zhang CL, Yin F (2012) Mechanisms of tumor necrosis factor-alpha-induced leaks in intes-tine epithelial barrier. Cytokine 59: 264-272

30. Heazlewood CK, Cook MC, Eri R, Price GR, Tauro SB, Taupin D, Thornton DJ, Png CW, Crockford TL, Cornall RJ, et al (2008) Aberrant mucin assembly in mice causes endoplasmic reticulum stress and spontaneous inflammation resembling ulcerative colitis. PLoS Med 5: e54

31. Helsens K, Colaert N, Barsnes H, Muth T, Flikka K, Staes A, Timmerman E, Wor-telkamp S, Sickmann A, Vandekerckhove J, et al (2010) ms_lims, a simple yet pow-erful open source laboratory information management system for MS-driven pro-teomics. Proteomics 10: 1261-1264

32. Huet E, Vallee B, Delbe J, Mourah S, Pruliere-Escabasse V, Tremouilleres M, Kado-matsu K, Doan S, Baudouin C, Menashi S, et al (2011) EMMPRIN modulates epi-thelial barrier function through a MMP-mediated occludin cleavage: implications in dry eye disease. Am J Pathol 179: 1278-1286

33. Inada M, Wang Y, Byrne MH, Rahman MU, Miyaura C, Lopez-Otin C, Krane SM (2004) Critical roles for collagenase-3 (Mmp13) in development of growth plate car-tilage and in endochondral ossification. Proc Natl Acad Sci USA 101: 17192-17197

34. Iwaya H, Maeta K, Hara H, Ishizuka S (2012) Mucosal permeability is an intrinsic factor in susceptibility to dextran sulfate sodium-induced colitis in rats. Exp Biol Med (Maywood) 237: 451-460

35. John LJ, Fromm M, Schulzke JD (2011) Epithelial barriers in intestinal inflamma-tion. Antioxid Redox Signal 15: 1255-1270

36. Kaser A, Flak MB, Tomczak MF, Blumberg RS (2011) The unfolded protein re-sponse and its role in intestinal homeostasis and inflammation. Exp Cell Res 317: 2772-2779

37. Kerensky TA, Gottlieb AB, Yaniv S, Au SC (2012) Etanercept: efficacy and safety for approved indications. Expert Opin Drug Safety 11: 121-139

38. Killar L, White J, Black R, Peschon J (1999) Adamalysins. A family of metzincins including TNF-alpha converting enzyme (TACE). Ann N Y Acad Sci 878: 442-452

39. Kitagawa H, Takeda F, Kohei H (1986) A simple method for estimation of gastric mucus and effects of antiulcerogenic agents on the decrease in mucus during water-immersion stress in rats. Arzneimittelforschung 36: 1240-1244

40. Le Gall SM, Bobe P, Reiss K, Horiuchi K, Niu XD, Lundell D, Gibb DR, Conrad D, Saftig P, Blobel CP (2009) ADAMs 10 and 17 represent differentially regulated components of a general shedding machinery for membrane proteins such as transforming growth factor alpha, L-selectin, and tumor necrosis factor alpha. Mol Biol Cell 20: 1785-1794

41. Lesuffleur T, Porchet N, Aubert JP, Swallow D, Gum JR, Kim YS, Real FX, Zweibaum A (1993) Differential expression of the human mucin genes MUC1 to MUC5 in relation to growth and differentiation of different mucus-secreting HT-29 cell subpopulations. J Cell Sci 106: 771-783

42. Li Q, Zhang Q, Zhang M, Wang C, Zhu Z, Li N, Li J (2008) Effect of n-3 polyunsaturated fatty acids on membrane microdomain localization of tight junction proteins in experimental colitis. FEBS J 275: 411-420

43. Li Q, Zhang Q, Wang C, Liu X, Li N, Li J (2009) Disruption of tight junctions during polymicrobial sepsis in vivo. J Pathol 218: 210-221

44. Lieberman JM, Sacchettini J, Marks C, Marks WH (1997) Human intestinal fatty acid binding protein: report of an assay with studies in normal volunteers and intestinal ischemia. Surgery 121: 335-342

45. Lu DY, Yu WH, Yeh WL, Tang CH, Leung YM, Wong KL, Chen YF, Lai CH, Fu WM (2009) Hypoxia-induced matrix metalloproteinase-13 expression in astrocytes enhances permeability of brain endothelial cells. J Cell Physiol 220: 163-173

46. Ma TY, Iwamoto GK, Hoa NT, Akotia V, Pedram A, Boivin MA, Said HM (2004) TNF-alpha-induced increase in intestinal epithelial tight junction permeability requires NF-kappa B activation. Am J Physiol Gastrointest Liver Physiol 286: G367-G376

47. Ma TY, Boivin MA, Ye D, Pedram A, Said HM (2005) Mechanism of TNF-{alpha} modulation of Caco-2 intestinal epithelial tight junction barrier: role of myosin light-chain kinase protein expression. Am J Physiol Gastrointest Liver Physiol 288: G422-G430

48. Marchiando AM, Shen L, Graham WV, Weber CR, Schwarz BT, Austin JR II, Raleigh DR, Guan Y, Watson AJ, Montrose MH, et al (2010) Caveolin-1-dependent occludin endocytosis is required for TNF-induced tight junction regulation in vivo. J Cell Biol 189: 111-126

49. McElroy SJ, Prince LS, Weitkamp JH, Reese J, Slaughter JC, Polk DB (2011) Tumor necrosis factor receptor 1-dependent depletion of mucus in immature small intestine: a potential role in neonatal necrotizing enterocolitis. Am J Physiol Gastrointest Liver Physiol 301: G656-G666

50. McGuckin MA, Linden SK, Sutton P, Florin TH (2011) Mucin dynamics and enteric pathogens. Nat Rev Microbiol 9: 265-278

51. Mueller C, Corazza N, Trachsel-Loseth S, Eugster HP, Buhler-Jungo M, Brunner T, Imboden MA (1999) Noncleavable transmembrane mouse tumor necrosis factor-

alpha (TNFalpha) mediates effects distinct from those of wild-type TNFalpha in vitro and in vivo. J Biol Chem 274: 38112-38118

52. Murthy S, Flanigan A, Coppola D, Buelow R (2002) RDP58, a locally active TNF inhibitor, is effective in the dextran sulphate mouse model of chronic colitis. Inflamm Res 51: 522-531

53. Myers KJ, Murthy S, Flanigan A, Witchell DR, Butler M, Murray S, Siwkowski A, Goodfellow D, Madsen K, Baker B (2003) Antisense oligonucleotide blockade of tumor necrosis factor-alpha in two murine models of colitis. J Pharmacol Exp Ther 304: 411-424

54. Niessen CM (2007) Tight junctions/adherens junctions: basic structure and function. J Invest Dermatol 127: 2525-2532

55. Nusrat A, Parkos CA, Verkade P, Foley CS, Liang TW, Innis-Whitehouse W, Eastburn KK, Madara JL (2000) Tight junctions are membrane microdomains. J Cell Sci 113: 1771-1781

56. Ocampo SM, Romero C, Avino A, Burgueno J, Gassull MA, Bermudez J, Eritja R, Fernandez E, Perales JC (2012) Functionally enhanced siRNA targeting TNFalpha attenuates DSS-induced colitis and TLR-mediated immunostimulation in mice. Mol Ther 20: 382-390

57. Overall CM, Blobel CP (2007) In search of partners: linking extracellular proteases to substrates. Nat Rev Mol Cell Biol 8: 245-257

58. Overall CM, Lopez-Otin C (2002) Strategies for MMP inhibition in cancer: innovations for the post-trial era. Nat Rev Cancer 2: 657-672

59. Rath T, Roderfeld M, Graf J, Wagner S, Vehr AK, Dietrich C, Geier A, Roeb E (2006) Enhanced expression of MMP-7 and MMP-13 in inflammatory bowel disease: a precancerous potential? Inflamm Bowel Dis 12: 1025-1035

60. Rath T, Roderfeld M, Halwe JM, Tschuschner A, Roeb E, Graf J (2010) Cellular sources of MMP-7, MMP-13 and MMP-28 in ulcerative colitis. Scand J Gastroenterol 45: 1186-1196

61. Rittirsch D, Huber-Lang MS, Flierl MA, Ward PA (2009) Immunodesign of experimental sepsis by cecal ligation and puncture. Nat Protoc 4: 31-36

62. Schmitz H, Fromm M, Bentzel CJ, Scholz P, Detjen K, Mankertz J, Bode H, Epple HJ, Riecken EO, Schulzke JD (1999) Tumor necrosis factor-alpha (TNFalpha) regulates the epithelial barrier in the human intestinal cell line HT-29/B6. J Cell Sci 112: 137-146

63. Shukla A, Barrett TF, Nakayama KI, Nakayama K, Mossman BT, Lounsbury KM (2006) Transcriptional up-regulation of MMP12 and MMP13 by asbestos occurs via a PKCdelta-dependent pathway in murine lung. FASEB J 20: 997-999

64. Smirnova MG, Kiselev SL, Birchall JP, Pearson JP (2001) Up-regulation of mucin secretion in HT29-MTX cells by the pro-inflammatory cytokines tumor necrosis factor-alpha and interleukin-6. Eur Cytokine Netw 12: 119-125

65. Staes A, Impens F, Van Damme P, Ruttens B, Goethals M, Demol H, Timmerman E, Vandekerckhove J, Gevaert K (2011) Selecting protein N-terminal peptides by combined fractional diagonal chromatography. Nat Protoc 6: 1130-1141

66. Swank GM, Deitch EA (1996) Role of the gut in multiple organ failure: bacterial translocation and permeability changes. World J Surg 20: 411-417

67. Takaishi H, Kimura T, Dalal S, Okada Y, D'Armiento J (2008) Joint diseases and matrix metalloproteinases: a role for MMP-13. Curr Pharm Biotechnol 9: 47-54
68. Tam EM, Morrison CJ, Wu YI, Stack MS, Overall CM (2004) Membrane protease proteomics: isotope-coded affinity tag MS identification of undescribed MT1-matrix metalloproteinase substrates. Proc Natl Acad Sci USA 101: 6917-6922
69. Turner JR (2009) Intestinal mucosal barrier function in health and disease. Nat Rev Immunol 9: 799-809
70. Umeda K, Ikenouchi J, Katahira-Tayama S, Furuse K, Sasaki H, Nakayama M, Matsui T, Tsukita S, Furuse M (2006) ZO-1 and ZO-2 independently determine where claudins are polymerized in tight-junction strand formation. Cell 126: 741-754
71. Van der Sluis M, De Koning BAE, De Bruijn ACJM, Velcich A, Meijerink JPP, Van Goudoever JB, Buller HA, Dekker J, Van Seuningen I, Renes IB, et al (2006) Muc2-deficient mice spontaneously develop colitis, indicating that Muc2 is critical for colonic protection. Gastroenterology 131: 117-129
72. Van Hauwermeiren F, Vandenbroucke RE, Libert C (2011) Treatment of TNF mediated diseases by selective inhibition of soluble TNF or TNFR1. Cytokine Growth Factor Rev 22: 311-319
73. Vandenbroucke RE, Dejager L, Libert C (2011a) The first MMP in sepsis. EMBO Mol Med 3: 367-369
74. Vandenbroucke RE, Dejonckheere E, Libert C (2011b) A therapeutic role for matrix metalloproteinase inhibitors in lung diseases? Eur Respir J 38: 1200-1214
75. Vandenbroucke RE, Dejonckheere E, Van Lint P, Demeestere D, Van Wonterghem E, Vanlaere I, Puimege L, Van Hauwermeiren F, De Rycke R, Mc Guire C, et al (2012) Matrix metalloprotease 8-dependent extracellular matrix cleavage at the blood-CSF barrier contributes to lethality during systemic inflammatory diseases. J Neurosci 32: 9805-9816
76. Vandesompele J, De Preter K, Pattyn F, Poppe B, Van Roy N, De Paepe A, Speleman F (2002) Accurate normalization of real-time quantitative RT-PCR data by geometric averaging of multiple internal control genes. Genome Biol 3: RESEARCH0034
77. Vanlaere I, Libert C (2009) Matrix metalloproteinases as drug targets in infections caused by gram-negative bacteria and in septic shock. Clin Microbiol Rev 22: 224-239 Table of Contents
78. Vizoso FJ, Gonzalez LO, Corte MD, Corte MG, Bongera M, Martinez A, Martin A, Andicoechea A, Gava RR (2006) Collagenase-3 (MMP-13) expression by inflamed mucosa in inflammatory bowel disease. Scand J Gastroenterol 41: 1050-1055
79. Williams KL, Fuller CR, Dieleman LA, DaCosta CM, Haldeman KM, Sartor RB, Lund PK (2001) Enhanced survival and mucosal repair after dextran sodium sulfate-induced colitis in transgenic mice that overexpress growth hormone. Gastroenterology 120: 925-937
80. Wlodarska M, Finlay BB (2010) Host immune response to antibiotic perturbation of the microbiota. Mucosal Immunol 3: 100-103
81. Wu MH, Lo JF, Kuo CH, Lin JA, Lin YM, Chen LM, Tsai FJ, Tsai CH, Huang CY, Tang CH (2012) Endothelin-1 promotes MMP-13 production and migration in human chondrosarcoma cells through FAK/PI3K/Akt/mTOR pathways. J Cell Physiol 227: 3016-3026

82. Yan Y, Kolachala V, Dalmasso G, Nguyen H, Laroui H, Sitaraman SV, Merlin D
     (2009) Temporal and spatial analysis of clinical and molecular parameters in dextran
     sodium sulfate induced colitis. PLoS ONE 4: e6073
83. Zitka O, Kukacka J, Krizkova S, Huska D, Adam V, Masarik M, Prusa R, Kizek R
     (2010) Matrix metalloproteinases. Curr Med Chem 17: 3751-3768

*There are several supplemental files that are not available in this version
of the article. To view this additional information, please use the citation
information cited on the first page of this chapter.*

PART IV

NUTRITION'S EFFECT ON THE MICROBIOME

CHAPTER 9

IMPACT OF A SYNBIOTIC FOOD ON THE GUT MICROBIAL ECOLOGY AND METABOLIC PROFILES

BEATRICE VITALI, MAURICE NDAGIJIMANA,
FEDERICA CRUCIANI, PAOLA CARNEVALI, MARCO CANDELA,
MARIA ELISABETTA GUERZONI, and PATRIZIA BRIGIDI

9.1 BACKGROUND

Humans can be considered as "superorganisms" with an internal ecosystem of diverse symbiotic microorganisms and parasites that have interactive metabolic processes. Their homeostatic balance is dependent upon the interactions between the host and its microbial components [1]. The human intestine is home to some 100 trillion microorganisms of at least 1000 species. The density of bacterial cells in the colon has been estimated at 10^{11} to 10^{12} per ml, which makes it one of the most densely populated microbial habitats known [2,3]. This microbial ecosystem serves numerous important functions for the human host, including protection against pathogens, nutrient processing, stimulation of angiogenesis, modulation

This chapter was originally published under the Creative Commons Attribution License. Vitali B, Ndagijimana M, Cruciani F, Carnevali P, Candela M,Guerzoni ME and Brigidi P. Impact of a Synbiotic Food on the Gut Microbial Ecology and Metabolic Profiles. BMC Microbiology *10,4 (2010). doi:10.1186/1471-2180-10-4.*

of intestinal immune response and regulation of host fat storage [4,5]. The composition of the adult gastrointestinal microbiota has been intensely studied, using both cultivation and, more recently, culture-independent, small subunit (SSU) ribosomal DNA (rDNA) sequence-based methods [6-8]. Members of the anaerobic genera *Bacteroides, Eubacterium, Clostridium, Ruminococcus*, and *Faecalibacterium* have typically been found to comprise a large majority of the human adult gut microbial community. In healthy adults, the gut microbiota consists of a stable individual core of colonizing microorganisms surrounded by temporal visitors [9,10]. Fluctuations around this core of phylotypes are due to host genotype, diet, age, sex, organic disease and drugs (especially antibiotics) [11]. It has been shown that the microbiota structure strongly influences the gut metabolic phenotype [12,13]. On short time scales, the host-specific effects are relatively constant and changes in the gut microbiome composition and activities are closely influenced by dietary variations.

An increasing awareness of the potential of gut microorganisms to influence human health has led to widespread investigation of the relationship between the gut microbiota and nutrients, particularly probiotics [14] and prebiotics [15] and their impact on the digestive system. Members of the genera *Bifidobacterium* and *Lactobacillus*, natural components of the colonic microbiota, are the most commonly used probiotic bacteria in many functional foods and dietary supplements [16]. Postulated health advantages associated to bifidobacteria and lactobacilli include the inhibition of pathogenic microorganisms, improvement of lactose digestion, reduction of serum cholesterol levels, prevention of cancer and enhancement of the host's immune system [17,18]. Several oligosaccharides have been studied as potential prebiotics, including lactulose, galactooligosaccharides and fructooligosaccharides (FOS) [19]. Dietary supplements of prebiotics increase the content and proportion of bifidobacteria [20] and exert positive effects on absorption of nutrients and minerals, synthesis of vitamins, prevention of constipation, colon cancer, and improvement of blood sugar and lipid profile [21]. Another possibility in the microbiota modulation is the use of synbiotics, in which probiotics and prebiotics are used in combination. This combination improves the survival of the probiotic strains, because specific substrates are readily available for their fermentation, and results in advantages to the host that the live microorganisms and prebiotics offer [11].

The inadequacy of conventional culture techniques to reflect the microbial diversity of the intestinal ecosystem has triggered the development of culture-independent 16S rRNA gene-based techniques for the evaluation of the effects of functional food administration in humans [22,23]. The latest frontier in the characterization of uncultured and complex microbial communities is the high-throughput technology of pyrosequencing, which achieves hundreds of thousands of sequences of a specific variable region within the small subunit of rRNA gene, consequently revealing the full diversity of an ecosystem [24,25]. However, since this approach is extremely labor intensive and time consuming, PCR-DGGE and real-time PCR represent population fingerprinting methods, commonly used to analyze the intestinal microbiota upon dietary intervention. PCR-DGGE allows the visualization of the predominant genetic diversity without prior knowledge of the composition or complexity of the microbial ecosystem present in the sample [23,26]. Real-time PCR enables specific intestinal bacterial populations to be directly quantified by using DNA isolated from fecal material [23,27-29].

Gene expression profiling and proteomic approaches have been applied to elucidate the molecular mechanisms underlying symbiotic host-bacterial relationships [30-32]. However, gene expression and proteomic data might only indicate the potential for physiological changes because many pathway feedback mechanisms are simply not reflected in protein concentration or gene expression. On the other hand, metabolite concentrations and their kinetic variations in tissues or biological matrixes represent real end-points of physiological regulatory processes [1,33]. Metabonomics is defined as "the quantitative measurement of the dynamic multiparametric metabolic response of living systems to pathophysiological stimuli or genetic modification" [34]. Metabonomics provides a systems approach to understand global metabolic regulation of an organism and its commensal and symbiotic partners [1]. Recently, complementary metabonomic approaches have been employed for the biochemical characterization of metabolic changes triggered by gut microbiota, dietary variation and stress interactions [35-39]. Solid phase microextraction followed by gaschromatography and mass spectrometry represents a novel method for studying metabolic profiles of biological samples. This approach has been used to compare neonates and adult feces [40] and to identify volatile markers of gastrointestinal disease [41].

In the present study, we characterized the impact of the intake of a synbiotic snack on the gut microbiota composition and metabolic profiles of healthy subjects. The synbiotic snack contained the substrate FOS, whose prebiotic effects are widely documented [42], and the probiotic strains *Lactobacillus helveticus* Bar13 and *Bifidobacterium longum* Bar33, which were selected on the basis of their adhesion and immune-regolation properties, as assessed by both in vitro [43] and in vivo studies on animal models [44]. Co-variations were searched between the gut microbiome structure, as reflected by community DNA fingerprints derived from PCR-DGGE and real-time PCR data, and host metabolic phenotypes, as detected by GC-MS/SPME.

9.2 RESULTS

9.2.1 EFFECTS OF THE SYNBIOTIC FOOD ON COMPOSITION OF THE GUT MICROBIOTA

PCR-DGGE analysis with universal primers targeting the V2-V3 region of the 16S rRNA gene was used to monitor the impact of the synbiotic food intake on the predominant bacterial population (Figure 1A). Population fingerprint profiles were compared and numerically analyzed by FPQuest Software. DGGE band profiles (mean of bands: 15.3) were stable for each subject over a month of feeding with the functional food. Only a slight difference in band richness was found between the time points of the study (T0, mean of bands: 15.8; T1, mean of bands: 14.8). DGGE bands were subjected to Mann-Whitney U-test in order to search for significant differences in the intensities between T0 and T1. No band showed a significant variation, indicating that the consumption of the synbiotic food did not alter the concentration of any major species of intestinal microbiota. Pearson correlation was used to calculate the similarity index (SI) between

DGGE band profiles related to the time points T0 and T1 for each healthy volunteer (Table 1). The high median value of SI (67.1%) revealed that the dominant bacterial composition remained constant over the treatment. Only 3 subjects presented SIs lower than 50% (subjects 8, 12 and 20). No subject showed significant variations between DGGE band profiles related to T0 and T1, as evaluated using the Pearson correlation analysis ($P > 0.05$).

TABLE 1: Similarity index (SI) of DGGE profiles related to T0 and T1

Subject	SI (%)
1	71.8
2	60.6
3	79.2
4	54.1
5	91.3
6	55.9
7	77.5
8	47.7
9	65.0
10	89.3
11	80.9
12	38.2
13	76.1
14	64.7
15	66.6
16	59.4
17	80.3
18	64.3
19	72.1
20	46.4

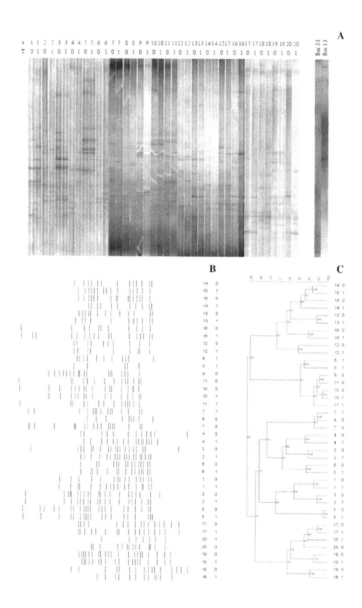

FIGURE 1: DGGE analysis of the fecal samples recovered from 20 healthy volunteers (s1-s20) before (T0) and after (T1) one month of the synbiotic intake. A: DGGE profiles related to fecal samples and *L. helveticus* Bar13 and *B. longum* Bar33 probiotic strains. B: line graph. C: Cluster analysis (Pearson correlation was used to calculate the similarity in DGGE profiles).

Cluster analysis of DGGE population profiling confirmed the stability of the overall structure of the microbiome, revealing no grouping according to the feeding (Figure 1B-C). T0 and T1 banding patterns were closely related for all the volunteers, except for the subject 8 (SI: 47.7%). Among different subjects, considerable variation in the composition of the population fingerprints could be observed. Both qualitative (presence or absence of a band) or quantitative (variable intensity of a band) variations did occur. These inter-individual variations were higher than changes elicited by the functional food consumed.

9.2.2 QUANTITATIVE VARIATIONS OF BIFIDOBACTERIA AND LACTOBACILLI

In order to evaluate the effect of the prebiotic component on modulation of bifidobacteria and lactobacilli populations and the capability of the probiotic bacteria to pass through the gut of the healthy host, quantitative variations of *Bifidobacterium* and *Lactobacillus* genera were determined by real-time PCR and compared to the variations of the species *B. longum* and *L. helveticus* (Table 2). All volunteers naturally harbored strains belonging to *Bifidobacterium* and *Lactobacillus*, as demonstrated by the presence of these genera in all stool samples recovered before the beginning of the feeding trial. *B. longum* was also found in all healthy subjects at the time point T0, in accordance with previous studies reporting *B. longum* as one of the major bifidobacterial species in the intestinal microbiota of human adults [29]. Differently, *L. helveticus* was detected only in 8 subjects at the time point T0, showing a frequency of 40%. *L. helveticus* is not a normal inhabitant of the intestinal microbiota, but strains belonging to this species are used as starter cultures in the manufacturing of a variety of fermented dairy products, to modulate flavor. Thus, presence of *L. helveticus* in fecal samples can be related to a diet rich in yogurt and cheese [45]. Table 2 highlights different trends of variation of *Bifidobacterium*, *Lactobacillus*, *B. longum* and *L. helveticus* concentrations among the subjects enrolled in the trial, suggesting a specific individual response to the dietary intervention. This variability is particularly evident for *L. helveticus*. In the majority of the volunteers, the synbiotic intake was associated to an increase or to the appearance of this species. In 2 subjects (4 and 9) no variation was found at the time point T1. In 4 subjects (6, 8, 19 and 20) *L. helveticus* did not appear after the feeding period and in the subject 20 it disappeared at the time point T1. These results indicate that the capability of *L. helveticus* Bar 13 to persist in the gastrointestinal tract is related to the specific characteristics of the host gut environment.

In order to assess the global impact of the functional food consumption on the bifidobacteria and lactobacilli populations, a statistical elaboration of the real-time PCR data was performed. Box plots in Figure 2 show the amounts of 16S rrn operons of *Bifidobacterium* (A), *B. longum* (B), *Lactobacillus* (C) and *L. helveticus* (D) detected at the time points T0 and T1 of the feeding study. The intake of the synbiotic food did not cause significant variations in the median value of *Bifidobacterium* (T0: 2.6×10^7; T1: 2.2×10^7), *B. longum* (T0: 4.7×10^6; T1: 5.1×10^6) and *Lactobacillus* (T0: 8.5×10^5; T1: 6.5×10^5). On the contrary, a significant increase ($P < 0.05$) of *L. helveticus* DNA was observed after the administration of the functional food (T0 median value: 0; T1 median value: 6.6×10^2), demonstrating the ability of *L. helveticus* Bar13 to pass through the gut of healthy humans. The significant increase of *L. helveticus* was directly linked to the low incidence of this species in the intestine of the human host. Analogously, the absence of significant variations in *Bifidobacterium, Lactobacillus* and *B. longum* could be related to the high T0 amounts of these bacterial groups, natural inhabitants of the gut microbiota of healthy humans. Amounts of *L. helveticus* were evaluated by real-time PCR in stool samples recovered from 10 subjects after a wash-out period of 20 days. Concentration of this species returned to a median value of 0, supporting the hypothesis of a transient persistence of the probiotic strain Bar13 during the feeding period (data not shown).

Figure 3 shows the relationship between the variation of *B. longum* species, expressed as the ratio of T1 and T0 16S rrn operons, and the basal concentration of *B. longum*, expressed as the number of 16S rrn operons measured at the time point T0. The trend of the curve indicates a strong influence of the initial concentration of *B. longum* on the variation of *B. longum* population after the feeding period. An evident increase of *B. longum* was observed in subjects 11, 12 and 18, who showed T0 amount of this species minor or equal to 1.0×10^6 16S rrn operons per µg of total

TABLE 2: Real-time PCR quantification of bifidobacteria and lactobacilli

Sub-ject	Time point	16S rrn operons/µg fecal genomic DNA (mean ± SD)			
		Bifidobacterium	*B. longum*	*Lactobacillus*	*L. helveticus*
1	T0	$9.4 \times 10^6 \pm 3.7 \times 10^6$	$3.2 \times 10^6 \pm 1.5 \times 10^6$	$2.6 \times 10^6 \pm 9.6 \times 10^5$	0.0 ± 0.0
	T1	$4.1 \times 10^6 \pm 8.3 \times 10^5$	$1.1 \times 10^6 \pm 2.9 \times 10^5$	$1.9 \times 10^6 \pm 9.9 \times 10^5$	$4.5 \times 10^2 \pm 2.9 \times 10^2$
2	T0	$8.9 \times 10^7 \pm 3.1 \times 10^7$	$4.2 \times 10^7 \pm 3.6 \times 10^7$	$1.1 \times 10^5 \pm 5.6 \times 10^4$	$9.0 \times 10^1 \pm 6.2 \times 10^1$
	T1	$1.6 \times 10^7 \pm 5.0 \times 10^6$	$4.7 \times 10^6 \pm 2.9 \times 10^5$	$5.1 \times 10^5 \pm 2.4 \times 10^5$	$2.6 \times 10^3 \pm 2.8 \times 10^2$
3	T0	$4.0 \times 10^8 \pm 3.6 \times 10^7$	$8.6 \times 10^6 \pm 2.6 \times 10^6$	$5.6 \times 10^4 \pm 3.5 \times 10^4$	0.0 ± 0.0
	T1	$2.4 \times 10^8 \pm 2.5 \times 10^7$	$2.4 \times 10^7 \pm 2.9 \times 10^6$	$2.6 \times 10^5 \pm 1.6 \times 10^5$	$2.8 \times 10^3 \pm 1.8 \times 10^3$
4	T0	$2.6 \times 10^8 \pm 2.8 \times 10^7$	$2.3 \times 10^7 \pm 2.9 \times 10^6$	$1.6 \times 10^5 \pm 1.0 \times 10^3$	$2.1 \times 10^3 \pm 8.7 \times 10^1$
	T1	$5.8 \times 10^8 \pm 1.2 \times 10^7$	$3.7 \times 10^7 \pm 3.1 \times 10^6$	$1.2 \times 10^5 \pm 2.7 \times 10^4$	$1.6 \times 10^3 \pm 2.2 \times 10^2$
5	T0	$3.1 \times 10^6 \pm 8.6 \times 10^5$	$9.8 \times 10^5 \pm 2.8 \times 10^5$	$1.9 \times 10^4 \pm 5.8 \times 10^3$	0.0 ± 0.0
	T1	$2.4 \times 10^6 \pm 7.3 \times 10^5$	$9.5 \times 10^5 \pm 3.4 \times 10^5$	$6.1 \times 10^4 \pm 3.4 \times 10^4$	$3.5 \times 10^2 \pm 2.3 \times 10^2$
6	T0	$1.7 \times 10^8 \pm 3.8 \times 10^7$	$6.5 \times 10^6 \pm 2.4 \times 10^5$	$2.7 \times 10^5 \pm 1.2 \times 10^5$	0.0 ± 0.0
	T1	$6.2 \times 10^8 \pm 4.2 \times 10^7$	$3.5 \times 10^7 \pm 2.0 \times 10^5$	$1.7 \times 10^5 \pm 1.1 \times 10^5$	0.0 ± 0.0
7	T0	$6.4 \times 10^7 \pm 4.8 \times 10^6$	$3.4 \times 10^7 \pm 1.2 \times 10^6$	$4.0 \times 10^5 \pm 1.7 \times 10^5$	$9.0 \times 10^1 \pm 8.2 \times 10^1$
	T1	$7.5 \times 10^7 \pm 1.2 \times 10^6$	$4.6 \times 10^7 \pm 5.5 \times 10^6$	$9.2 \times 10^5 \pm 4.9 \times 10^5$	$1.4 \times 10^4 \pm 3.2 \times 10^3$
8	T0	$1.8 \times 10^6 \pm 5.8 \times 10^5$	$6.0 \times 10^5 \pm 3.6 \times 10^5$	$1.0 \times 10^6 \pm 1.0 \times 10^6$	0.0 ± 0.0
	T1	$4.1 \times 10^6 \pm 8.5 \times 10^5$	$1.3 \times 10^6 \pm 9.7 \times 10^5$	$1.7 \times 10^5 \pm 1.7 \times 10^5$	0.0 ± 0.0
9	T0	$4.4 \times 10^6 \pm 2.8 \times 10^5$	$3.0 \times 10^6 \pm 2.3 \times 10^6$	$9.2 \times 10^5 \pm 9.0 \times 10^5$	$3.0 \times 10^3 \pm 1.1 \times 10^3$
	T1	$5.6 \times 10^6 \pm 1.4 \times 10^5$	$3.8 \times 10^6 \pm 1.3 \times 10^6$	$2.0 \times 10^6 \pm 1.0 \times 10^6$	$1.8 \times 10^3 \pm 1.7 \times 10^3$
10	T0	$1.0 \times 10^8 \pm 1.8 \times 10^7$	$7.0 \times 10^7 \pm 4.5 \times 10^7$	$7.7 \times 10^5 \pm 7.6 \times 10^5$	0.0 ± 0.0
	T1	$3.3 \times 10^8 \pm 7.7 \times 10^7$	$4.3 \times 10^7 \pm 2.5 \times 10^7$	$1.3 \times 10^6 \pm 1.2 \times 10^6$	$3.2 \times 10^3 \pm 2.7 \times 10^3$

TABLE 2: *Cont.*

Sub- ject	Time point	16S rrn operons/µg fecal genomic DNA (mean ± SD)			
		Bifidobacterium	*B. longum*	*Lactobacillus*	*L. helveticus*
11	T0	$4.1 \times 10^6 \pm 7.5 \times 10^5$	$1.2 \times 10^6 \pm 2.5 \times 10^5$	$5.1 \times 10^5 \pm 4.1 \times 10^5$	$6.0 \times 10^2 \pm 3.8 \times 10^2$
	T1	$3.4 \times 10^7 \pm 6.2 \times 10^5$	$3.1 \times 10^7 \pm 1.0 \times 10^7$	$7.8 \times 10^5 \pm 7.7 \times 10^5$	$1.7 \times 10^4 \pm 3.1 \times 10^3$
12	T0	$3.4 \times 10^5 \pm 7.6 \times 10^4$	$7.5 \times 10^2 \pm 3.0 \times 10^1$	$1.7 \times 10^7 \pm 1.1 \times 10^7$	0.0 ± 0.0
	T1	$1.3 \times 10^6 \pm 7.0 \times 10^5$	$2.0 \times 10^5 \pm 9.3 \times 10^4$	$5.8 \times 10^5 \pm 5.6 \times 10^5$	$3.6 \times 10^3 \pm 6.4 \times 10^2$
13	T0	$3.5 \times 10^7 \pm 1.6 \times 10^6$	$1.2 \times 10^7 \pm 2.6 \times 10^5$	$1.8 \times 10^5 \pm 1.0 \times 10^5$	0.0 ± 0.0
	T1	$2.3 \times 10^7 \pm 3.8 \times 10^6$	$4.6 \times 10^6 \pm 4.4 \times 10^5$	$2.5 \times 10^5 \pm 1.8 \times 10^5$	$1.8 \times 10^2 \pm 4.3 \times 10^1$
14	T0	$1.1 \times 10^7 \pm 6.9 \times 10^5$	$2.3 \times 10^6 \pm 1.6 \times 10^6$	$1.1 \times 10^6 \pm 1.8 \times 10^5$	0.0 ± 0.0
	T1	$5.4 \times 10^7 \pm 1.7 \times 10^7$	$1.0 \times 10^7 \pm 6.5 \times 10^6$	$7.2 \times 10^5 \pm 6.4 \times 10^5$	$3.0 \times 10^2 \pm 3.0 \times 10^1$
15	T0	$6.1 \times 10^7 \pm 7.4 \times 10^6$	$1.7 \times 10^7 \pm 8.3 \times 10^6$	$3.9 \times 10^5 \pm 2.9 \times 10^5$	$1.8 \times 10^1 \pm 1.6 \times 10^1$
	T1	$2.5 \times 10^7 \pm 5.3 \times 10^6$	$1.0 \times 10^7 \pm 5.8 \times 10^6$	$2.5 \times 10^5 \pm 2.2 \times 10^5$	$3.2 \times 10^2 \pm 1.4 \times 10^2$
16	T0	$1.3 \times 10^9 \pm 4.5 \times 10^8$	$4.0 \times 10^7 \pm 1.2 \times 10^7$	$2.0 \times 10^6 \pm 1.1 \times 10^6$	0.0 ± 0.0
	T1	$1.3 \times 10^9 \pm 2.0 \times 10^8$	$2.2 \times 10^7 \pm 3.8 \times 10^6$	$1.0 \times 10^6 \pm 8.2 \times 10^5$	$8.3 \times 10^2 \pm 1.4 \times 10^1$
17	T0	$1.6 \times 10^7 \pm 1.6 \times 10^6$	$5.0 \times 10^6 \pm 3.2 \times 10^6$	$1.3 \times 10^7 \pm 2.9 \times 10^6$	$1.3 \times 10^2 \pm 1.1 \times 10^2$
	T1	$2.2 \times 10^7 \pm 1.9 \times 10^6$	$4.0 \times 10^6 \pm 2.7 \times 10^6$	$1.5 \times 10^7 \pm 2.0 \times 10^5$	$6.6 \times 10^2 \pm 9.5 \times 10^1$
18	T0	$1.1 \times 10^5 \pm 3.1 \times 10^6$	$1.4 \times 10^3 \pm 4.4 \times 10^2$	$3.1 \times 10^7 \pm 2.7 \times 10^7$	0.0 ± 0.0
	T1	$3.7 \times 10^5 \pm 8.9 \times 10^4$	$1.7 \times 10^5 \pm 7.3 \times 10^4$	$3.0 \times 10^6 \pm 1.2 \times 10^6$	$6.5 \times 10^2 \pm 1.2 \times 10^2$
19	T0	$5.2 \times 10^7 \pm 1.7 \times 10^7$	$4.3 \times 10^5 \pm 1.8 \times 10^5$	$2.5 \times 10^6 \pm 1.9 \times 10^6$	0.0 ± 0.0
	T1	$2.0 \times 10^7 \pm 8.0 \times 10^6$	$1.5 \times 10^5 \pm 9.4 \times 10^4$	$2.0 \times 10^6 \pm 1.5 \times 10^6$	0.0 ± 0.0
20	T0	$6.6 \times 10^6 \pm 5.2 \times 10^6$	$4.4 \times 10^6 \pm 2.2 \times 10^6$	$1.0 \times 10^7 \pm 8.4 \times 10^6$	$1.8 \times 10^3 \pm 2.6 \times 10^2$
	T1	$7.0 \times 10^6 \pm 3.3 \times 10^5$	$5.5 \times 10^6 \pm 3.3 \times 10^6$	$2.7 \times 10^5 \pm 2.6 \times 10^5$	0.0 ± 0.0

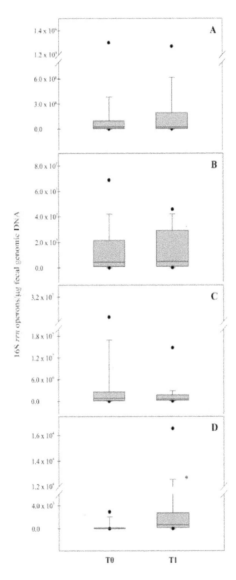

FIGURE 2: Real-time PCR evaluation of 16S rrn operons of Bifidobacterium (A), *B. longum* (B), Lactobacillus (C) and *L. helveticus* (D) related to the time points (T0 and T1) of the feeding study. Data are expressed as number of operons in 1 μg of total bacterial DNA extracted from the feces. The box represents the interquartile range (25-75th percentile) and the line within the box is the median value. The bottom and top bars indicate the 10th and 90th percentiles, respectively. Outlier values are indicated (black circles). * indicates a significant difference (P < 0.05).

bacterial DNA. Notably, subject 12, presenting the lowest *B. longum* concentration at the time point T0 (7.5×10^2), showed the highest variation of *B. longum* (T1/T0: 2.6×10^2) after the synbiotic intake. The same subject presented the lowest SI (38.2%) between DGGE band profiles related to the time points T0 and T1. These data suggest the capability of *B. longum* Bar33 to pass through the human gastrointestinal tract, but this property can be detected only in subjects harboring low basal level of *B. longum* species.

9.2.3 CHANGES IN INTESTINAL METABOLIC PROFILES

In this investigation about 130 different metabolites belonging to the families of alcohols, ketones, aldehydes, sulfur compounds, nitrogen compounds and SCFA were detected in feces by means of GC-MS/SPME analysis (see Additional file 1). A two-tailed Mann-Whitney test was performed on the metabolic data matrix in order to identify the molecules significantly affected by the consumption of the functional food. A CAP analysis performed on the selected molecules evidenced that metabolites whose changes were positively correlated with the synbiotic administration principally belonged to the families of ketones (methyl-5-hepten-2-one, 2-propanone, 2-butanone, 2-pentanone, 2,3-butanedione) and SCFA (acetic and valeric acid). Differently, the concentration of 1-octanol, thiophene and nonanone decreased significantly after the feeding period. These results are showed in the Figure 4, which reports the loadings plot obtained from the CAP analysis. The scores plot (canonical axe) obtained from the same supervised method showed a perfect classification of the samples, on the basis of the synbiotic food intake (Figure 5). The application of the CAP analysis on metabolites data set characterized by GC-MS/SPME resulted in classification and predictive abilities of 100% (see Additional file 2), as evaluated by the leave-four-out procedure used, using only a reduced number of experimental chromatographic peaks as input variables.

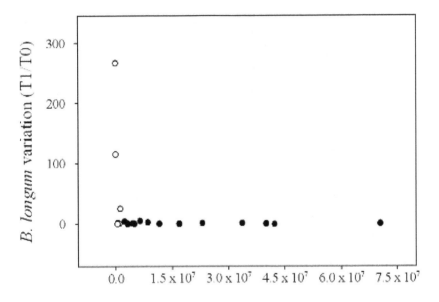

FIGURE 3: Relationship between *B. longum* variations (T1/T0 16S rrn operons) and *B. longum* amount before the feeding trial (T0 16S rrn operons). Empty circles indicate subjects with T0 value minor or equal to 1.0×10^6 16S rrn operons per μg of total bacterial DNA. Filled circles indicate subjects with T0 value higher than 1.0×10^6 16S rrn operons per μg of total bacterial DNA.

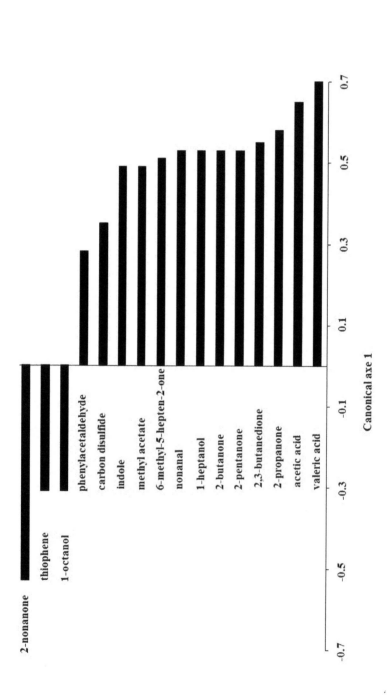

FIGURE 4: CAP loadings plot of metabolites whose concentration was significantly affected by the intake of the synbiotic food (P < 0.05). Positive and negative coefficients indicate the increase or decrease of metabolite amounts following the feeding period.

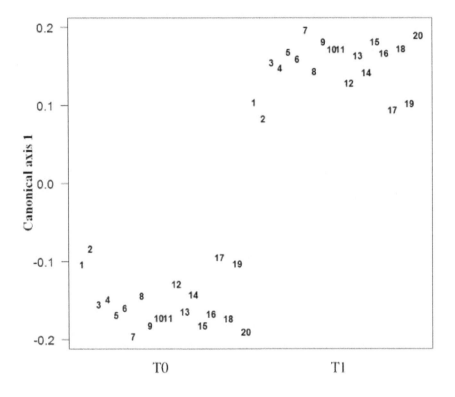

FIGURE 5: CAP scores plot of the stool samples collected from the twenty volunteers before (T0) and after (T1) the synbiotic food intake.

9.3 DISCUSSION

The significant involvement of the gut microbiota in the human health suggests that modulation of commensal microbial composition and metabolism through combinations of probiotics and prebiotics could be a dietary strategy to prevent diverse diseases, such as obesity, diabetes, non-alcoholic fatty liver disease, inflammatory bowel disease, and even cancers [4].

In the present study, the impact of a synbiotic food supplement on the gut microbiota structure of healthy humans was evaluated by using an integrated molecular approach based on PCR-DGGE and real-time PCR.

DGGE profiles of the predominant fecal microbiota generated complex but overall relatively stable and unique profiles for each individual. Elaboration of DGGE data revealed high SI values between T0 and T1 profiles, and no clustering of banding patterns according to the feeding. These results demonstrated that no significant change in the structure of the gut microbiota of healthy subjects did occur following dietary intervention, confirming previous findings regarding the subject specificity of the predominant fecal communities and their stability over time and resistance to perturbations [9,23]. Notably, we cannot exclude an effect of the synbiotic intake on minor bacterial species, an effect that could be investigated using high-throughput sequencing techniques. However, the impact on the dominant colonic microbiota represents the main parameter to evaluate the clinical relevance for the use of a functional food.

Because DGGE can be considered a semiquantitative tool for monitoring the dynamics of the predominant bacterial species of an ecosystem, additional analysis with real-time PCR was performed to obtain a quantitative estimation of the effect of the synbiotic intake on bifidobacteria and lactobacilli populations. In particular, variations in amounts of *B. longum* and *L. helveticus* were evaluated in order to assess the capability of the probiotic species included in the synbiotic food to pass through the gastrointestinal tract of the human host. Only *L. helveticus* concentration increased significantly after the ingestion of the functional food, demonstrating the gut persistence of the probiotic *L. helveticus* strain during the feeding period. Since *L. helveticus* species is not a natural inhabitant of the human intestine and its presence in feces is diet related [45], this result was not surprising and suggests that low abundant species could be optimal models for studying the gut colonization of probiotic bacteria. On the other hand, visualization of the gut colonization of a high abundant species, such as *B. longum*, is strictly related to its basal concentration. For this reason, we observed the *B. longum* increase only in subjects with the lowest concentration of *B. longum* species at the time point T0.

The intake of the synbiotic food resulted in significant changes in some gut metabolic activities, as highlighted by the CAP analysis of the fecal metabolic profiles, which pointed out a separation of fecal samples of the subjects on the basis of the synbiotic food intake. Surprisingly little is known about volatile organic compounds formed in the gut. GC-MS/SPME, detecting volatile molecules with high sensitivity, represents a suitable approach to identify microbial metabolites in fecal samples, such as SCFAs, ketones, esters and sulfur compounds [46].

Two SCFAs, acetic and valeric acids, were the metabolites showing the highest increase after the synbiotic administration. Although a general increase was observed also for butyric acid, this variation was not statistically significant due to the high variability of the measures. SCFAs are very common in the gut environment, arising from metabolism of undigested carbohydrates, such as dietary fiber and prebiotics, by colonic bacteria. The increase of SCFAs is particularly interesting, as they play a role in regulation of cell proliferation and differentiation of the colonic epithelial cells. Increases in SCFA production have been associated with decreased pH, which may reduce potential pathogenic clostridia, decreased solubility of bile acids, increased absorption of minerals, and reduced ammonia absorption by the protonic dissociation of ammonia and other amines [47]. Other metabolites whose changes were positively and significantly correlated with the synbiotic intake belonged to the family of methylketones (methyl-5-hepten-2-one, 2-propanone, 2-butanone, 2-pentanone, 2,3-butanedione). In particular, the significant increase of 2-pentanone can be regarded as the most interesting effect associated with the synbiotic food intake. In fact, 2-pentanone, which is a naturally occurring compound in fruits, vegetables and fermented foods, has anti-inflammatory and chemopreventive properties. According to Pettersson et al. [48], it inhibits the prostaglandin production and COX-2 protein expression in human colon cancer cells. The increase of 2,3-butanedione is interesting since it may have health benefits by impacting on the growth of some bacteria, such as *L. delbrueckii* subsp. *bulgaricus* and *Streptococcus thermophilus* [41]. Furthermore, during glucose catabolism 2,3-butanedione serves as an electron acceptor and can be reduced to 2,3-butanediol via acetoin. This pathway was shown to be important in the removal of toxic amounts of pyruvate and in maintenance of pH homeostasis [49]. A diverse range of sulfur compounds has been identified in stool samples [41]. The usual source of sulfur compounds is the microbial breakdown of sulfur containing amino acids and the increase of these compounds suggests an abundance or metabolic activity of bacteria able to breakdown cystein and methionine. In our study, a significant increase of carbon disulfide was observed following the feeding period. Carbon disulfide may be produced by carbonation of hydrogen sulphide as a detoxification mechanism exerted by colonic bacteria. According to Garner et al. [41], carbon disulfide has been found in 100% of the samples from healthy donors and absent in many samples of patients with *Campylobacter jejuni* and *Clostridium difficile*. Various esters were detected in all fecal samples. In particular, a significant increase of methyl acetate, ester of methanol and acetic acid, was evident after the synbiotic intake. Methanol is rarely found as free alcohol in the gut, where it is generated from the breakdown of macromolecules including pectins, bran and aspartame. In general, free alcohols and endogenous fatty acids are metabolized into fatty acid esters in liver, pancreas and intestine [50]. At the intestinal site, esterification of alcohols by colonic bacteria can be regarded as a microbial strategy to remove or trap toxic molecules such as fatty acids and alcohols.

To sum up, the investigation of the fecal volatile metabolites by GC-MS/SPME allowed to correlate the consumption of the synbiotic food with the stimulation of health-promoting metabolic activities of the gut microbiota, such as regulation of the colonic epithelial cell proliferation and differentiation, anti-inflammatory and chemopreventive properties and detoxification processes.

9.3 CONCLUSION

In the current study molecular fingerprinting techniques (PCR-DGGE and real-time PCR) were integrated to the GC-MS/SPME analysis of the metabolic profiles to investigate the global impact of a dietary intervention on the gut ecology and metabolism in healthy humans. In particular, the major findings of this study are the following: (i) the synbiotic food does not modify the overall structure of the gut microbiome, as detected by DGGE; (ii) the gut survival of the probiotic strains may be supposed on the basis of the increase of *B. longum* and *L. helveticus* after the synbiotic consumption; (iii) the perturbation of the gut metabolism triggered by a synbiotic food intake generates significant changes in the GC-MS/SPME profiles; (iv) changes in metabolic phenotypes seem to indicate potential implications of the synbiotic food in health maintenance and prevention of diverse diseases.

In order to better investigate the mechanistic basis of the probiotics and prebiotics action on gut microbial activities and the outcomes on human health, it will be necessary to integrate the GC-MS/SPME and/or NMR profiles of feces with simultaneous analysis of different biofluids, including urine and plasma.

9.4 METHODS

9.4.1 STUDY POPULATION

Twenty randomly selected healthy volunteers (11 women and 9 men) aged between 20 and 50 (mean: 35) participated in the study. The Ethics Committee of the University of Bologna (Italy) approved the study, and all subjects gave informed consent. None of the subjects had a history of gastrointestinal or metabolic disease or previous surgery (apart from appendectomy). The subjects did not receive antibiotic treatment or any other medical treatment influencing intestinal microbiota during 3 months before the start of the study. Subjects maintained their usual diet during the study period. All the volunteers had normal weight with a body mass index in the range 18.5-24.9. The volunteers received one dose of a synbiotic snack (Barilla, Parma, Italy), twice a day for a period of 1 month. The synbiotic bar consisted of a biscuit covered by chocolate. The biscuit contained 500 mg of FOS (Actilight® 950P, Marckolsheim, France) and the chocolate included a mixture of the probiotic strains *B. longum* Bar33 and

L. helveticus Bar13 (Barilla culture collection). 10^9 CFU of each probiotic strain were present in a dose of the synbiotic bar.

9.4.2 EXTRACTION OF DNA FROM FECAL SAMPLES

Stool samples were collected from volunteers before the start of the feeding study (T0) and at the end of the ingestion period (T1) and immediately frozen at -80°C until use. Total DNA was extracted from 230 mg of feces by using QIAamp DNA Stool Mini Kit (Qiagen, Hilden, Germany), according to the manufacturer's instructions.

9.4.3 PCR-DGGE AND CLUSTER ANALYSIS

Amplification of the V2-V3 region of the bacterial 16S rRNA gene was carried out using the universal eubacterial primers GCclamp-HDA1 and HDA2 [51], supplied by M-Medical (Milan, Italy). The amplification reactions were performed in a Biometra Thermal Cycler T Gradient (Biometra, Göttingen, Germany). AmpliTaq Gold DNA Polymerase (Applied Biosystem, Foster City, CA) was used as thermostable DNA polymerase. The reaction mixture contained 0.5 μM of each primer, 200 μM of each dNTP, 0.5 U of DNA Polymerase, and 4 μl of the bacterial DNA template in a final volume of 50 μl. The thermocycle program consisted of the following time and temperature profile: 95°C for 15 min; 30 cycles of 95°C for 60 s, 56°C for 30 s, 72°C for 30 s; and 72°C for 8 min. A volume of 15-20 μl of PCR samples was used for DGGE analysis, which was performed by using the D-Code Universal Mutation System Apparatus (Bio-Rad, Los Angeles, CA), as previously described [52]. Briefly, the sequence-specific separation of the PCR fragments was obtained in 8% (w/v) polyacrylamide gels, containing a 30% to 50% gradient of urea and formamide. Electrophoresis was started at a voltage of 250 V for 5 minutes and continued at constant voltage of 90 V and temperature of 60°C for 16 h. Following electrophoresis, the gel was silver stained [53] and scanned using a Molecular Imager Gel Doc XR System (Bio-Rad). DGGE gel images were analyzed using the FPQuest Software Version 4.5 (Bio-Rad). In order to compensate for gel-to-gel differences and external distortion to electrophoresis, the DGGE patterns were aligned and normalized using an external reference ladder, containing PCR amplicons from pure cultures of intestinal bacterial species. A cluster analysis of the DGGE patterns was performed using the FPQuest Software. The similarity in the profiles was calculated on the basis of the Pearson correlation coefficient with the Ward clustering algorithm.

9.4.4 DEVELOPMENT OF L. HELVETICUS SPECIES-SPECIFIC PRIMERS

By using 16S and 16S-23S rRNA sequences obtained from the DDBJ and EMBL databases, multiple alignments of sequences related to *L. helveticus* and reference organisms were constructed with the program Clustal W http://www.ebi.ac.uk/Tools/clustalw2. Potential target sites for specific detection of the species *L. helveticus* were identified and the following primers were designed: F_Hel (5'-GTGCCATCCTAAGAGATTAGGA-3') and R_Hel (5'-TATCTCTACTCTCCATCACTTC-3'). A Blast search http://www.ncbi.nlm.nih.gov/BLAST was carried out to test the virtual specificity of the primers. Validation of specificity was performed by PCR experiments against different species of *Lactobacillus* (*L. acidophilus, L. casei, L. plantarum, L. bulgaricus, L. reuteri, L. gasseri, L. johnsonii*) and other intestinal genera (*Bifidobacterium, Streptococcus, Escherichia*). The primers were synthesized by M-Medical (Milan, Italy) and optimal annealing temperature was established by gradient PCR.

9.4.5 REAL-TIME QUANTITATIVE PCR

Quantitative PCR was performed in a LightCycler instrument (Roche, Mannheim, Germany) and SYBR Green I fluorophore was used to correlate the amount of PCR product with the fluorescence signal. The following genus- and species-specific primers sets, targeted to 16S or 16S-23S rRNA sequences, were used: Bif164/Bif662 (Bifidobacterium [54]); Lac1/Lab0677r (*Lactobacillus* [55,56]); BiLON1/BiLON2 (B. longum

[29]); F_Hel/R_Hel (*L. helveticus* [this work]). Three sub-samples of each DNA extract were amplified in a final volume of 20 µl containing 4 mM of MgCl$_2$, 0.5 µM of each primer, 2 µl of LightCycler-FastStart DNA Master SYBR Green I (Roche), and either 2 µl of template or water (no-template control). The thermal cycling conditions were as follows: an initial denaturation step at 95°C for 10 min followed by 40 cycles of denaturation at 95°C for 15 s; primer annealing at 60°C (*Bifidobacterium*), 65°C (*Lactobacillus* and *B. longum)* and 63°C (*L. helveticus*) for 25 s; extension at 72°C for 25 s (*Bifidobacterium*), 20 s (*Lactobacillus*), 45 s (*B. longum*) and 10 s (*L. helveticus*) and a fluorescence acquisition step at 90°C (*Bifidobacterium* and *B. longum*) or 85°C (*Lactobacillus* and *L. helveticus*) for 5 s. For each step the temperature transition rate was 20°C/s. Quantification of rrn operons of *Bifidobacterium, Lactobacillus* and *B. longum* was done by using standard curves made from known concentrations of genomic DNA from the sequenced strains *B. longum* NCC2705 [30] and *L. acidophilus* NCFM [57]. For *L. helveticus* species the probiotic strain included in the synbiotic was used as standard and the number of rrn operons in the genome was deduced from the sequenced genome of *L. helveticus* DPC 4571 [58]. Chromosomal DNA of the strains used as standards was extracted by using DNeasy Tissue Kit (Qiagen) and serially diluted from 10^5 to 10^1 molecules/µl. Results obtained by PCR were converted to the average estimate of total rrn operons from each group present in 1 µg of total DNA, and standard deviations (SD) were calculated.

9.4.6 GC-MS/SPME

A carboxen-polydimethylsiloxane coated fiber (85 µm) and a manual SPME holder (Supelco, Bellefonte, PA) were used in this study after preconditioning according to the manufacturer's instruction manual. Before each head space sampling, the fiber was exposed to the GC inlet for 5 min for thermal desorption at 250°C in a blank sample. Five ml of fecal slurries (20%) were placed in 10 ml glass vials, added with 4-methyl-2-pentanol (4 mg/l) as internal standard. The samples were then equilibrated for 10 min at 45°C. The SPME fiber was exposed to each sample for 40 min and then was inserted into the injection port of the GC for a 5 min sample desorption. GC-MS analyses were performed on an Agilent 7890A gas-chromatograph (Agilent Technologies, Palo Alto, CA) coupled to an Agilent 5975C mass selective detector operating in electron impact mode (ionization voltage 70 eV). A Supelcowax 10 capillary column (60 m length, 0.32 mm ID) was used (Supelco). The temperature program was: 50°C for 1 min, then programmed at 4.5°C/min to 65°C and finally at 10°C/min to 230°C which was maintained for 25 min. Injector, interface and ion source temperatures were 250, 250 and 230°C, respectively. The mass-to-charge ratio interval was 30-350 Da at 2.9 scans per second. Injections were performed in splitless mode and helium (1 ml/min) was used as carrier gas. The identification of all the molecules detected in fecal samples was based on comparison of their retention times and spectral data with those of pure compounds (Sigma-Aldrich, Milan, Italy) analyzed in the same conditions. The identification was further confirmed by comparing mass spectra of all compounds with those contained in available databases (NIST version 2005 and Wiley version 1996) and in literature [41]. Quantitative data of the identified compounds were obtained by interpolation of the relative areas versus the internal standard area, in calibration curves built with pure reference compounds. The concentration of volatile compounds, for which there were no pure references, was obtained by using the same calibration graphs of the compounds with the most similar chemical structure.

9.4.7 STATISTICAL ANALYSES

For each subject, variations of the DGGE profiles related to the time points T0 and T1 were analyzed by Pearson correlation. Significant differences in the intensity of each DGGE band among all fecal samples were searched by using Mann-Whitney U-test. Mann-Whitney U-test was also used to analyze differences in total rrn operons of target genera and species and to determine metabolites significantly affected by the synbiotic food intake. A P value below 0.05 was considered statistically significant. Metabolites with a P value below 0.05 were then used in further multivariate analysis. These selected metabolites formed a matrix containing two kinds of information: the effects of the synbiotic food intake (within-individual variability) and the natural differences between individuals (between-individuals variability). These two kinds of information were separated following the method of Jansen et al. [59]. A CAP analysis was then performed on the within-individual variability matrix [60]. The CAP constrained ordination procedure can be summarized as follows: the data were reduced by performing a principal coordinate analysis (PCO) on the parameters using a dissimilarity measure based on Euclidean distances; an appropriate number of PCOs were chosen non-arbitrarily, which maximize the number of observations correctly classified [61,60]. The robustness of the model obtained was established by a 4-fold cross validation method, repeatedly leaving out a fourth of the samples and predicting them back into the model [62]. Finally a traditional canonical analysis on the first three PCOs was performed. The hypothesis of no significant difference in multivariate location among the groups was tested by using a permutation test based on 9999 permutations.

Statistical analyses were performed using the software SigmaStat (Systat Sofware Inc., San Jose, CA) and the package Canoco for Windows 4.5 (Microcomputer Power, Ithaca, NY).

REFERENCES

1. Rezzi S, Ramadan Z, Fay LB, Kochhar S: Nutritional metabonomics: applications and perspectives. J Proteome Res 2007, 6:513-525.
2. Eckburg PB, Bik EM, Bernstein CN, Purdom E, Dethlefsen L, Sargent M, Gill SR, Nelson KE, Relman DA: Diversity of the human intestinal microbial flora. Science 2005, 308:1635-1638.
3. Ley RE, Peterson DA, Gordon JI: Ecological and evolutionary forces shaping microbial diversity in the human intestine. Cell 2006, 124:837-848.
4. Bäckhed F, Ley RE, Sonnenburg JL, Peterson DA, Gordon JI: Host-bacterial mutualism in the human intestine. Science 2005, 307:1915-1920.
5. Palmer C, Bik EM, Digiulio DB, Relman DA, Brown PO: Development of the human infant intestinal microbiota. PLoS Biol 2007, 5:1556-1573.
6. Vaughan EE, Schut F, Heilig HG, Zoetendal EG, de Vos WM, Akkermans AD: A molecular view of the intestinal ecosystem. Curr Issues Intest Microbiol 2000, 1:1-12.
7. Gill SR, Pop M, Deboy RT, Eckburg PB, Turnbaugh PJ, Samuel BS, Gordon JI, Relman DA, Fraser-Liggett CM, Nelson KE: Metagenomic analysis of the human distal gut microbiome. Science 2006, 312:1355-1359.
8. Palmer C, Bik EM, Eisen MB, Eckburg PB, Sana TR, Wolber PK, Relman DA, Brown PO: Rapid quantitative profiling of complex microbial populations. Nucleic Acids Res 2006, 34:e5.

9. Zoetendal EG, Akkermans AD, de Vos WM: Temperature gradient gel electrophoresis analysis of 16S rRNA from human fecal samples reveals stable and host-specific communities of active bacteria. Appl Environ Microbiol 1998, 64:3854-3859.

10. Zoetendal EG, Rajilic-Stojanovic M, de Vos WM: High-throughput diversity and functionality analysis of the gastrointestinal tract microbiota. Gut 2008, 57:1605-1615.

11. Collins MD, Gibson GR: Probiotics, prebiotics, and synbiotics: approaches for modulating the microbial ecology of the gut. Am J Clin Nutr 1999, 69(Suppl):1052-1057.

12. Li M, Wang B, Zhang M, Rantalainen M, Wang S, Zhou H, Zhang Y, Shen J, Pang X, Zhang M, Wei H, Chen Y, Lu H, Zuo J, Su M, Qiu Y, Jia W, Xiao C, Smith LM, Yang S, Holmes E, Tang H, Zhao G, Nicholson JK, Li L, Zhao L: Symbiotic gut microbes modulate human metabolic phenotypes. Proc Natl Acad Sci USA 2008, 105:2117-2122.

13. Nicholson JK, Holmes E, Wilson ID: Gut microorganisms, mammalian metabolism and personalized health care. Nat Rev Microbiol 2005, 3:431-438.

14. Fuller R: A review: probiotics in man and animals. J Appl Bacteriol 1989, 66:365-378.

15. Gibson GR, Roberfroid MB: Dietary modulation of the human colonic microbiota: introducing the concept of prebiotics. J Nutr 1995, 125:1401-1412.

16. Guarner F, Malagelada JR: Gut flora in health and disease. Lancet 2003, 361:512-519.

17. Parvez S, Malik KA, Ah Kang S, Kim HY: Probiotics and their fermented food products are beneficial for health. J Appl Microbiol 2006, 100:1171-1185.

18. Farnworth ER: The evidence to support health claims for probiotics. J Nutr 2008, 138(suppl):1250-1254.

19. Cummings JH, Macfarlane GT, Englyst HN: Prebiotic digestion and fermentation. Am J Clin Nutr 2001, 73(suppl):415-420.

20. Gibson GR: Dietary modulation of the human gut microflora using prebiotics. Br J Nutr 1998, 80(suppl):209-212.

21. Goetze O, Fruehauf H, Pohl D, Giarrè M, Rochat F, Ornstein K, Menne D, Fried M, Thumshirn M: Effect of a prebiotic mixture on intestinal comfort and general wellbeing in health. Br J Nutr 2008, 100:1077-1085.

22. Suau A, Bonnet R, Sutren M, Godon JJ, Gibson GR, Collins MD, Doré J: Direct analysis of genes encoding 16S rRNA from complex communities reveals many novel molecular species within the human gut. Appl Environ Microbiol 1999, 65:4799-4807.

23. Vanhoutte T, De Preter V, De Brandt E, Verbeke K, Swings J, Huys G: Molecular monitoring of the fecal microbiota of healthy human subjects during administration of lactulose and Saccharomyces boulardii. Appl Environ Microbiol 2006, 72:5990-5997.

24. Andersson AF, Lindberg M, Jakobsson H, Bäckhed F, Nyrén P, Engstrand L: Comparative analysis of human gut microbiota by barcoded pyrosequencing. PLoS One 2008, 3:e2836.

25. Armougom F, Raoult D: Use of pyrosequencing and DNA barcodes to monitor variations in Firmicutes and Bacteroidetes communities in the gut microbiota of obese humans. BMC Genomics 2008, 9:576.

26. Tannock GW, Munro K, Bibiloni R, Simon MA, Hargreaves P, Gopal P, Harmsen H, Welling G: Impact of consumption of oligosaccharide-containing biscuits on the fecal microbiota of humans. Appl Environ Microbiol 2004, 70:2129-2136.

27. Malinen E, Kassinen A, Rinttilä T, Palva A: Comparison of real-time PCR with SYBR Green I or 5'-nuclease assays and dot-blot hybridization with rDNA-targeted oligonucleotide probes in quantification of selected faecal bacteria. Microbiology 2003, 149:269-277.

28. Bartosch S, Fite A, Macfarlane GT, McMurdo ME: Characterization of bacterial communities in feces from healthy elderly volunteers and hospitalized elderly patients by using real-time PCR and effects of antibiotic treatment on the fecal microbiota. Appl Environ Microbiol 2004, 70:3575-3581.

29. Matsuki T, Watanabe K, Fujimoto J, Kado Y, Takada T, Matsumoto K, Tanaka R: Quantitative PCR with 16S rRNA-gene-targeted species-specific primers for analysis of human intestinal bifidobacteria. Appl Environ Microbiol 2004, 70:167-173.

30. Schell MA, Karmirantzou M, Snel B, Vilanova D, Berger B, Pessi G, Zwahlen MC, Desiere F, Bork P, Delley M, Pridmore RD, Arigoni F: The genome sequence of Bifidobacterium longum reflects its adaptation to the human gastrointestinal tract. Proc Natl Acad Sci USA 2002, 99:14422-14427.

31. Xu J, Bjursell MK, Himrod J, Deng S, Carmichael LK, Chiang HC, Hooper LV, Gordon JI: A genomic view of the human-Bacteroides thetaiotaomicron symbiosis. Science 2003, 299:2074-2076.

32. Pridmore RD, Berger B, Desiere F, Vilanova D, Barretto C, Pittet AC, Zwahlen MC, Rouvet M, Altermann E, Barrangou R, Mollet B, Mercenier A, Klaenhammer T, Arigoni F, Schell MA: The genome sequence of the probiotic intestinal bacterium Lactobacillus johnsonii NCC 533. Proc Natl Acad Sci USA 2004, 101:2512-2517.

33. Holmes E, Wilson ID, Nicholson JK: Metabolic phenotyping in health and disease. Cell 2008, 134:714-717.

34. Nicholson JK, Lindon JC, Holmes E: Metabonomics: understanding the metabolic responses of living systems to pathophysiological stimuli via multivariate statistical analysis of biological NMR spectroscopic data. Xenobiotica 1999, 29:1181-1189.

35. Wang Y, Tang H, Nicholson JK, Hylands PJ, Sampson J, Holmes E: A metabonomic strategy for the detection of the metabolic effects of chamomile (Matricaria recutita L.) ingestion. J Agric Food Chem 2005, 53:191-196.

36. Marchesi JR, Holmes E, Khan F, Kochhar S, Scanlan P, Shanahan F, Wilson ID, Wang Y: Rapid and noninvasive metabonomic characterization of inflammatory bowel disease. J Proteome Res 2007, 6:546-551.

37. Martin FP, Dumas ME, Wang Y, Legido-Quigley C, Yap IK, Tang H, Zirah S, Murphy GM, Cloarec O, Lindon JC, Sprenger N, Fay LB, Kochhar S, van Bladeren P, Holmes E, Nicholson JK: A top-down systems biology view of microbiome-mammalian metabolic interactions in a mouse model. Mol Syst Biol 2007, 3:112.

38. Martin FP, Wang Y, Sprenger N, Holmes E, Lindon JC, Kochhar S, Nicholson JK: Effects of probiotic Lactobacillus paracasei treatment on the host gut tissue metabolic profiles probed via magic-angle-spinning NMR spectroscopy. J Proteome Res 2007, 6:1471-1481.

39. Martin FP, Wang Y, Sprenger N, Yap IK, Lundstedt T, Lek P, Rezzi S, Ramadan Z, van Bladeren P, Fay LB, Kochhar S, Lindon JC, Holmes E, Nicholson JK: Probiotic modulation of symbiotic gut microbial-host metabolic interactions in a humanized microbiome mouse model. Mol Syst Biol 2008, 4:157.

40. De Lacy Costello B, Ewen R, Ewer AK, Garner CE, Probert CSJ, Ratcliffe NM, Smith S: An analysis of volatiles in the headspace of the faeces of neonates. J Breath Res 2008, 2:1-8.

41. Garner EC, Smith S, Costello BL, White P, Spencer R, Probert CSJ, Ratcliffe NM: Volatile organic compounds from feces and their potential for diagnosis of gastrointestinal disease. Faseb J 2007, 21:1675-1688.

42. Probert HM, Gibson GR: Investigating the prebiotic and gas-generating effects of selected carbohydrates on the human colonic microflora. Lett Appl Microbiol 2002, 35:473-480.

43. Candela M, Perna F, Carnevali P, Vitali B, Ciati R, Gionchetti P, Rizzello F, Campieri M, Brigidi P: Interaction of probiotic Lactobacillus and Bifidobacterium strains with human intestinal epithelial cells: adhesion properties, competition against enteropathogens and modulation of IL-8 production. Int J Food Microbiol 2008, 125:286-292.

44. Roselli M, Finamore A, Nuccitelli S, Carnevali P, Brigidi P, Vitali B, Nobili F, Rami R, Garaguso I, Mengheri E: Prevention of TNBS-induced colitis by different Lactobacillus and Bifidobacterium strains is associated with an expansion of gammadeltaT and regulatory T cells of intestinal intraepithelial lymphocytes. Inflamm Bowel Dis 2009, 15:1526-1536.

45. Saito Y, Sakamoto M, Takizawa S, Benno Y: Monitoring the cell number and viability of Lactobacillus helveticus GCL1001 in human feces by PCR methods. FEMS Microbiol Lett 2004, 231:125-130.

46. Ndagijimana M, Vallicelli M, Cocconcelli PS, Cappa F, Patrignani F, Lanciotti R, Guerzoni ME: Two 2[5H]-furanones as possible signaling molecules in Lactobacillus helveticus. Appl Environ Microbiol 2006, 72:6053-6061.

47. Wong JMW, Jenkins DJA: Carbohydrate digestibility and metabolic effects. J Nutr 2007, 137(suppl):2539-2546.

48. Pettersson J, Karlsson PC, Göransson U, Rafter JJ, Bohlin L: The flavouring phytochemical 2-pentanone reduces prostaglandin production and COX-2 expression in colon cancer cells. Biol Pharm Bull 2008, 31:534-537.

49. Ott A, Germond JE, Chaintreau A: Vicinal diketone formation in yogurt: 13C precursors and effect of branched-chain amino acids. J Agric Food Chem 2000, 48:724-731.

50. Diczfalusy MA, Björkhem I, Einarsson C, Hillebrant CG, Alexson SE: Characterization of enzymes involved in formation of ethyl esters of long-chain fatty acids in humans. J Lipid Res 2001, 42:1025-1032.

51. Walter J, Tannock GW, Tilsala-Timisjarvi A, Rodtong S, Loach DM, Munro K, Alatossava T: Detection and identification of gastrointestinal Lactobacillus species by using denaturing gradient gel electrophoresis and species-specific PCR primers. Appl Environ Microbiol 2000, 66:297-303.

52. Vitali B, Pugliese C, Biagi E, Candela M, Turroni S, Bellen G, Donders GGG, Brigidi P: Dynamics of vaginal bacterial communities in women developing bacterial

vaginosis, candidiasis, or no infection, analyzed by PCR-denaturing gradient gel electrophoresis and real-time PCR. Appl Environ Microbiol 2007, 73:5731-5741.

53. Bassam BJ, Caetano-Anollés G, Gresshoff PM: Fast and sensitive silver staining of DNA in polyacrylamide gels. Anal Biochem 1991, 196:80-83.

54. Kok RG, de Waal A, Schut F, Welling GW, Weenk G, Hellingwerf KJ: Specific detection and analysis of a probiotic Bifidobacterium strain in infant feces. Appl Environ Microbiol 1996, 62:3668-3672.

55. Walter J, Hertel C, Tannock GW, Lis CM, Munro K, Hammes WP: Detection of Lactobacillus, Pediococcus, Leuconostoc and Weissella species in human feces by using group-specific PCR primers and denaturing gradient gel electrophoresis. Appl Environ Microbiol 2001, 67:2578-2585.

56. Heilig HGHJ, Zoetendal EG, Vaughan EE, Marteau P, Akkermans ADL, de Vos WM: Molecular diversity of Lactobacillus spp. and other lactic acid bacteria in the human intestine as determined by specific amplification of 16S ribosomal DNA. Appl Environ Microbiol 2002, 68:114-123.

57. Altermann E, Russel WM, Azcarate-Peril MA, Barrangou R, Buck BL, McAuliffe O, Souther N, Dobson A, Duong T, Callanan M, Lick S, Hamrick A, Cano R, Klaenhammer TR: Complete genome sequence of the probiotic lactic acid bacterium Lactobacillus acidophilus NCFM. Proc Natl Acad Sci USA 2005, 102:3906-3912.

58. Callanan M, Kaleta P, O'Callaghan J, O'Sullivan O, Jordan K, McAuliffe O, Sangrador-Vegas A, Slattery L, Fitzgerald GF, Beresford T, Ross RP: Genome sequence of Lactobacillus helveticus, an organism distinguished by selective gene loss and insertion sequence element expansion. J Bacteriol 2008, 190:727-735.

59. Jansen JJ, Hoefsloot HCJ, Greef J, Timmerman ME, Smilde AK: Multilevel component analysis of time-resolved metabolic fingerprint data. Anal Chim Acta 2005, 530:173-183.

60. Anderson MJ, Willis TJ: Canonical analysis of principal coordinates: a useful method of constrained ordination for ecology. Ecology 2003, 84:511-525.

61. Anderson MJ, Robinson J: Generalized discriminant analysis based on distances. Aust Nz J Stat 2003, 45:301-318.

62. Lindon JC, Nicholson JK, Holmes E, Keun HC, Craig A, Pearce JT, Bruce SJ, Hardy N, Sansone SA, Antti H, Jonsson P, Daykin C, Navarange M, Beger RD, Verheij ER, Amberg A, Baunsgaard D, Cantor GH, Lehman-McKeeman L, Earll M, Wold S, Johansson E, Haselden JN, Kramer K, Thomas C, Lindberg J, Schuppe-Koistinen I, Wilson ID, Reily MD, Robertson DG, Senn H, Krotzky A, Kochhar S, Powell J, Ouderaa F, Plumb R, Schaefer H, Spraul M: Summary recommendations for standardization and reporting of metabolic analyses. Nat Biotechnol 2005, 23:833-838.

There are several supplemental files that are not available in this version of the article. To view this additional information, please use the citation information cited on the first page of this chapter.

CHAPTER 10

DIET-MICROBIOTA INTERACTIONS AND THEIR IMPLICATIONS FOR HEALTHY LIVING

IAN B. JEFFERY AND PAUL W. O'TOOLE

10.1 INTRODUCTION

The gastrointestinal tract contains a diverse microbial community, which is predominantly bacterial and which is referred to as the gut microbiota. Over the last decade, the microbial composition of the gut has been the subject of increasingly intense research, much due to its demonstrated impact upon various health conditions. The Human Microbiome Project (HMP), MetaHIT (Metagenome of Human Intestinal Tract) and the smaller ELDERMET project, as well as numerous labs around the world (Table 1), have taken advantage of new high-throughput technologies to thoroughly characterise the human microbiome from multiple body sites at every stage of life. A number of these projects employed whole-community shotgun sequencing to study the gene content of the microbial populations. Through these studies, it has become apparent that these microorganisms are not just passive residents of the gut, but carry out a range of biological functions that are important in the nutrition and well-being of the individual.

This chapter was originally published under the Creative Commons Attribution License. Jeffery IB and O'Toole PW. Diet-Microbiota Interactions and Their Implications for Healthy Living. Nutrients *5 (2013); pp. 234-252. doi:10.3390/nu5010234.*

TABLE 1: Microbiome consortiums

Program	Duration	Funding Organization	Conditions of Interest
NIH Jumpstart Program	2007–2008	NIH, USA	Generate 200 complete bacterial genome sequences and perform compositional analysis of various body regions.
NIH Human Microbiome Project	2007	NIH Roadmap Program, USA	Characterize the microbes on the human body and correlate the changes in these microbial populations with human health.
DACC—Data Analysis and Coordination Center	2008–2013	NIH Human Microbiome Project (HMP), USA	Assist in standardization of data pipelines (storage, analysis and display of data) and provide access to data.
MetaHIT, Metagenomics of the Human Intestinal Tract	2008–2011	European Commission (FP7)	Describe the role of the microbiota in Inflammatory Bowel Disease (IBD) and obesity, and generate a reference catalogue of intestinal microbial genes.
Canadian Human Microbiome Initiative	2009	Canadian Institutes of Health Research (CIHR), Canada	A number of projects relating to human microbial interactions and their effect on health.
The Australian Jumpstart Human Microbiome Project	2009	Commonwealth Scientific and Industrial Research Organisation (CSIRO), Australia	Sequencing of specific bacterial strains and the application of metagenomics techniques to investigate the interaction between intestinal microbes and their host.
MicroObes, Human Intestinal Microbiome in Obesity and Nutritional Transition	2008–2010	French National Agency for Research (ANR), France	Identify metagenomic signatures that characterise the relationship between the intestinal microbiota and the nutritional and metabolic status of the host.
Korean Microbiome Diversity Using Korean Twin Cohort Project	2010–2015	National Research Foundation of Korea, Korea	Determine the microbiomes on various epithelial sites of the human body using Korean Twin Cohort and investigate the relationship between human microbiomes and disease. To establish a dedicated centre for Korean microbiome information and analysis.
ELDERMET Project	2007–2013	National Development Food Research Health Initiative and Science Foundation Ireland	Characterize the faecal microbiota associated with ageing and correlate diversity, composition, and metabolic potential of the faecal microbial metagenome with health, diet and lifestyle.

The most heavily studied part of the gut is the distal colon, through the use of high-throughput next-generation technologies and phylochips to characterise faecal derived populations. In adults, this population is characterised by the predominance of two phyla, *Bacteroidetes* and *Firmicutes,* with minor contributions from the *Proteobacteria* and *Actinobacteria* [1]. However, it is known that the microbial content of the gut changes along its length, with the small intestine containing a higher relative abundance of members of the *Actinobacteria* and *Streptococcaceae* [2]. Autochthonous bacteria have evolved within the gut to form a mutually beneficial relationship with their human hosts. Considering the size of the human gut and the density of bacteria that it contains, the nature of this relationship is very relevant. The bacteria in the gut have developed a number of adaptations for living in this unique environment, such as mechanisms for avoiding or modulating inflammatory responses [3]. On the other side of this interaction paradigm, evolution in the host has taken the form of Toll-like receptors (TLR) that are used to identify bacteria (and other antigens) and to respond appropriately as part of an innate and adaptive immune system [4]. The host also produces a complex polymeric barrier or mucin layer that separates the bacteria from the epithelium [5,6]. A number of studies have examined the core human microbiota within the gut, which may be operationally defined as those microbes that are found in a majority of individuals [7]. Qin et al. (2010) [8] found that there are 1000 to 1150 prevalent bacterial species, with each individual harbouring at least 160 species. This translated to 3.3 million non-host-encoded genes of which 99% were of bacterial origin, with ~536,000 prevalent unique bacterial genes in each individual of which 40% would be shared with at least half of the individuals in their cohort. Annotation suggests that these microbial genes are involved in the production of essential metabolites and the degradation and utilisation of complex carbohydrates and biosynthesis of vitamins [8,9].

There are significant inter-individual differences in the presence and absence of the bacterial species found in the gastrointestinal tract. There are a number of highly abundant species that are present in the majority of a population, but the overall composition of the gut depends on the age, health, diet and even geographical location of the individual [10]. These bacteria have a substantial scope to modify the phenotype of the individual though production of metabolites and through interaction with the physiology of the individual in a diverse number of ways. Thus, dietary modulation of the gut microbiota composition and function will have implications for the host phenotype.

10.2 MICROBIOTA AND DIET

A number of studies have examined the relationship between the faecal microbiota and diet. De Filippo et al. (2011) [11] showed that the faecal microbiota in a cohort of Italian children was different to that found in children in a rural village in Burkina Faso. Similar to the different microbial populations reported by the ELDERMET consortium [12], Italian children, who consume less plant-based foods, harboured more *Bacteroides* and *Alistipes* in their microbiota. The microbiota of the rural Burkina Faso children had an abundance of bacteria from the genus *Prevotella,* similar to the healthier diet individuals in the ELDERMET cohort. The Burkina Faso children also harboured significantly higher levels of faecal short-chain fatty acid producers than the Italian children. Interestingly *Xylanibacter*, which was absent in the ELDERMET and Italian microbiota communities, but was present in the Burkina Faso children, is known to contain a set of genes for cellulose and xylan hydrolysis. The main fibres that reach the distal colon and are utilized by the gut microbiota and their enzymes are carbohydrates and proteins that are refractory to host digestion. The level of metabolic activity in the microbiota will depend on how much of these materials are making it down into the gut. Although the microbiota will respond to short-term changes in the diet, the long-term changes seem to define what type of microbial population is present and this in turn determines the metabolites produced and the potential impact on the health of the host [13].

Filippo et al. (2011) [11] hypothesized that the gut microbiota co-evolved with the polysaccharide-rich diet of Burkina Faso individuals, allowing them to maximize energy intake from dietary fibre, while also dampening inflammation and protecting them from non-infectious colonic diseases. Wu et al. (2011) [13] also found that the microbiota composition was strongly associated with long-term diet, with *Bacteroides* being associated with diets enriched in animal products. The *Prevotella* genus was associated with diets that contained more plant-based foods. All three studies (older persons—ELDERMET [12]; Burkina Faso versus Italian children [11]; and American adults [13]) found similar microbiota-diet associations at three different stages of life, showing that the diet modulates the microbiota regardless of gender or other confounding factors.

A study performed in the mouse model also showed that switching from a low-fat, plant polysaccharide diet to a high fat, high sugar, Western-style diet lead to alterations in the microbiome and its metabolic function [14]. The high plant polysaccharide diets are full of resistant starch and oligosaccharides that the microbiota can utilise [15] and have been shown to affect the abundances of a number of microbes [16]. Subjects fed resistant starch type 2 from high amylose maize showed an increased abundance of *Ruminococcus* spp. and *Eubacterium rectale*, while consumption of resistant starch type 3 (water-insoluble semi-crystalline structures formed from amylose) promoted the growth of *Eubacterium rectale, Roseburia* spp. and *Ruminococcus bromii*. These species are able to bind directly to insoluble starch particles and to degrade them and may be the key species in bacterial food chains that target starch [17]. A detailed description on the mechanisms involved in the breakdown of fibre is beyond the scope of this review, but has been recently described [15].

10.3 AGE-RELATED GUT MICROBIOTA CHANGES

The microbiota composition is not stable over the whole life-time of an individual. At the extremities of life, a number of discernible patterns of microbiota change have been recorded. Since the microbiota and its metabolic activities react and change according to diet, some of these age-related microbiota composition changes may be attributable to diet. The diet in elderly individuals can change for a number of reasons, including loss of sensation of taste and smell, tooth loss and chewing difficulties. These changes may result in an increased consumption of high sugar/high fat foods and a reduction in the proportion of plant-based foods consumed. Although diet-related microbiota changes undoubtedly occur at all life stages, the majority of the research performed to date has been focused on healthy or diseased adults, with fewer investigations having been carried out on children and the elderly. However, in the younger and older subjects in the population, the observed microbial changes can be more dramatic, and so these are an excellent source of information on associations between health and the microbiota. This is particularly true for the study of the development and decline of microbial populations. How these populations change depends on how they are modulated. A recent study by the ELDERMET consortium has focused on elderly individuals, whose dietary patterns were found to change for a number of reasons, one of the most dramatic being the change in diet going into long-term residential care [12]. Within and between the community living subjects and those in long-term care, we uncovered an association between an increase in the microbiota diversity in the gut and a diet rich in healthy foods, as defined by the Healthy Food Diversity index (HFD [18]). Conversely, diets with a low HFD score were associated with microbiota populations that were less diverse and had predicted reduced functionality and so potentially conferring fewer benefits to the respective individual. As well as a difference in diversity levels, there were differences in the dominant genera present in the different subject groups. The microbiota associated with diets rich in plant-based foods were abundant in *Prevotella*, while the individuals with a lower HFD harboured more *Bacteroides*. A further reduction in the HFD scores associated with individuals living in long-term care resulted in *Parabacteroides* and *Alistipes* becoming the dominant *Bacteroidetes* genera. These microbiota alterations were associated with changes in frailty, inflammation and altered abundances of short chain fatty acids (SCFAs) producers, as well as correlations with other clinical markers [12].

Intestinal microbiota composition may also vary in elderly subjects independently of diet for a number of physiological and immunological factors, such as a reduction in the immune system functionality [19–21]. This is indicated in the reduced abundance of *Ruminococcus* and *Blautia* spp. and the increased abundance of *Escherichia* in the elderly when compared to young controls [12]. It has been previously reported that the microbiota associated with elderly individuals has a reduced abundance of several butyrate producers (Key members of *Clostridium* cluster XIVa and *Clostridium* cluster IV) when compared to younger individuals [22,23]. This was confirmed in the ELDERMET study, where it was shown that the oldest and frailest individuals had significantly lower copy numbers of genes related to butyrate, acetate and propionate production in the faecal metagenome [12]. The age-related increase in the proportion of facultative anaerobes, including *Escherichia* amongst other genera, has also been noted in previous studies. These bacteria are present at low levels in healthy young adults, but are present in increased abundances in the inflamed gut [22,24,25].

10.4 DIETARY MODULATION

As global life expectancy increases, it is important to maintain quality of life and independence in the elderly. The study of older persons is starting to provide a wealth of information and more complete understanding of their diet-microbiota interactions. This provides the possibility of modulating the microbiota to benefit health. The mechanisms of dietary modulation of the microbiota include the physical ability of high fibre diets to increase faecal bulk, which is one of the factors that affects transit time along the gut. Jumpertz et al. (2011) [26] have shown that the human gut microbiota can undergo long-term changes that occur over a couple of days when there is a significant increase in the calorie intake of the individual. Transit time itself affects the composition of the human faecal microbiota because, as the transit time decreases, there is a decrease in the proportions of slow growing species, such as methanogens, and an increase in sulphate reducing bacteria counts, while concentrations of total SCFAs are increased, leading to a lowering of faecal pH [27]. But, more importantly, the macronutrient composition of the ingested food determines which species flourish and which taxa will be able to colonise the gut and, so, determines the eventual composition of the microbiota.

For new taxa to become established and abundant in a stable gut ecosystem, their functionality must permit them to thrive in the presence of other organisms that are competing for resources. At the most basic level, this functionality is conferred by the presence and absence of genes. Autochthonous bacteria have coevolved with the human host and each other to perform important roles in nutrient and energy extraction and energy regulation that the host would otherwise be unable to accomplish. There are numerous positive interspecies associations in the gut [12,28], probably due to adaptation to similar substrate-availability and flow-rate environments and to cross-feeding between different organisms [29]. The importance of cross-feeding between different organisms was demonstrated by Samuel and Gordon [30] when they investigated the utilization of polysaccharides by *Bacteroides thetaiotaomicron* in germ-free mice colonized in the presence and absence of *Methanobrevibacter smithii* or the sulphate-reducing bacterium *Desulfovibrio piger.* They found that *M. smithii* directs *B. thetaiotaomicron* to focus on fermentation of dietary fructans to acetate, whereas *B. thetaiotaomicron*-derived formate is used by *M. smithii* for methanogenesis. *B. thetaiotaomicron–M. smithii* co-colonization resulted in increased weight gain and energy harvest when compared to mice colonised by *B. thetaiotaomicron* alone or by *B. thetaiotaomicron* and *D. piger.* Indeed, this type of crossfeeding is an important and widespread phenomenon [12,28,31]. This suggests that targeted dietary modulation of species will affect populations of microbes within the microbiota and, so, modulate energy harvest, storage and expenditure. The microbiota also affects energy balance through metabolites that its members produce. The produced metabolic outputs from the community will depend on what species/genes are present and expressed and what substrates are available to the microbiota [32].

10.5 PRODUCTION OF METABOLITES

The gut microbiota performs many functions in the breakdown of complex carbohydrates and the generation of beneficial metabolites. This is made possible by the large array of genes that encode enzymes that are essential to these processes. Germ-free animals that do not contain a microbiota/microbiome still survive and reproduce, but their diet must contain a higher quantity and diversity of essential nutrients to maintain their health [33].

In conventional mice and normal humans, resistant starch and oligosaccharides that are undigested in the small intestine may be utilised in the large intestine by bacteria to produce SCFAs. There are a number of SCFAs that are produced; the most abundant being acetate, propionate and butyrate [34]. These are taken up by the host and may provide up to 10%

of its energy requirements. Butyrate is absorbed by colonocytes and other cells of the colonic epithelium [35], thus providing energy to the host from dietary components that would otherwise pass undigested through the gut. In fact, if colonocytes are deprived of butyrate, they undergo autophagy [36]. Acetate and propionate are taken up by the circulatory system and, so, are utilized by the general physiology, i.e., not just the intestine. Acetate is oxidized in the citric acid cycle [37], and propionate is incorporated into glucose metabolism. As well as being absorbed by the host, SCFAs have been shown to affect transit time through modulation of gut motility [38,39] and to affect insulin sensitivity and energy expenditure, giving them a link to metabolic syndrome [40].

High amounts of SCFAs may decrease the intestinal pH [41] and prevent the growth of potentially pathogenic bacteria, such as *E. coli* and other members of the *Enterobacteriaceae* [42]. While a number of gut bacteria are tolerant of lower pH values, such as a number of the *Firmicutes* species, especially those belonging to *Clostridium* cluster XIVa [43], this low pH tolerance is not a feature of many *Bacteroidetes* spp. and *Bifidobacterium* spp. [43], thus making SCFA production a potential modulator of these taxa. The increased concentration of SCFAs may also help in the absorption of minerals, such as calcium, by increasing their solubility and increasing the expression of calcium binding proteins [44]. Butyrate also exerts an anti-inflammatory [45] and anti-carcinogenic effect [46] in these cells. SCFAs may also be involved in the control of appetite, as they can be detected by receptors expressed in the gut called free fatty acid receptor 2 (FFAR2) and free fatty acid receptor 3 (FFAR3) [47]. These, in turn, regulate hormones involved in appetite control; thus, the microbiota and its production of SCFAs may have a role to play in food intake of an individual [47].

The microbiota is involved in the production and absorption of essential vitamins and micronutrients. It has been established that the levels of essential vitamins, such as folate and biotin, may be higher in individuals than their diet would suggest/support. This can be attributed to microbial production of folate and biotin, as well as a number of vitamins, including other water soluble B vitamins and vitamin K [48]. It was assumed that, as these vitamins were produced in the colon, they would not be absorbed, but excreted. This notion was challenged with the discovery of colonic transporters for biotin [49], thiamine [50], riboflavin [51], pyridoxine [52] and folate [53].

Folate is important in synthesis, repair and methylation of DNA and is necessary for cell division and growth. The primary mechanism for dietary folate absorption is its deconjugation to monoglutamates and subsequent absorption by active transport carriers in the small intestine, but evidence suggests that a similar mucosal transport mechanism operates in the colon [53]. Many microorganisms in the large intestine are capable of synthesizing folate. Furthermore, it has been shown that the infant colon contains pools of readily absorbed monoglutamylated folate [54]. A number of studies have indicated that resistant carbohydrate is utilized by the bacteria in the colon in the biosynthesis of folate, particularly *Bifidobacterium bifidum* and *Bifidobacterium longum* subsp. *infantis* [55–57]. A number of other B-group vitamins that are synthesised by members of the microbiota and that may be produced in the gut include riboflavin, vitamin B12, niacin and pyridoxine [58].

Vitamin K is a group of structurally similar, fat-soluble compounds that are important co-factors in the post-translational modification of certain proteins required for blood coagulation and in metabolic pathways. Microbial conversion of the plant derived vitamin K1 (phylloquinone) to vitamin K2 (menaquinone) is believed to be facilitated by a number of species in the human gut [59–61].

10.6 DIET, MICROBIOTA AND FUNCTIONAL BOWEL DISORDERS

There is growing interest in the concept of dietary modulation of the microbiota for improving health. In modern society, disorders with plausible links to microbiota alterations are increasing, such as Irritable Bowel Syndrome (IBS) and obesity [14,62–64]. Irritable Bowel Syndrome (IBS) is the most common of the functional bowel disorders and affects a significant percentage of the population of the industrial world [65]. Although originally thought to be a psychosomatic disorder, it is now regarded as multi-factorial, with genetic, neurological and psychosocial elements, all potentially contributing to symptomology [66]. It is becoming increasingly recognised that low-grade inflammation [67,68] and changes in the gut microbiota are present in a majority of patients, reinforced by observations that probiotic and antibiotic intervention may be effective in reducing the severity of the IBS symptoms [69,70]. A microbiota re-configuration associated with the majority of IBS-related microbiotas has been confirmed by several studies using high throughput technologies to determine the alterations of the microbiota of the distal bowel in IBS compared to healthy subjects [63,71–73].

Dietary modulation of the microbiota in IBS and functional bloating is of particular interest due to the reported decrease in symptoms associated with the use of the Low FODMAP diet in the treatment of IBS [74]. FODMAP is an acronym derived from Fermentable, Oligo-, Di-, Mono-saccharides and Polyols [75]. This diet focuses on reducing the consumption of rapidly fermentable, short-chain carbohydrates that are poorly absorbed in the small intestine, namely fructose (monosaccharide), lactose (disaccharide), fructans and galactans (oligosaccharides) and polyols, such as sorbitol, maltitol, xylitol and mannitol [76]. Poor absorption occurs for a number of reasons; (a) fructose is only slowly absorbed due to low-capacity transport mechanisms across the epithelium [77]; (b) there is a lack of hydrolases of fructans and galactans; and (c) there are no specific transporters for polyols and these molecules are too large for uptake by passive diffusion. For lactose, a proportion of the population is unable to hydrolase the molecule, but this proportion depends on ethnicity [78].

The FODMAPs diet removes these rapidly fermentable substrates altogether or uses breath tests to stratify individuals based on their absorption of fructose and lactose [79]. Interestingly, this test has been also used to detect small intestinal bacterial overgrowth (SIBO; [80]), the eradication of which has been shown to alleviate the symptoms of IBS [65]. There is limited data to suggest that fructose malabsorption and SIBO might have a bidirectional cause-effect relationship, but nevertheless, upon the administration of fructose, there is an increase in the hydrogen produced as measured by the breath test and an increase in the concentration of acetate found in the blood [76], which may be produced by *E. coli* [81]. It has been shown that a diet that contains no substrates for bacteria to ferment alleviates IBS symptoms in 85% of cases, accompanied by a normalisation of the lactulose breath test, an indicator of SIBO [82].

At the time of writing, there is no information on how consumption of a FODMAPs diet would affect the microbiota signature detected in faecal samples of IBS subjects. It has been shown that when individuals are fed a high FODMAP diet, a significant proportion of the substrates will pass through the small intestine to the proximal colon [83]. This increased substrate in the proximal colon may explain the reported increased microbial production of SCFAs by the microbiota of IBS subjects [84–86]. Many of the faecal microbiota taxa that have been shown to be associated with IBS, such as *Ruminococcaceae* and *Clostridium* cluster XIVa, are known to be enriched for species that produce SCFAs [87]. As described previously, SCFAs are essential to the normal functioning of the gut, but there is some evidence that abnormally high levels of butyrate can promote visceral hypersensitivity [88] and high levels of SCFAs can cause powerful contractions in the terminal ileum [89]. These observations are of clinical relevance, given the association of IBS with visceral hypersensitivity and dysmotility.

The FODMAPs diet alleviates the symptoms of IBS better than other healthy eating advice, with the majority of individuals on the diet reporting improved symptoms [90]. It has not been shown that the diet normalises the individual, and we may speculate that a resumption of the normal diet will result in a resumption of the original symptoms. However, the FODMAPs diet has been shown to be an effective way to alleviate symptoms of functional gastrointestinal disorders.

With regard to food related issues that may have a causative effect, there is a perception among IBS sufferers that they may suffer from food intolerance or allergy, and this leads many IBS subjects to initiate a variety of dietary changes [91]. Altering of diets in this regard is common, with 20%–70% of IBS sufferers self-reporting one or more food intolerances [92]. Despite this, clinically validated food hypersensitivity appears to be relatively uncommon in IBS [93], but, when detected, the removal of the offending foods has been associated with a reduction or a complete elimination of symptoms [94,95]. However, the mechanism of action of the FODMAPs diet may explain why IBS symptoms may be eased by a gluten free diet [96], because this diet is low in content of cereals that contain high levels of FODMAP substrates.

10.7 OBESITY AND METABOLIC DISORDER

Although the development of obesity and insulin resistance is complex, with many genetic and environmental factors involved [97–103], it is associated with the presence of chronic inflammation in visceral adipose tissue, which is believed to be a leading promoter of insulin resistance in obesity. Studies, primarily in animals, have demonstrated that a number of microbial factors may be associated with the development of metabolic disorder and diabetes [104]. Cani et al. (2008) [105] showed that genetically obese ob/ob mice, which are characterised by obesity and insulin resistance, showed an improvement in insulin sensitivity and inflammatory parameters when treated with antibiotics.

Turnbaugh et al. (2009) [106] reported that obesity is associated with microbial compositional changes at the phylum level. They found that individuals with high BMIs had a lower proportion of *Bacteroidetes* and a higher proportion of *Actinobacteria* when compared to leaner individuals. This agreed with their previous study on obese mice, where they found a 50% reduction in the abundance of *Bacteroidetes* and a proportional increase in Firmicutes [107] and also agreed with major findings of another study of humans in 2006, where they detected a decreased relative proportion of *Bacteroidetes* in obese individuals [108]. However, a number of studies have failed to confirm these associations and have reported the opposite association [109] or found no association at all [26,110].

Studies have shown that the composition of the diet and the amount of calories consumed are strong modifiers of the microbiota. Zhang et al. (2010) [111] examined genetic susceptibility, diet and weight gain and how they affect the microbiota in Apoa-1 knockout mice compared to wild-type and reported that the majority of the microbiota changes that were detected were associated with the diet [111]. This dietary effect was almost five-times the effect of the genetic susceptibility, reinforcing the traditional view of the dietary impact on weight. However, without a microbiota, germ-free animals are resistant to high-fat diet-induced obesity and metabolic syndrome [112] and genetically identical animals respond differently to a high fat diet [113]. This phenotypic independent association of the microbiota was demonstrated using Sprague-Dawley rats that were found to be obesity-prone or obesity-resistant, depending on their microbiota composition. The obesity-prone rats exhibited increased TLR4 activation, which was associated with ileal inflammation [114], as well as a decrease in intestinal alkaline phosphatase, a luminal enzyme that detoxifies lipopolysaccharide (LPS). This resulted in increased localization of occludin in the cytoplasm of epithelial cells and phosphorylation of the myosin light chain, which is associated with increased intestinal permeability [114]. Furthermore, there were increased concentrations of plasma LPS in the circulatory systems of the rats. It was concluded that the consumption of a high-fat diet induces the changes in the gut microbiota, but the development of inflammation was associated with the appearance of hyperphagia and an obese phenotype. This was confirmed in a subsequent study, where it was shown that infusing a low level of LPS for four weeks caused weight gain and insulin resistance without a high-fat diet [115]. Further evidence was provided by Serino et al. (2012) [116], who showed that when genetically identical mice were fed a fat-enriched carbohydrate-free diet, not all mice developed insulin resistance. The subgroup of mice that did show a marked change in insulin sensitivity also presented with a modified gut microbiota. This microbiota (and the increased insulin resistance) was associated with increased gut permeability, increased endotoxaemia and systemic/adipose tissue inflammation. The associated global microbiota changes can be summarised as an inverted *Bacteroidetes* to *Firmicutes* ratio with a reduction in the proportional abundance of the *Lachnospiracaea* family and *Oscillibacter* genus in the insulin resistant subgroup. Qin et al. (2012) [117] described a decrease in the abundance of butyrate-producing bacteria and an increase in various opportunistic pathogens, as well as an enrichment of other microbial functions conferring sulphate reduction and oxidative stress resistance in diabetic individuals. They did not, however, comment on the association with diet.

The microbiota also affects the expenditure and storage of the nutrients through the expression of genes in the host, such as fasting-induced adipocyte factor (Fiaf). Fiaf is a circulating lipoprotein lipase inhibitor that induces circulating lipoprotein lipase to hydrolyse circulating triacylglycerols to free fatty acids [118]. Bäckhed et al. (2007) [112] investigated obesity associated with a western-style, high fat, high sugar diet in mice and showed that mice responded with increased adiposity, but that animals that were germ-free were protected from obesity. This resistance disappeared in germ-free knockout mice lacking the Fiaf gene and, so, were not protected from the diet-induced obesity. This evidence points to an unfavourable dietary modification of the microbiota being related to the onset of hyperphagia, obesity, insulin resistance and metabolic syndrome.

10.8 CONCLUSION

Although it has been known for some time that the microbiota performs numerous biological functions that affect the metabolic functions of the host, it is only within the last number of years that the importance of this is becoming apparent. Our intestinal microbial community can affect the rate of deposition and utilization of fat, insulin resistance and diabetes and our inflammation state, as well as our general health and wellbeing. Over recent years, large observational studies and animals trials in combination with high throughput technologies have been used to identify and understand the impact of environmental factors, such as diet and genotype, on controlling the microbiota. The importance of the association of the microbiota and its functions with diet cannot be over-stated in the light of the monumental shifts in diets that have occurred in a very short evolutionarily timeframe. These diets are continuing to change, and it is now estimated that in the United States, a sizeable proportion of individuals consume very little vegetables, with less than half of individuals reporting eating vegetables at dinner. Even less of these individuals include vegetables in lunch foods, like sandwiches and wraps [119]. It may be that our consumption of processed foods, widespread use of antibiotics and disinfectants and our modern lifestyle may have forever altered our ancient gut microbiome. We may never be able to identify or restore our microbiomes to their ancestral state, but dietary modulation to manipulate specific gut microbial species or groups of species may offer new therapeutic approaches to conditions that are prevalent in modern society, such as functional gastrointestinal disorders, obesity and maybe even age-related under-nutrition. We predict that this will become an increasingly important area of health research.

REFERENCES

1. Eckburg, P.B.; Bik, E.M.; Bernstein, C.N.; Purdom, E.; Dethlefsen, L.; Sargent, M.; Gill, S.R.; Nelson, K.E.; Relman, D.A. Diversity of the human intestinal microbial flora. Science 2005, 308, 1635–1638.

2. Frank, D.N.; St Amand, A.L.; Feldman, R.A.; Boedeker, E.C.; Harpaz, N.; Pace, N.R. Molecular-phylogenetic characterization of microbial community imbalances in human inflammatory bowel diseases. Proc. Natl. Acad. Sci. USA 2007, 104, 13780–13785.

3. Mathis, D.; Benoist, C. Microbiota and autoimmune disease: The hosted self. Cell Host Microbe 2011, 10, 297–301.

4. Hooper, L.V.; Macpherson, A.J. Immune adaptations that maintain homeostasis with the intestinal microbiota. Nat. Rev. Immunol. 2010, 10, 159–169.

5. Hansson, G.C.; Johansson, M.E. The inner of the two Muc2 mucin-dependent mucus layers in colon is devoid of bacteria. Gut Microbes 2010, 1, 51–54.

6. Johansson, M.E.; Phillipson, M.; Petersson, J.; Velcich, A.; Holm, L.; Hansson, G.C. The inner of the two Muc2 mucin-dependent mucus layers in colon is devoid of bacteria. Proc. Natl. Acad. Sci. USA 2008, 105, 15064–15069.

7. Tap, J.; Mondot, S.; Levenez, F.; Pelletier, E.; Caron, C.; Furet, J.-P.; Ugarte, E.; Muñoz-Tamayo, R.; Paslier, D.L.; Nalin, R.; et al. Towards the human intestinal microbiota phylogenetic core. Environ. Microbiol. 2009, 11, 2574–2584.

8. Qin, J.; Li, R.; Raes, J.; Arumugam, M.; Burgdorf, K.S.; Manichanh, C.; Nielsen, T.; Pons, N.; Levenez, F.; Yamada, T.; et al. A human gut microbial gene catalogue established by metagenomic sequencing. Nature 2010, 464, 59–65.

9. Human Microbiome Project Consortium. Structure, function and diversity of the healthy human microbiome. Nature 2012, 486, 207–214.

10. Yatsunenko, T.; Rey, F.E.; Manary, M.J.; Trehan, I.; Dominguez-Bello, M.G.; Contreras, M.; Magris, M.; Hidalgo, G.; Baldassano, R.N.; Anokhin, A.P.; et al. Human gut microbiome viewed across age and geography. Nature 2012, 486, 222–227.

11. De Filippo, C.; Cavalieri, D.; di Paola, M.; Ramazzotti, M.; Poullet, J.B.; Massart, S.; Collini, S.; Pieraccini, G.; Lionetti, P. Impact of diet in shaping gut microbiota revealed by a comparative study in children from Europe and rural Africa. Proc. Natl. Acad. Sci. USA 2010, 107, 14691–14696.

12. Claesson, M.J.; Jeffery, I.B.; Conde, S.; Power, S.E.; O'Connor, E.M.; Cusack, S.; Harris, H.M.B.; Coakley, M.; Lakshminarayanan, B.; O'Sullivan, O.; et al. Gut microbiota composition correlates with diet and health in the elderly. Nature 2012, 488, 178–184.

13. Wu, G.D.; Chen, J.; Hoffmann, C.; Bittinger, K.; Chen, Y.-Y.; Keilbaugh, S.A.; Bewtra, M.; Knights, D.; Walters, W.A.; Knight, R.; et al. Linking long-term dietary patterns with gut microbial enterotypes. Science 2011, 334, 105–108.

14. Turnbaugh, P.J.; Ley, R.E.; Mahowald, M.A.; Magrini, V.; Mardis, E.R.; Gordon, J.I. An obesity-associated gut microbiome with increased capacity for energy harvest. Nature 2006, 444, 1027–1131.

15. Flint, H.J.; Scott, K.P.; Duncan, S.H.; Louis, P.; Forano, E. Microbial degradation of complex carbohydrates in the gut. Gut Microbes 2012, 3, 289–306.

16. Flint, H.J. The impact of nutrition on the human microbiome. Nutr. Rev. 2012, 70, S10–S13.
17. Leitch, E.C.; Walker, A.W.; Duncan, S.H.; Holtrop, G.; Flint, H.J. Selective colonization of insoluble substrates by human faecal bacteria. Environ. Microbiol. 2007, 9, 667–679.
18. Drescher, L.S.; Thiele, S.; Mensink, G.B. A new index to measure healthy food diversity better reflects a healthy diet than traditional measures. J. Nutr. 2007, 137, 647–651.
19. Guigoz, Y.; Doré, J.; Schiffrin, E.J. The inflammatory status of old age can be nurtured from the intestinal environment. Curr. Opin. Clin. Nutr. Metab. Care 2008, 11, 13–20.
20. Tiihonen, K.; Ouwehand, A.C.; Rautonen, N. Human intestinal microbiota and healthy ageing. Ageing Res. Rev. 2010, 9, 107–116.
21. Ostan, R.; Bucci, L.; Capri, M.; Salvioli, S.; Scurti, M.; Pini, E.; Monti, D.; Franceschi, C. Immunosenescence and immunogenetics of human longevity. Neuroimmunomodulation 2008, 15, 224–240.
22. Biagi, E.; Nylund, L.; Candela, M.; Ostan, R.; Bucci, L.; Pini, E.; Nikkïla, J.; Monti, D.; Satokari, R.; Franceschi, C.; et al. Through ageing, and beyond: Gut microbiota and inflammatory status in seniors and centenarians. PLoS One 2010, 5, e10667.
23. Mäkivuokko, H.; Tiihonen, K.; Tynkkynen, S.; Paulin, L.; Rautonen, N. The effect of age and non-steroidal anti-inflammatory drugs on human intestinal microbiota composition. Br. J. Nutr. 2010, 103, 227–234.
24. Mueller, S.; Saunier, K.; Hanisch, C.; Norin, E.; Alm, L.; Midtvedt, T.; Cresci, A.; Silvi, S.; Orpianesi, C.; Verdenelli, M.C.; et al. Differences in fecal microbiota in different European study populations in relation to age, gender, and country: A cross-sectional study. Appl. Environ. Microbiol. 2006, 72, 1027–1033.
25. Mariat, D.; Firmesse, O.; Levenez, F.; Guimarães, V.; Sokol, H.; Doré, J.; Corthier, G.; Furet, J.-P. The Firmicutes/Bacteroidetes ratio of the human microbiota changes with age. BMC Microbiol. 2009, 9, doi:10.1186/1471-2180-9-123.
26. Jumpertz, R.; Le, D.S.; Turnbaugh, P.J.; Trinidad, C.; Bogardus, C.; Gordon, J.I.; Krakoff, J. Energy-balance studies reveal associations between gut microbes, caloric load, and nutrient absorption in humans. Am. J. Clin. Nutr. 2011, 94, 58–65.
27. El Oufir, L.; Flourié, B.; Bruley des Varannes, S.; Barry, J.L.; Cloarec, D.; Bornet, F.; Galmiche, J.P. Relations between transit time, fermentation products, and hydrogen consuming flora in healthy humans. Gut 1996, 38, 870–877.
28. Faust, K.; Sathirapongsasuti, J.F.; Izard, J.; Segata, N.; Gevers, D.; Raes, J.; Huttenhower, C. Microbial co-occurrence relationships in the human microbiome. PLoS Comput. Biol. 2012, 8, e1002606.
29. Flint, H.J.; Duncan, S.H.; Scott, K.P.; Louis, P. Interactions and competition within the microbial community of the human colon: Links between diet and health. Environ. Microbiol. 2007, 9, 1101–1111.
30. Samuel, B.S.; Gordon, J.I. A humanized gnotobiotic mouse model of host-archaeal-bacterial mutualism. Proc. Natl. Acad. Sci. USA 2006, 103, 10011–10016.
31. Jeffery, I.B.; Claesson, M.J.; O'Toole, P.W.; Shanahan, F. Categorization of the gut microbiota: Enterotypes or gradients? Nat. Rev. Microbiol. 2012, 10, 591–592.

32. Louis, P.; Scott, K.P.; Duncan, S.H.; Flint, H.J. Understanding the effects of diet on bacterial metabolism in the large intestine. J. Appl. Microbiol. 2007, 102, 1197–1208.

33. Marks, T.; Farkas, W.R. Effects of a diet deficient in tyrosine and queuine on germ-free mice. Biochem. Biophys. Res. Commun. 1997, 230, 233–237.

34. Topping, D.L.; Clifton, P.M. Short-chain fatty acids and human colonic function: Roles of resistant starch and nonstarch polysaccharides. Physiol. Rev. 2001, 81, 1031–1064.

35. Soergel, K.H.; Ruppin, H.; Bar-Meir, S.; Wood, C.M.; Schmitt, M.G., Jr. N-butyrate absorption in the human colon. Dig. Dis. Sci. 1982, 27, 90–92.

36. Donohoe, D.R.; Garge, N.; Zhang, X.; Sun, W.; O'Connell, T.M.; Bunger, M.K.; Bultman, S.J. The microbiome and, butyrate regulate energy metabolism and autophagy in the mammalian colon. Cell Metab. 2011, 13, 517–526.

37. Skutches, C.L.; Sigler, M.H.; Teehan, B.P.; Cooper, J.H.; Reichard, G.A. Contribution of dialysate acetate to energy metabolism: Metabolic implications. Kidney Int. 1983, 23, 57–63.

38. Scheppach, W. Effects of short chain fatty acids on gut morphology and function. Gut 1994, 35, S35–S38.

39. Lewis, S.J.; Heaton, K.W. Increasing, butyrate concentration in the distal colon by accelerating intestinal transit. Gut 1997, 41, 245–251.

40. Gao, Z.; Yin, J.; Zhang, J.; Ward, R.E.; Martin, R.J.; Lefevre, M.; Cefalu, W.T.; Ye, J. Butyrate improves insulin sensitivity and increases energy expenditure in mice. Diabetes 2009, 58, 1509–1517.

41. Ghosh, S.; Dai, C.; Brown, K.; Rajendiran, E.; Makarenko, S.; Baker, J.; Ma, C.; Halder, S.; Montero, M.; Ionescu, V.A.; et al. Colonic microbiota alters host susceptibility to infectious colitis by modulating inflammation, redox status, and ion transporter gene expression. Am. J. Physiol. Gastrointest. Liver Physiol. 2011, 301, G39–G49.

42. Zimmer, J.; Lange, B.; Frick, J.-S.; Sauer, H.; Zimmermann, K.; Schwiertz, A.; Rusch, K.; Klosterhalfen, S.; Enck, P. A vegan or vegetarian diet substantially alters the human colonic faecal microbiota. Eur. J. Clin. Nutr. 2012, 66, 53–60.

43. Duncan, S.H.; Louis, P.; Thomson, J.M.; Flint, H.J. The role of pH in determining the species composition of the human colonic microbiota. Environ. Microbiol. 2009, 11, 2112–2122.

44. Scholz-Ahrens, K.E.; Ade, P.; Marten, B.; Weber, P.; Timm, W.; Açil, Y.; Glüer, C.-C.; Schrezenmeir, J. Prebiotics, probiotics, and synbiotics affect mineral absorption, bone mineral content, and bone structure. J. Nutr. 2007, 137, 838S–846S.

45. Ogawa, H.; Rafiee, P.; Fisher, P.J.; Johnson, N.A.; Otterson, M.F.; Binion, D.G. Butyrate modulates gene and protein expression in human intestinal endothelial cells. Biochem. Biophys. Res. Commun. 2003, 309, 512–519.

46. Whitehead, R.H.; Young, G.P.; Bhathal, P.S. Effects of short chain fatty acids on a new human colon carcinoma cell line (LIM1215). Gut 1986, 27, 1457–1463.

47. Sleeth, M.L.; Thompson, E.L.; Ford, H.E.; Zac-Varghese, S.E.; Frost, G. Free fatty acid receptor 2 and nutrient sensing: A proposed role for fibre, fermentable carbohydrates and short-chain fatty acids in appetite regulation. Nutr. Res. Rev. 2010, 23, 135–145.

48. Hill, M.J. Intestinal flora and endogenous vitamin synthesis. Eur. J. Cancer Prev. 1997, 6, S43–S45.
49. Said, H.M.; Ortiz, A.; McCloud, E.; Dyer, D.; Moyer, M.P.; Rubin, S. Biotin uptake by human colonic epithelial NCM460 cells: A carrier-mediated process shared with pantothenic acid. Am. J. Physiol. 1998, 275, C1365–C1371.
50. Said, H.M.; Ortiz, A.; Subramanian, V.S.; Neufeld, E.J.; Moyer, M.P.; Dudeja, P.K. Mechanism of thiamine uptake by human colonocytes: Studies with cultured colonic epithelial cell line NCM460. Am. J. Physiol. Gastrointest. Liver Physiol. 2001, 281, G144–G150.
51. Said, H.M.; Ortiz, A.; Moyer, M.P.; Yanagawa, N. Riboflavin uptake by human-derived colonic epithelial NCM460 cells. Am. J. Physiol. Cell Physiol. 2000, 278, C270–C276.
52. Said, Z.M.; Subramanian, V.S.; Vaziri, N.D.; Said, H.M. Pyridoxine uptake by colonocytes: A specific and regulated carrier-mediated process. Am. J. Physiol. Cell Physiol. 2008, 294, C1192–C1197.
53. Dudeja, P.K.; Torania, S.A.; Said, H.M. Evidence for the existence of a carrier-mediated folate uptake mechanism in human colonic luminal membranes. Am. J. Physiol. 1997, 272, G1408–G1415.
54. Kim, T.H.; Yang, J.; Darling, P.B.; O'Connor, D.L. A large pool of available folate exists in the large intestine of human infants and piglets. J. Nutr. 2004, 134, 1389–1394.
55. Pompei, A.; Cordisco, L.; Amaretti, A.; Zanoni, S.; Matteuzzi, D.; Rossi, M. Folate production by bifidobacteria as a potential probiotic property. Appl. Environ. Microbiol. 2007, 73, 179–185.
56. Pompei, A.; Cordisco, L.; Amaretti, A.; Zanoni, S.; Raimondi, S.; Matteuzzi, D.; Rossi, M. Administration of folate-producing bifidobacteria enhances folate status in Wistar rats. J. Nutr. 2007, 137, 2742–2746.
57. Strozzi, G.P.; Mogna, L. Quantification of folic acid in human feces after administration of Bifidobacterium probiotic strains. J. Clin. Gastroenterol. 2008, 42, S179–S184.
58. Leblanc, J.G.; Milani, C.; de Giori, G.S.; Sesma, F.; van Sinderen, D.; Ventura, M. Bacteria as vitamin suppliers to their host: A gut microbiota perspective. Curr. Opin. Biotechnol. 2012, in press.
59. Mathers, J.C.; Fernandez, F.; Hill, M.J.; McCarthy, P.T.; Shearer, M.J.; Oxley, A. Dietary modification of potential vitamin K supply from enteric bacterial menaquinones in rats. Br. J. Nutr. 1990, 63, 639–652.
60. Morishita, T.; Tamura, N.; Makino, T.; Kudo, S. Production of menaquinones by lactic acid bacteria. J. Dairy Sci. 1999, 82, 1897–1903.
61. Ramotar, K.; Conly, J.M.; Chubb, H.; Louie, T.J. Production of menaquinones by intestinal anaerobes. J. Infect. Dis. 1984, 150, 213–218.
62. Duchmann, R.; Kaiser, I.; Hermann, E.; Mayet, W.; Ewe, K.; Meyer zum Büschenfelde, K.H. Tolerance exists towards resident intestinal flora, but is broken in active inflammatory bowel disease (IBD). Clin. Exp. Immunol. 1995, 102, 448–455.
63. Jeffery, I.B.; O'Toole, P.W.; Öhman, L.; Claesson, M.J.; Deane, J.; Quigley, E.M.; Simrén, M. An irritable bowel syndrome subtype defined by species-specific alterations in faecal microbiota. Gut 2012, 61, 997–1006.

64. Isolauri, E. Development of healthy gut microbiota early in life. J. Paediatr. Child. Health 2012, 48, 1–6.
65. Pimentel, M.; Chow, E.J.; Lin, H.C. Eradication of small intestinal bacterial over-growth reduces symptoms of irritable bowel syndrome. Am. J. Gastroenterol. 2000, 95, 3503–3506.
66. Chang, L. The role of stress on physiological responses and clinical symptoms in irritable bowel syndrome. Gastroenterology 2011, 140, 761–765.
67. Brint, E.K.; MacSharry, J.; Fanning, A.; Shanahan, F.; Quigley, E.M. Differential expression of toll-like receptors in patients with irritable bowel syndrome. Am. J. Gastroenterol. 2011, 106, 329–336.
68. Langhorst, J.; Junge, A.; Rueffer, A.; Wehkamp, J.; Foell, D.; Michalsen, A.; Musial, F.; Dobos, G.J. Elevated human beta-defensin-2 levels indicate an activation of the innate immune system in patients with irritable bowel syndrome. Am. J. Gastroen-terol. 2009, 104, 404–410.
69. Pimentel, M.; Lembo, A.; Chey, W.D.; Zakko, S.; Ringel, Y.; Yu, J.; Mareya, S.M.; Shaw, A.L.; Bortey, E.; Forbes, W.P. Rifaximin therapy for patients with irritable bowel syndrome without constipation. N. Engl. J. Med .2011, 364, 22–32.
70. Quigley, E.M. Therapies aimed at the gut microbiota and inflammation: antibiotics, prebiotics, probiotics, synbiotics, anti-inflammatory therapies. Gastroenterol. Clin. North Am. 2011, 40, 207–222.
71. Rajilić-Stojanović, M.; Biagi, E.; Heilig, H.G.; Kajander, K.; Kekkonen, R.A.; Tims, S.; de Vos, W.M. Global and deep molecular analysis of microbiota signatures in fecal samples from patients with irritable bowel syndrome. Gastroenterology 2011, 141, 1792–1801.
72. Salonen, A.; de Vos, W.M.; Palva, A. Gastrointestinal microbiota in irritable bowel syndrome: Present state and perspectives. Microbiology 2010, 156, 3205–3215.
73. Jeffery, I.B.; Quigley, E.M.; Ohman, L.; Simrén, M.; O'Toole, P.W. The microbiota link to irritable bowel syndrome: An emerging story. Gut Microbes 2012, 3, 572–576.
74. Gibson, P.R.; Shepherd, S.J. Evidence-based dietary management of functional gas-trointestinal symptoms: The FODMAP approach. J. Gastroenterol. Hepatol. 2010, 25, 252–258.
75. Gibson, P.R.; Shepherd, S.J. Personal view: Food for thought—Western lifestyle and susceptibility to Crohn's disease. The FODMAP hypothesis. Aliment. Pharmacol. Ther. 2005, 21, 1399–1409.
76. Rumessen, J.J.; Gudmand-Høyer, E. Fructans of chicory: Intestinal transport and fermentation of different chain lengths and relation to fructose and sorbitol malab-sorption. Am. J. Clin. Nutr. 1998, 68, 357–364.
77. Gibson, P.R.; Newnham, E.; Barrett, J.S.; Shepherd, S.J.; Muir, J.G. Review article: Fructose malabsorption and the bigger picture. Aliment. Pharmacol. Ther. 2007, 25, 349–363.
78. Itan, Y.; Jones, B.L.; Ingram, C.J.; Swallow, D.M.; Thomas, M.G. A worldwide corre-lation of lactase persistence phenotype and genotypes. BMC Evol. Biol. 2010, 10, 36.
79. Bate, J.P.; Irving, P.M.; Barrett, J.S.; Gibson, P.R. Benefits of breath hydrogen test-ing after lactulose administration in analysing carbohydrate malabsorption. Eur. J. Gastroenterol. Hepatol. 2010, 22, 318–326.

80. Rana, S.V.; Sharma, S.; Kaur, J.; Sinha, S.K.; Singh, K. Comparison of lactulose and glucose breath test for diagnosis of small intestinal bacterial overgrowth in patients with irritable bowel syndrome. Digestion 2012, 85, 243–247.

81. Luli, G.W.; Strohl, W.R. Comparison of growth, acetate production, and acetate inhibition of Escherichia coli strains in batch and fed-batch fermentations. Appl. Environ. Microbiol. 1990, 56, 1004–1011.

82. Pimentel, M.; Constantino, T.; Kong, Y.; Bajwa, M.; Rezaei, A.; Park, S. A 14-day elemental diet is highly effective in normalizing the lactulose breath test. Dig. Dis. Sci. 2004, 49, 73–77.

83. Barrett, J.S.; Gearry, R.B.; Muir, J.G.; Irving, P.M.; Rose, R.; Rosella, O.; Haines, M.L.; Shepherd, S.J.; Gibson, P.R. Dietary poorly absorbed, short-chain carbohydrates increase delivery of water and fermentable substrates to the proximal colon. Aliment. Pharmacol. Ther. 2010, 31, 874–882.

84. Mortensen, P.B.; Andersen, J.R.; Arffmann, S.; Krag, E. Short-chain fatty acids and the irritable bowel syndrome: The effect of wheat bran. Scand. J. Gastroenterol. 1987, 22, 185–192.

85. Treem, W.R.; Ahsan, N.; Kastoff, G.; Hyams, J.S. Fecal short-chain fatty acids in patients with diarrhea-predominant irritable bowel syndrome: In vitro studies of carbohydrate fermentation. J. Pediatr. Gastroenterol. Nutr. 1996, 23, 280–286.

86. Malinen, E.; Rinttilä, T.; Kajander, K.; Mättö, J.; Kassinen, A.; Krogius, L.; Saarela, M.; Korpela, R.; Palva, A. Analysis of the fecal microbiota of irritable bowel syndrome patients and healthy controls with real-time PCR. Am. J. Gastroenterol. 2005, 100, 373–382.

87. Louis, P.; Young, P.; Holtrop, G.; Flint, H.J. Diversity of human colonic, butyrate-producing bacteria revealed by analysis of the, butyryl-CoA:acetate CoA-transferase gene. Environ. Microbiol. 2010, 12, 304–314.

88. Bourdu, S.; Dapoigny, M.; Chapuy, E.; Artigue, F.; Vasson, M.-P.; Dechelotte, P.; Bommelaer, G.; Eschalier, A.; Ardid, D. Rectal instillation of, butyrate provides a novel clinically relevant model of noninflammatory colonic hypersensitivity in rats. Gastroenterology 2005, 128, 1996–2008.

89. Kamath, P.S.; Phillips, S.F.; Zinsmeister, A.R. Short-chain fatty acids stimulate ileal motility in humans. Gastroenterology 1988, 95, 1496–1502.

90. Staudacher, H.M.; Whelan, K.; Irving, P.M.; Lomer, M.C. Comparison of symptom response following advice for a diet low in fermentable carbohydrates (FODMAPs) versus standard dietary advice in patients with irritable bowel syndrome. J. Hum. Nutr. Diet. 2011, 24, 487–495.

91. Monsbakken, K.W.; Vandvik, P.O.; Farup, P.G. Perceived food intolerance in subjects with irritable bowel syndrome—Etiology, prevalence and consequences. Eur. J. Clin. Nutr. 2006, 60, 667–672.

92. El-Salhy, M. Diet and effects of diet management on quality of life and symptoms in patients with irritable bowel syndrome. Mol. Med. Rep. 2012, 5, 1382–1390.

93. Vighi, G.; Marcucci, F.; Sensi, L.; di Cara, G.; Frati, F. Allergy and the gastrointestinal system. Clin. Exp. Immunol. 2008, 153, 3–6.

94. Carroccio, A.; Brusca, I.; Mansueto, P.; Soresi, M.; D'Alcamo, A.; Ambrosiano, G.; Pepe, I.; Iacono, G.; Lospalluti, M.L.; La Chiusa, S.M.; di Fede, G. Fecal assays detect hypersensitivity to cow's milk protein and gluten in adults with irritable bowel syndrome. Clin. Gastroenterol. Hepatol. 2011, 9, 965–971.

95. Guo, H.; Jiang, T.; Wang, J.; Chang, Y.; Guo, H.; Zhang, W. The value of eliminating foods according to food-specific immunoglobulin G antibodies in irritable bowel syndrome with diarrhoea. J. Int. Med. Res. 2012, 40, 204–210.

96. Biesiekierski, J.R.; Newnham, E.D.; Irving, P.M.; Barrett, J.S.; Haines, M.; Doecke, J.D.; Shepherd, S.J.; Muir, J.G.; Gibson, P.R. Gluten causes gastrointestinal symptoms in subjects without celiac disease: A double-blind randomized placebo-controlled trial. Am. J. Gastroenterol. 2011, 106, 508–514.

97. Frayling, T.M.; Timpson, N.J.; Weedon, M.N.; Zeggini, E.; Freathy, R.M.; Lindgren, C.M.; Perry, J.R.; Elliott, K.S.; Lango, H.; Rayner, N.W.; et al. A common variant in the FTO gene is associated with body mass index and predisposes to childhood and adult obesity. Science 2007, 316, 889–894.

98. Cecil, J.E.; Tavendale, R.; Watt, P.; Hetherington, M.M.; Palmer, C.N. An obesity-associated FTO gene variant and increased energy intake in children. N. Engl. J. Med. 2008, 359, 2558–2566.

99. Chambers, J.C.; Elliott, P.; Zabaneh, D.; Zhang, W.; Li, Y.; Froguel, P.; Balding, D.; Scott, J.; Kooner, J.S. Common genetic variation near MC4R is associated with waist circumference and insulin resistance. Nat. Genet. 2008, 40, 716–718.

100. Loos, R.J.; Lindgren, C.M.; Li, S.; Wheeler, E.; Zhao, J.H.; Prokopenko, I.; Inouye, M.; Freathy, R.M.; Attwood, A.P.; Beckmann, J.S.; et al. Common variants near MC4R are associated with fat mass, weight and risk of obesity. Nat. Genet. 2008, 40, 768–775.

101. Meyre, D.; Delplanque, J.; Chèvre, J.-C.; Lecoeur, C.; Lobbens, S.; Gallina, S.; Durand, E.; Vatin, V.; Degraeve, F.; Proença, C.; et al. Genome-wide association study for early-onset and morbid adult obesity identifies three new risk loci in European populations. Nat. Genet. 2009, 41, 157–159.

102. Thorleifsson, G.; Walters, G.B.; Gudbjartsson, D.F.; Steinthorsdottir, V.; Sulem, P.; Helgadottir, A.; Styrkarsdottir, U.; Gretarsdottir, S.; Thorlacius, S.; Jonsdottir, I.; et al. Genome-wide association yields new sequence variants at seven loci that associate with measures of obesity. Nat. Genet. 2009, 41, 18–24.

103. Willer, C.J.; Speliotes, E.K.; Loos, R.J.; Li, S.; Lindgren, C.M.; Heid, I.M.; Berndt, S.I.; Elliott, A.L.; Jackson, A.U.; Lamina, C.; et al. Six new loci associated with body mass index highlight a neuronal influence on body weight regulation. Nat. Genet. 2009, 41, 25–34.

104. Tilg, H.; Kaser, A. Gut microbiome, obesity, and metabolic dysfunction. J. Clin. Invest. 2011, 121, 2126–2132.

105. Cani, P.D.; Bibiloni, R.; Knauf, C.; Waget, A.; Neyrinck, A.M.; Delzenne, N.M.; Burcelin, R. Changes in gut microbiota control metabolic endotoxemia-induced inflammation in high-fat diet-induced obesity and diabetes in mice. Diabetes 2008, 57, 1470–1481.

106. Turnbaugh, P.J.; Hamady, M.; Yatsunenko, T.; Cantarel, B.L.; Duncan, A.; Ley, R.E.; Sogin, M.L.; Jones, W.J.; Roe, B.A.; Affourtit, J.P.; et al. A core gut microbiome in obese and lean twins. Nature 2009, 457, 480–484.

107. Ley, R.E.; Bäckhed, F.; Turnbaugh, P.; Lozupone, C.A.; Knight, R.D.; Gordon, J.I. Obesity alters gut microbial ecology. Proc. Natl. Acad. Sci. USA 2005, 102, 11070–11075.

108. Ley, R.E.; Turnbaugh, P.J.; Klein, S.; Gordon, J.I. Microbial ecology: Human gut microbes associated with obesity. Nature 2006, 444, 1022–1023.

109. Schwiertz, A.; Taras, D.; Schäfer, K.; Beijer, S.; Bos, N.A.; Donus, C.; Hardt, P.D. Microbiota and SCFA in lean and overweight healthy subjects. Obesity (Silver Spring) 2010, 18, 190–195.

110. Duncan, S.H.; Lobley, G.E.; Holtrop, G.; Ince, J.; Johnstone, A.M.; Louis, P.; Flint, H.J. Human colonic microbiota associated with diet, obesity and weight loss. Int. J. Obes. (Lond.) 2008, 32, 1720–1724.

111. Zhang, C.; Zhang, M.; Wang, S.; Han, R.; Cao, Y.; Hua, W.; Mao, Y.; Zhang, X.; Pang, X.; Wei, C.; et al. Interactions between gut microbiota, host genetics and diet relevant to development of metabolic syndromes in mice. ISME J. 2010, 4, 232–241.

112. Bäckhed, F.; Manchester, J.K.; Semenkovich, C.F.; Gordon, J.I. Mechanisms underlying the resistance to diet-induced obesity in germ-free mice. Proc. Natl. Acad. Sci. USA 2007, 104, 979–984.

113. De La Serre, C.B.; Ellis, C.L.; Lee, J.; Hartman, A.L.; Rutledge, J.C.; Raybould, H.E. Propensity to high-fat diet-induced obesity in rats is associated with changes in the gut microbiota and gut inflammation. Am. J. Physiol. Gastrointest. Liver Physiol. 2010, 299, G440–G448.

114. Shen, L.; Black, E.D.; Witkowski, E.D.; Lencer, W.I.; Guerriero, V.; Schneeberger, E.E.; Turner, J.R. Myosin light chain phosphorylation regulates barrier function by remodeling tight junction structure. J. Cell Sci. 2006, 119, 2095–2106.

115. Cani, P.D.; Amar, J.; Iglesias, M.A.; Poggi, M.; Knauf, C.; Bastelica, D.; Neyrinck, A.M.; Fava, F.; Tuohy, K.M.; Chabo, C.; et al. Metabolic endotoxemia initiates obesity and insulin resistance. Diabetes 2007, 56, 1761–1772.

116. Serino, M.; Luche, E.; Gres, S.; Baylac, A.; Bergé, M.; Cenac, C.; Waget, A.; Klopp, P.; Iacovoni, J.; Klopp, C.; et al. Metabolic adaptation to a high-fat diet is associated with a change in the gut microbiota. Gut 2012, 61, 543–553.

117. Qin, J.; Li, Y.; Cai, Z.; Li, S.; Zhu, J.; Zhang, F.; Liang, S.; Zhang, W.; Guan, Y.; Shen, D.; et al. A metagenome-wide association study of gut microbiota in type 2 diabetes. Nature 2012, 490, 55–60.

118. Bäckhed, F.; Ding, H.; Wang, T.; Hooper, L.V.; Koh, G.Y.; Nagy, A.; Semenkovich, C.F.; Gordon, J.I. The gut microbiota as an environmental factor that regulates fat storage. Proc. Natl. Acad. Sci. USA 2004, 101, 15718–15723.

119. Satia, J.A.; Kristal, A.R.; Patterson, R.E.; Neuhouser, M.L.; Trudeau, E. Psychosocial factors and dietary habits associated with vegetable consumption. Nutrition 2002, 18, 247–254.

PART V

USING THE MICROBIOME TO IDENTIFY AND CURE DISEASE

CHAPTER 11

PREBIOTICS, FECAL TRANSPLANTS AND MICROBIAL NETWORK UNITS TO STIMULATE BIODIVERSITY OF THE HUMAN GUT MICROBIOME

PIETER VAN DEN ABBEELE, WILLY VERSTRAETE, SAHAR EL AIDY, ANNELIES GEIRNAERT, AND TOM VAN DE WIELE

11.1 INTRODUCTION

Over the last decades, specific mechanisms of how the human gut microbiome determines human health or disease states have been elucidated (Round and Mazmanian, 2009). It has become clear that the dynamic interaction with these intestinal microbes can be divided in different stages over the human lifespan (Fig. 1). Drastic changes occur during the first years of life as the newborn gut progresses from a sterile environment to a densely populated microbial habitat. This gut ecosystem exerts restrictive selection on its microbial inhabitants as only microbes that are capable of establishing a mutualistic relation with the host are maintained (Backhed et al., 2005; Ley et al., 2008). In human infancy and early childhood, the complex microbial ecosystem is formed through the successive establishment of different bacterial groups; aerotolerant bacteria establish first,

This chapter was originally published under the Creative Commons Attribution License. Van den Abbeele P, Verstraete W, El Aidy S, Geirnaert A, and Van de Wiele T. Prebiotics, Faecal Transplants and Microbial Network Units to Stimulate Biodiversity of the Human Gut Microbiome. Microbial Biotechnology 6:4 (2013); pp. 335–340. doi:10.1111/1751-7915.12049.

followed by more and more strict anaerobes, as observed in ex-germfree reductionist animal models (Adlerberth and Wold, 2009). As a result, the infant gastrointestinal microbiota is quite variable in its composition and relatively unstable over time. On average, 3 years after birth the microbial community consists of a mixture of microbes that is largely similar to that found in the adult intestine (Yatsunenko etal., 2012). At that time, the complex microbiota is predominantly colonized by obligate anaerobes to provide a strong barrier against the establishment and proliferation of new bacterial groups, in a phenomena known as colonization resistance (Vollaard and Clasener, 1994). The colonizing microbes can rapidly shape themselves in response to changes in host environment. Likewise, when the host environment changes, the immune system and metabolic profile must adjust to these fluctuations in order to keep a mutualistic relationship with its microbiota. Although individual-specific and relatively stable in younger healthy adults, the microbiota in elderly displays greater inter-individual variation (Claesson etal., 2011). Such high variation correlates with immunosenescence, which characterizes the ageing process (Claesson etal., 2012). Moreover, once its symbiotic coexistence is disrupted during acute (e.g. invasion of pathogens or antibiotic treatment) or chronic conditions (e.g. inflammatory bowel diseases and obesity), the microbial community may become a major threat to the host.

This raises the question of how to restore the microbial dysbiosis and the resulting imbalance in the host–microbe symbiotic relationship when things go wrong. Existing approaches to manage the human gut microbiome include functional foods such as probiotics, prebiotics and synbiotics. While probiotics are beneficial live microorganisms (FAO/WHO, 2002), prebiotics are indigestible food compounds that selectively stimulate specific beneficial microbial genus(era)/species already present in the gut (Gibson and Roberfroid, 1995; Roberfroid etal., 2010). Unfortunately, antibiotics are still commonly prescribed causing severe disturbances in the microbiome. A very promising therapeutic approach is the use of faecal transplants, which allows to install a healthy, diverse gut microbiome in a human subject that suffered from a severely dysbiosed gut microbiota. In this mini-review, we emphasize the importance of biodiversity and, in this context, re-define the current prebiotic concept. We also propose a novel ecosystem-based approaches to restore host–microbial imbalances in

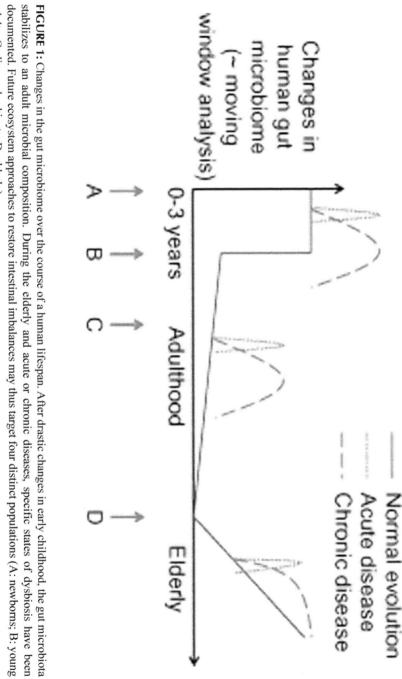

FIGURE 1: Changes in the gut microbiome over the course of a human lifespan. After drastic changes in early childhood, the gut microbiota stabilizes to an adult microbial composition. During the elderly and acute or chronic diseases, specific states of dysbiosis have been documented. Future ecosystem approaches to restore intestinal imbalances may thus target four distinct populations (A: newborns; B: young adults; C: diseased subjects; D: elderly).

disease based on the success of faecal transplants, i.e. by providing specific microbial network units.

11.2 THE BIODIVERSITY CONCEPT

Biodiversity is generally considered crucial for the well-functioning of an ecosystem. This is also valid for the microbial ecosystem of the human gut where a decreased diversity has been correlated with disease states such as recurrent Clostridium difficile infection (Chang et al., 2008), Crohn's disease (Manichanh et al., 2006) and obesity (Turnbaugh et al., 2009). A recent study by Yatsunenko and colleagues (2012) elucidated that US residents have a markedly less diverse microbiota than human subjects living in ancient geographic locations.

This lower microbial diversity is caused by several typical Western society practices. Everything starts at birth, as caesarean sections are becoming a common mode of delivery. In 2010, almost one-third of the births in the USA was through caesarean delivery (Martin et al., 2012). This deprives the newborn from being exposed to a broad spectrum of vaginal microbes resulting in lower intestinal microbial diversity in the gut microbiome of the newborn (Biasucci et al., 2008). Moreover, breast-feeding is often replaced by formula milk despite the fact that breast milk is essential for the early microbial development by providing nutrients for early-life symbionts (e.g. bifidobacteria) (Sela and Mills, 2010) and even by providing live bacteria (Cabrera-Rubio et al., 2012). Misuse of antibiotic treatments (Dethlefsen et al., 2008) further contributes to the decreased microbial diversity in the human gut microbiome. Another microbial exposure route that has been decreasing in the last decades is exposure via the drinking water. In most countries, drinking water is sterilized by the addition of chlorine. In countries such as the Netherlands and Switzerland water is not disinfected. Although drinking water may not contain real gut commensals, drinking chlorinated water instead of non-disinfected water raises questions regarding immune system education capacity. The question is often raised whether public health, fitness or capacity to excel might relate to the issue of natural versus chlorinated water, but is still not documented properly. This issue certainly deserves appropriate study.

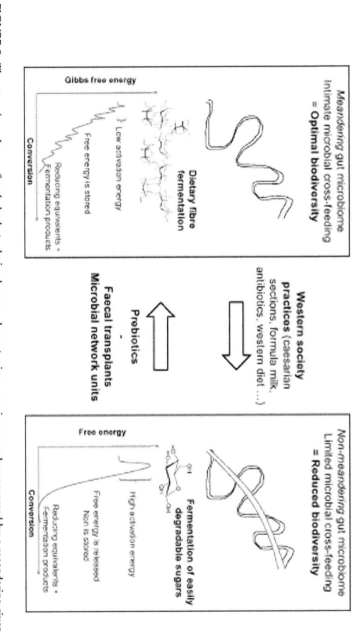

FIGURE 2: The stepwise release of carbohydrate-derived energy by gut microorganisms can be compared by a meandering river in which the water potential energy is gradually lowered. Such an environment creates many functional niches thereby selecting for a high microbial diversity, similar to a high biological diversity in meandering river ecosystem. Shortcuts through microbial metabolic meanders in the human gut can be compared with the canalization of a meandering river. Such environment entails a limited amount of functional niches thereby selecting for a limited microbial diversity.

The Western diet that is unbalanced and too homogeneous in composition also contributes to a lower microbial diversity and eventually does not support the co-evolved host–microbe partnership (De Filippo et al., 2010). The non-digestible fraction consists of substrates that do not require complex metabolic interactions between members of the gut microbial ecosystem. This results in rapid release of nutritional energy by a limited amount of microbes. In contrast, diets that have a high dietary fibre content do support microbial diversity as this stimulates microbial interactions through which nutrient-derived energy is harvested in different stages by different microbial members. This can be compared with the dissipation of potential energy over several meanders in a river system. We therefore state that a healthy well-structured microbiome is characterized by a meandering metabolism (Fig. 2). Such slow release of nutritional energy is characteristic for high fibre diets which may protect against inflammation and non-infectious colonic diseases (De Filippo et al., 2010). In contrast, the typical Western diet results in dissipation of the nutrient-derived energy through shortcuts in such metabolic meanders. In terms of the ecological r/K-selection theory (Pianka, 1970), this selects for a higher abundance of r-strategists: microorganisms that have a low substrate affinity but that display high growth rates when easily degradable substrates are abundantly available. This also results in a depletion of K-strategists: microorganisms that have a high substrate affinity but that display low growth rates as they rely on other microbial members that participate in the metabolic "meandering" network.

Starting at birth, the human body is exposed to a lower diversity of microbial antigens as a consequence of the reported typical Western society practices. This results in a weakened immune regulation that depletes the gut mucosal barrier and predisposes the human host to Western diseases that have been increasing since the beginning of the 20th century.

11.3 TOWARDS ECOSYSTEM APPROACHES TO RESTORE THE DIVERSITY OF THE HUMAN MICROBIOME: PREBIOTICS, FAECAL TRANSPLANTS AND MICROBIAL NETWORK UNITS

Given the importance of biodiversity in the gut microbiome for human health, therapeutic strategies that aim at improving health should incorporate this biodiversity concept. Besides redefining existing concepts such as the prebiotic concept, this may lead to novel ecosystem-based approaches such as supplementation of essential microbial network units.

TABLE 1: Complex polysaccharides that arrive in the colon [such as long-chain arabinoxylans (LC-AX) or inulin (IN)] increase the abundance of specific primary degraders but importantly, they also increase a similar cohort of secondary degraders that benefit through cross-feeding. This increases the microbial diversity of the human microbiome.

Higher taxonomic group	Bacterial group	Percentual abundance (%)		
		Control	LC-AX	IN
Clostridium cluster IV	*Subdoligranulum variable*-like	0.50 ± 0.06^a	1.44 ± 0.37^b	1.59 ± 0.29^b
Clostridium cluster XIVa	*Clostridium colinum*-like	0.62 ± 0.04^a	3.20 ± 0.10^b	3.65 ± 0.37^b
	Clostridium sphenoides-like	1.63 ± 0.27^a	3.36 ± 0.17^b	3.23 ± 0.21^b
	Eubacterium rectale-like	0.96 ± 0.16^a	4.72 ± 0.36^b	5.95 ± 0.69^b
	Lachnospira pectinoschiza-like	0.98 ± 0.11^a	2.54 ± 0.18^b	3.16 ± 0.19^c
	Lachnobacillus bovis-like	1.06 ± 0.21^a	2.72 ± 0.60^{ab}	3.11 ± 0.47^b
	Roseburia intestinalis-like	0.54 ± 0.05^a	4.43 ± 1.10^b	5.90 ± 1.11^b

This table contains an example of such a cohort of secondary degraders, as identified during a study with humanized rats, treated with LC-AX or IN Van den Abbeele et al., 2011). The abundance (%) of bacterial groups (belonging to higher taxonomic groups) are based on the HITChip analysis. Values indicated with a different superscript are significantly different (a, b or c; n=4).

First, the concept of prebiotic compounds may need to be revised. Prebiotics have been defined as "indigestible food compounds that selectively stimulate the growth and/or activity of one or a limited number of microbial genus(era)/species in the gut that confer(s) health benefits to the host" (Gibson and Roberfroid, 1995; Roberfroid et al., 2010). While stimulation of bifidobacteria or lactobacilli is generally regarded as beneficial, this concept seems too narrow. A new, more accurate definition for a prebiotic compound may be "an indigestible food compound that stimulates the ecological biodiversity in the human gut microbiome." Indeed, a recent study using a novel molecular tool with high-phylogenetic resolution indicated that prebiotic compounds such as inulin (IN) and long-chain arabinoxylans (LC-AX) both increase the abundance of specific primary degraders. Despite the very different structure of IN and LC-AX, both compounds also increased a similar spectrum of secondary degraders that benefit through cross-feeding with the primary degrader (Table 1) (Van den Abbeele et al., 2011). Such microbes that increased in both treatments mostly belonged to relatives from the *Clostridium* clusters IV and XIVa. Although primary degraders are essential to initiate the breakdown of the specific polysaccharides, the stimulation of these microbial networks/meanders increases the microbial diversity and may be more beneficial than the increase of a specific primary degrader.

A second approach to restore microbial diversity when a human microbiota is severely disturbed is a faecal transplantation (Shahinas et al., 2012). This approach has already been applied to treat *C. difficile*-associated disease (Khoruts et al., 2010; Guo et al., 2012), which is thought to result from persistent disruption of the commensal gut microbiota and which is considered as an important cause of antibiotic-induced diarrhoea and colitis. Moreover, faecal transplantation from lean individuals to individuals suffering from metabolic syndrome, displayed increased insulin sensitivity corresponding with stimulation of microbial groups that are known to benefit from cross-feeding (metabolic meandering) such as butyrate-producing microbes of the *Clostridium* clusters IV and XIVa (Vrieze et al., 2012). Faecal transplants thus seem to be promising techniques to restore microbial diversity in microbial communities that are severely dysbiosed. However, given the high microbial complexity of human faeces, faecal samples require thorough risk assessment before they can be applied as a faecal transplant. Therefore, faecal transplants are only applied in severe cases while otherwise antibiotics are still a common practice. To guarantee a more stable and diverse microbial composition during such antibiotic treatments, the current recommendation is to consume yogurt or cheese (often containing a single microbial species) during these treatments. The current state of the art should allow to go beyond these recommendations and design much better products.

Therefore, based on the concept of faecal transplants, we introduce a third concept to remediate a dysbiosed microbiota or to assist microbiome development during different stages of a human lifespan: intestinal microbial network units. Such a network unit contains a consortium of microbes that is capable of performing a specific function, as we will demonstrate according to three different examples: degradation of specific complex polysaccharides (e.g. starch, LC-AX or mucins), induction of specific immune pathways (e.g. Treg cells) or a mixture of essential symbionts for a specific human life stage (e.g. microbial mix for newborns).

The first example considers the fermentation of otherwise indigestible polysaccharides to health-promoting short-chain fatty acids. This microbial metabolic function is so beneficial that it is assumed to be the main evolutionary driving force to include microorganisms in the gastrointestinal tract and to acquire carefully designed defence mechanisms (McFall-Ngai, 2007). The diverse spectrum of glycans, which is present in the human colon, is derived from the diet (resistant starch, LC-AX, IN) or the host (mucins). To construct a microbial network unit for these specific glycans, one needs to consider the concept of a king and his court. First, there is the specific primary degrader or keystone species for this glycan ("king"). For many of the diverse spectrum of glycans that are present in the colon, such keystone species have been proposed. As an example, resistant starch requires the presence of *Ruminococcus bromii* (Ze et al., 2012), LC-AX are specifically degraded by *Bifidobacterium longum* (Van den Abbeele et al., 2011) and *Akkermansia muciniphila* seems a crucial species for the initial breakdown of mucins (Belzer and de Vos, 2012). To produce an industrial product, i.e. an effective microbial network unit, one also needs to provide the primary degrader ("king") with its cross-feeding microbes ("court"). This may be achieved using conventional in vitro fermentors which can be inoculated with relevant keystone species and a mixture of cross-feeding microbes (e.g. relatives of the microbial groups listed in Table 1). After inoculation and stabilization, such a microbial network unit for specific functions can be attained and produced at large scale.

As a second example, microbial network units may also be constructed for specific immunomodulatory functions such as induction of the regulatory arm of colonic T cells. A recent study by El Aidy and colleagues (2012a) reported on the dynamic changes in the regulation of intestinal homeostasis during microbial colonization. During the process of microbial colonization in germfree mice, inflammatory tissue responses were avoided by the induction of the regulatory arm of T cells, including (among others) Foxp3 and Il10 markers for tolerance-promoting Tregs that were induced, especially during the later stage of colonization of the colon. The expression of these tolerance markers paralleled the colonization of several *Clostridium* cluster IV and XIVa species (El Aidy et al., 2012b). The latter bacterial groups were previously reported to stimulate the expression of Tregs (Atarashi et al., 2011), potentially related to their strong capacity to colonize the mucin-associated microbiota (Van den Abbeele et al., 2012). Moreover, these *Clostridium* cluster IV and XIVa species represent only a small proportion of the microbial community in the inflammatory bowel disease patients (Frank et al., 2007). Constructing a microbial network unit that contains these species may thus allow reaching a microbial network unit that specifically induces colonic Tregs that may be relevant for administration to inflammatory bowel disease patients.

Third, microbial network units may also be relevant with respect to the different stages of a human lifespan (Fig. 1). As discussed above, current Western society practices such as caesarean sections and the use of formula milk, contribute to early host–microbial imbalances. When designing a microbial mix for babies, it will be important that besides the presence of well-known early-life symbionts such as *Bifidobacterium* sp., also bacteria perceived as rather harmful should be administered (probably after sterilization). This was pointed out by a recent study of Mai and colleagues (2011) who investigated the early microbial factors that may cause necrotizing enterocolitis in preterm infants. The latter study is unique in its experimental set-up, as samples were collected before disease, rather than collecting samples when babies are already ill. Necrotizing enterocolitis went along with a bloom in the *Proteobacteria* but importantly the disease was preceded by lower-than-normal levels of *Proteobacteria* in the early microbial population of these babies. For a proper immune maturation, both beneficial and detrimental microbes are thus necessary. Similarly, microbial network units may be designed for 3-year-old children that should be colonized by an adult-like microbiota, while also the elderly may profit from a specific microbial consortium.

Finally, microbes that may be beneficial for the entire human population may be administered to the drinking water. Recently, there were already trials to apply "Effective Microorganisms (EM)" in water treatment as well as in other domains including agriculture and supplements for human consumption (Daiss et al., 2008; Ke et al., 2009). EM are mixed cultures of beneficial natural fermentative microorganisms that can be applied to increase the necessary microbial diversity needed for living. EM consist of a mixed culture of photosynthetic bacteria, lactic acid bacteria and yeast. While further research is still required to unravel the health consequences of consumption of disinfected versus undisinfected naturally colonized water, people consuming water treated with EM will presumably gain the benefit of the metabolites developed by these microorganisms, which act as substrates for increasing beneficial populations.

11.4 CONCLUSIONS

Past and ongoing research has allowed to appreciate the importance of biodiversity in the human gut microbiome, caused by the diverse metabolic interactions among different microbial species. Rather than stimulating single species, prebiotic compounds should enhance these metabolic interactions to support a biodiverse gut microbiome. Based on the already elucidated important microbial processes within the complex human gut microbiome, future research should further aim at the elucidation and the technical formulation, production and validation of specific microbial network units.

REFERENCES

1. Adlerberth, I., and Wold, A.E. (2009) Establishment of the gut microbiota in Western infants. Acta Paediatr 98: 229–238.
2. Atarashi, K., Tanoue, T., Shima, T., Imaoka, A., Kuwahara, T., Momose, Y., et al. (2011) Induction of colonic regulatory T cells by indigenous Clostridium species. Science 331: 337–341.

3. Backhed, F., Ley, R.E., Sonnenburg, J.L., Peterson, D.A., and Gordon, J.I. (2005) Host–bacterial mutualism in the human intestine. Science 307: 1915–1920.
4. Belzer, C., and de Vos, W.M. (2012) Microbes inside – from diversity to function: the case of Akkermansia. ISME J 6: 1449–1458.
5. Biasucci, G., Benenati, B., Morelli, L., Bessi, E., and Boehm, G. (2008) Cesarean delivery may affect the early biodiversity of intestinal bacteria. J Nutr 138: 1796S–1800S.
6. Cabrera-Rubio, R., Collado, M.C., Laitinen, K., Salminen, S., Isolauri, E., and Mira, A. (2012) The human milk microbiome changes over lactation and is shaped by maternal weight and mode of delivery. Am J Clin Nutr 96: 544–551.
7. Chang, J.Y., Antonopoulos, D.A., Kalra, A., Tonelli, A., Khalife, W.T., Schmidt, T.M., and Young, V.B. (2008) Decreased diversity of the fecal microbiome in recurrent Clostridium difficile-associated diarrhea. J Infect Dis 197: 435–438.
8. Claesson, M.J., Cusack, S., O'Sullivan, O., Greene-Diniz, R., de Weerd, H., Flannery, E., et al. (2011) Composition, variability, and temporal stability of the intestinal microbiota of the elderly. Proc Natl Acad Sci USA 108: 4586–4591.
9. Claesson, M.J., Jeffery, I.B., Conde, S., Power, S.E., O'Connor, E.M., Cusack, S., et al. (2012) Gut microbiota composition correlates with diet and health in the elderly. Nature 488: 178–184.
10. Daiss, N., Lobo, M.G., and Gonzalez, M. (2008) Changes in postharvest quality of Swiss chard grown using 3 organic preharvest treatments. J Food Sci 73: S314–S320.
11. De Filippo, C., Cavalieri, D., Di Paola, M., Ramazzotti, M., Poullet, J.B., Massart, S., et al. (2010) Impact of diet in shaping gut microbiota revealed by a comparative study in children from Europe and rural Africa. Proc Natl Acad Sci USA 107: 14691–14696.
12. Dethlefsen, L., Huse, S., Sogin, M.L., and Relman, D.A. (2008) The pervasive effects of an antibiotic on the human gut microbiota, as revealed by deep 16S rRNA sequencing. PLoS Biol 6: e280.
13. El Aidy, S., van Baarlen, P., Derrien, M., Lindenbergh-Kortleve, D.J., Hooiveld, G., Levenez, F., et al. (2012a) Temporal and spatial interplay of microbiota and intestinal mucosa drive establishment of immune homeostasis in conventionalized mice. Mucosal Immunol 5: 567–579.
14. El Aidy, S., Derrien, M., Merrifield, C.A., Levenez, F., Dore, J., Boekschoten, M.V., et al. (2012b) Gut bacteria-host metabolic interplay during conventionalisation of the mouse germfree colon. ISME J doi:10.1038/ismej.2012.1142.
15. FAO/WHO (2002) Guidelines for the Evaluation of Probiotics in Food: Report of a Joint FAO/WHO Working Group. London, Ontario, Canada: Food and Agriculture Organization of the United Nations and World Health Organization.
16. Frank, D.N., St. Amand, A.L., Feldman, R.A., Boedeker, E.C., Harpaz, N., and Pace, N.R. (2007) Molecular-phylogenetic characterization of microbial community imbalances in human inflammatory bowel diseases. Proc Natl Acad Sci USA 104: 13780–13785.
17. Gibson, G.R., and Roberfroid, M.B. (1995) Dietary modulation of the human colonic microbiota – introducing the concept of prebiotics. J Nutr 125: 1401–1412.

18. Guo, B., Harstall, C., Louie, T., van Zanten, S.V., and Dieleman, L.A. (2012) Systematic review: faecal transplantation for the treatment of Clostridium difficile-associated disease. Aliment Pharmacol Ther 35: 865–875.

19. Ke, B., Xu, Z.L., Ling, Y.F., Qiu, W.Y., Xu, Y.Y., Higa, T., and Aruoma, O.I. (2009) Modulation of experimental osteoporosis in rats by the antioxidant beverage effective microorganism-X (EM-X). Biomed Pharmacother 63: 114–119.

20. Khoruts, A., Dicksved, J., Jansson, J.K., and Sadowsky, M.J. (2010) Changes in the composition of the human fecal microbiome after bacteriotherapy for recurrent Clostridium difficile-associated diarrhea. J Clin Gastroenterol 44: 354–360.

21. Ley, R.E., Hamady, M., Lozupone, C., Turnbaugh, P.J., Ramey, R.R., Bircher, J.S., et al. (2008) Evolution of mammals and their gut microbes. Science 320: 1647–1651.

22. McFall-Ngai, M. (2007) Adaptive immunity: care for the community. Nature 445: 153–153.

23. Mai, V., Young, C.M., Ukhanova, M., Wang, X., Sun, Y., Casella, G., et al. (2011) Fecal microbiota in premature infants prior to necrotizing enterocolitis. PLoS ONE 6: e20647.

24. Manichanh, C., Rigottier-Gois, L., Bonnaud, E., Gloux, K., Pelletier, E., Frangeul, L., et al. (2006) Reduced diversity of faecal microbiota in Crohn's disease revealed by a metagenomic approach. Gut 55: 205–211.

25. Martin, J.A., Hamilton, B.E., Ventura, S.J., Osterman, M.J.K., Wilson, E.C., and Matthews, T.J. (2012) Births: final data for 2012. Natl Vital Stat Rep 61: 1–72.

26. Pianka, E.R. (1970) r-selection and K-selection. Am Nat 104: 592–597.

27. Roberfroid, M., Gibson, G.R., Hoyles, L., McCartney, A.L., Rastall, R., Rowland, I., et al. (2010) Prebiotic effects: metabolic and health benefits. Br J Nutr 104: S1–S63.

28. Round, J.L., and Mazmanian, S.K. (2009) The gut microbiota shapes intestinal immune responses during health and disease. Nat Rev Immunol 9: 313–323.

29. Sela, D.A., and Mills, D.A. (2010) Nursing our microbiota: molecular linkages between bifidobacteria and milk oligosaccharides. Trends Microbiol 18: 298–307.

30. Shahinas, D., Silverman, M., Sittler, T., Chiu, C., Kim, P., Allen-Vercoe, E., et al. (2012) Toward an understanding of changes in diversity associated with fecal microbiome transplantation based on 16S rRNA gene deep sequencing. mBio 3: e00338-12.

31. Turnbaugh, P.J., Hamady, M., Yatsunenko, T., Cantarel, B.L., Duncan, A., Ley, R.E.,

32. Van den Abbeele, P., Gérard, P., Rabot, S., Bruneau, A., El Aidy, S., Derrien, M., et al. (2011) Arabinoxylans and inulin differentially modulate the mucosal and luminal gut microbiota and mucin-degradation in humanized rats. Environ Microbiol 13: 2667–2680.

33. Van den Abbeele, P., Belzer, C., Goossens, M., Kleerebezem, M., De Vos, W.M., Thas, O., et al. (2012) Butyrate-producing Clostridium cluster XIVa species specifically colonize mucins in an in vitro gut model. ISME J doi:10.1038/ismej.2012.158.

34. Vollaard, E.J., and Clasener, H.A.L. (1994) Colonization resistance. Antimicrob Agents Chemother 38: 409–414.

35. Vrieze, A., Van Nood, E., Holleman, F., Salojärvi, J., Kootte, R.S., Bartelsman, J.F.W.M., et al. (2012) Transfer of intestinal microbiota from lean donors increases insulin sensitivity in individuals with metabolic syndrome. Gastroenterology 143: 913–916.e917.

36. Yatsunenko, T., Rey, F.E., Manary, M.J., Trehan, I., Dominguez-Bello, M.G., Contreras, M., et al. (2012) Human gut microbiome viewed across age and geography. Nature 486: 222–227.
37. Ze, X., Duncan, S.H., Louis, P., and Flint, H.J. (2012) Ruminococcus bromii is a keystone species for the degradation of resistant starch in the human colon. ISME J 6: 1535–1543.

CHAPTER 12

MICROBIOTA AND HEALTHY AGEING: OBSERVATIONAL AND NUTRITIONAL INTERVENTION STUDIES

HARALD BRÜSSOW

Microbiota and its impact on human health has become a topical area of microbiological research. However, health is a vast field as explored in a parallel minireview (Brüssow, submitted) and the role of the gut microbiota on human health has been discussed under many headings. In the present minireview, I will concentrate on one specific aspect. Our societies are ageing and if we want to avoid that our societies will suffer from an increasing burden of disease, we must also assure healthy ageing. This subject has not only a high societal priority, it has also a long tradition in microbiology.

This chapter was originally published under the Creative Commons Attribution License. Brüssow H. Microbiota and Healthy Ageing: Observational and Nutritional Intervention Studies. Microbial Biotechnology *6,4 (2013): pp. 326–334. doi:10.1111/1751-7915.12048.*

12.1 HEALTHY AGEING

In fact, the first association between microbes and healthy ageing was made by one of the founding fathers of modern microbiology and immunology, namely Elie Metchnikoff from Kharkov/Ukraine. He shared the Nobel Prize for Medicine with Paul Ehrlich in 1908 and published in the same year an influential book 'The Prolongation of Life' (Metchnikoff, 1908). As nicely described in a 1908 book review from the *New York Times* he developed in this book the idea that higher animals needed an increasingly complex intestine to struggle for existence. Unfortunately, the intestine became the breeding place for poisonous microbes. The ravages of these poisonous microbes are not only the cause of disease (Koch's germ theory of disease), but from the detrimental metabolism of some gut bacteria spring the debility of old age leading to earlier death. Metchnikoff distinguished two types of metabolism for gut bacteria: proteolytic bacteria lead to putrefaction with noxious metabolites as waste products and saccharolytic bacteria lead to fermentation with beneficial metabolic end-products like lactic acid. He suggested combating putrefaction in the gut by hygiene, diet and biologicals. He recommended the consumption of boiled food and drinks since microbes enter the digestive tract in vast numbers with raw food. He called for appropriate mastication (quick eating leaving food lumps in the intestine which become then heavily colonized by gut microbes) and particularly he made an argument for milk fermented by lactic acid bacteria as food. The fermentative metabolism of lactic acid bacteria would counterbalance putrefaction by the noxious gut bacteria and their toxic effect on our tissues. He backed this theory by the observation that population showing traditionally high yoghurt consumption also showed increased longevity.

This idea was picked up in Japan and developed there into an industrial product. The Japanese microbiologist Shirota isolated the first probiotic bacterium in 1930 and developed this *Lactobacillus casei* strain into a dairy drink which was introduced on the market in 1935. Over the decades this sole product was used to develop a substantial nutrition and health business. Despite this early industrialization, over the following decades the microbiota of the human gut and its relationship to human health met only limited interest from applied and environmental microbiologists.

12.2 GUT MICROBIOTA AND AGEING

A review on intestinal flora and ageing from the early 1990s reported that many factors in addition to ageing altered the composition of the gut microbiota (physiological state, drugs, disease, diet and stress) (Mitsuoka, 1992). The composition of the gut microbiota was known to affect physiological functions (e.g. digestion and absorption), drug efficacy, carcinogenesis, immune function and infection. Three groups of gut bacteria were distinguished. Symbiotic gut bacteria (*Bacteroidaceae, Eubacterium, Peptococcaceae, Bifidobacterium, Lactobacillus*), which are important for the maintenance of health via synthesis of vitamins, help in digestion, stimulation of immune function and their inhibition of pathogenic microbes. A second group comprised *Escherichia, Streptococcus* and *Veillonella*. Protein degradation by these bacteria leads to NH_3, H_2S, amines, phenols production and was linked—as originally proposed by Metchnikoff—to the production of toxic compounds and thereby possibly to ageing. The third group of gut bacteria were pathogens that induced infections. Research on the gut commensal *Escherichia coli* became a founding pillar of bacterial genetics and molecular microbiology. In contrast, until the mid-1990s, the gut microbiota in its ecological complexity was only investigated by a small research community using nearly exclusively culture-based methods. Since then a growing number of molecular methods were developed that allowed increasingly detailed, cheap and time-efficient approaches characterizing bacterial microbiota. Techniques like DGGE, T-RFLP, dot-blot hybridization, FISH, qPCR, phylogenetic microarrays and then particularly the sequencing of cloned 16S rRNA amplicons attracted many scientists to the field of gut microbiota (O'Toole and Claesson, 2010). In parallel, research into probiotic gut bacteria intensified (Woodmansey, 2007). With the current techniques of massive sequencing (454 pyrosequencing, Illumina technique) and the expanding arsenal of –omics techniques and major international research initiatives in the Human Microbiome Project, gut microbiota analyses and gut microbiota-human health studies reach top-ranking scientific journals (Clemente et al., 2012). This gut microbiome research is clearly exciting as an eye-opener for a previously unsuspected biological diversity in our body. It led to new ways of looking into human genetic diversity extending phenotype–genotype association studies from the few ten thousand human genes to the potentially million of genes encountered in our bacterial commensals. The field proposed widely quoted working hypotheses like the link between gut microbiome composition and human health: the most prominent being the association of the *Bacteroides/Firmicutes* ratio in gut microbiota with obesity. Overall, the field is, however, still in the state of botany in the 18th century when naturalists returned with countless new plants from expeditions into until then poorly explored parts of the world. A census was made and the diversity of plant life was described, but no theory was yet available to make sense out of this mind-boggling biological diversity. We are still in the census period of microbial diversity corresponding to the time of Linné in botany; instead of taxonomical methods we now use increasingly sophisticated statistical methods and hope to sort out associations which could lead us to new biological insight. The exciting progress of DNA sequence technologies and "–omics" approaches are also a temptation to run more and more descriptive census approaches simply because they are technologically feasible. However, we also need the elaboration of biological hypotheses about the meaning of commensalism, host–microbe interaction and microbial diversity which makes explicit predictions that are tested with experiments and surveys. To stay with the botany analogy, the contribution of Russel Wallace is still missing in the field.

Despite an explosion in gut microbiome literature, data on the changes of the gut microbiota with old age are still limited. On the basis of studies using culture methods, the mid-1990 research situation could be summarized as followed: bifidobacteria diminished with age, while clostridia, lactobacilli, streptococci and enterobacteria increased with age and *Bacteroides* remained stable. Over the last 10 years, a handful of studies re-investigated the question. A study compared the faecal colony counts of seven young adults with that of four elderly subjects using culture methods and biochemical markers for species definition. The small number of investigated subjects reflects the laborious aspect of this approach. The authors found that Bacteroides species diversity increased and that bifidobacterial species diversity decreased in the elderly subjects (Hopkins and MacFarlane, 2002). In another study the same authors reported again a marked decrease in bifidobacteria, a slight decrease in lactobacilli, but no change in viable counts for the *Bacteroides-Prevotella* group in elderly compared with young adults. The bifidobacteria in the healthy elderly showed either high or negligible counts resulting in wide standard errors (Hopkins et al., 2001). In a follow-up study by the same Gut Microbiology Group at the University of Dundee/UK, 12 healthy young adults were compared with six healthy elderly subjects for faecal bacterial counts. The researchers observed a decrease in *Bacteroides* species diversity in elderly, but no overall decrease in bifidobacteria. However, the species composition of bifidobacteria changed with age: *B. angulatum* and *B. longum*, respectively, were the most common isolates in elderly and younger adults. Both *Bacteroides* and bifidobacteria showed reduced numbers in the faeces of the elderly subjects. Facultative anaerobes increased with age (Woodmansey et al., 2004). From these three papers published by the same research group investigating local subjects for gut microbiota composition, it is apparent that substantial inter-individual differences will make it difficult to arrive at general conclusions. The high variability of the gut microbiota composition was also documented by another group using a different analytical technique, namely oligonucleotide probes for fluorescence in situ hybridization of faecal samples coupled with flow cytometry. Overall, 85 young adults were compared with 145 healthy elderly subjects from four European countries. The French and Swedish study arms showed no age-related microbiota changes. Age effects were only seen in the German and the Italian study groups. However, when considering the predominant bacterial groups (*Eubacterium-Clostridium, Bacteroides-Prevotella*), the German elderly subjects showed an increase while the Italian elderly participants showed a decrease in faecal number for these bacteria when compared with the corresponding local younger subjects. *Bifidobacteria* were high only in Italian subjects, and that in both age groups (Mueller et al., 2006).

A French study using qPCR methodology to assess five bacterial genera documented a marked change in the ratio of *Firmicutes* to *Bacteroidetes* from 11 to 0.6 when comparing young with elderly adults. Elderly subjects exhibited high levels of *E. coli* and *Bacteroidetes* (Mariat et al., 2009). Another group investigated the gut microbiota in 21 centenarians, 22 seniors (mean age 73 years) and 20 adults younger than 40 years from Europe using the Human Intestinal Tract Chip (HITChip) and qPCR technology. No significant difference was seen between the young and elderly subjects. Even the microbiota composition of the centenarians was still similar to that of young adults: the centenarians showed only an increase in bacilli and in facultative anaerobes, but neither were a dominant faecal population. Interestingly, the centenarians showed an increase in pathogens (*Klebsiella pneumoniae*) and a slight, but significant decrease in *Faecalibacterium prausnitzii* (a symbiont with anti-inflammatory properties) when compared with seniors. This shift in microbiota composition was associated with an increased inflammatory status as determined by plasma levels of pro-inflammatory cytokines. The group coined the term 'inflammageing' for this chronic low-grade inflammatory status which they suggested as one possible driver of the ageing process (Biagi et al., 2010).

In 2007 the ELDERMET consortium was established to investigate the role of the intestinal microbiota in 161 Irish subjects older than 65 years as an agent and indicator of health. When the faecal microbiota of the study participants was investigated by pyrosequencing of 16S rRNA and compared with that of nine younger control subjects, the researchers observed an increase in *Bacteroidetes* from 41% to 57% of the sequences and a concomitant decrease in *Firmicutes* from 51% to 40% in younger and older subjects respectively. However, averaging hides a dramatic inter-individual variability in the composition of the elderly gut microbiota. The proportion of *Bacteroidetes* ranged from 3% to 92% in the different elderly subjects and that of *Firmicutes* varied from 7% to 94%. When plotted as a histogram, an essential smooth distribution for the *Bacteroidetes/Firmicutes* ratio was observed between the two extremes. The same characteristic was observed when the ratio of clusters IV and XIV was investigated within the *Clostridium* group. The wide distribution of the data was also seen for other bacterial groups, e.g. *Faecalibacterium* showed a steady distribution between 16% and <1% prevalence. When the *Bacteroidetes* group was further differentiated, some differences between the young and elderly adults could be identified. Microbiota compositional differences were—as expected—greater between individuals than between individuals who were sampled twice (Claesson et al., 2011).

12.3 AGEING AND AILING

In the previous section, we have seen that ageing (except perhaps for extreme ageing) does not leave a consistent imprint on the gut microbiota. In fact, this observation is not surprising. When you have great inter-individual variability for a given parameter in a population as it is the case for gut microbiota, you need more precisely defined or quite drastic conditions to expect consistent changes in gut microbiota. Old age alone is apparently not a sufficiently strong disturbing factor to upset the gut microbiota composition, it might need addition events like antibiotic treatment (Bartosch et al., 2004; Woodmansey et al., 2004) or *Clostridium difficile* infection (Hopkins et al., 2001; Hopkins and MacFarlane, 2002) to get significant and consistent signal changes in elderly subjects. One study compared faecal microbiota in hospitalized elderly patients receiving and not receiving antibiotic treatment. Only a marginal reduction in total 16S rRNA gene copy numbers was seen in the antibiotic treated patients, but significant reductions in *Bifidobacterium, F. prausnitzii* and *Desulfovibrio* were induced by antibiotic treatment (Bartosch et al., 2004). Another study from the Dundee group showed a significant increase in total facultative anaerobe counts upon antibiotic treatment in elderly patients. The higher number of proteolytic bacteria in the stool of antibiotic-treated elderlies was also associated with an increased proteolytic species diversity particularly in fusobacteria, clostridia and propionibacteria (Woodmansey et al., 2004). The Dundee researchers compared also healthy elderlies with elderlies suffering from *Clostridium difficile*-associated diarrhoea (CDAD). CDAD patients showed reduced numbers of bifidobacteria and bacteroides, but increased numbers of enterobacteria (Hopkins et al., 2001). A follow-up study of the Dundee group comparing healthy with CDAD elderly subjects confirmed these conclusions (Hopkins and MacFarlane, 2002).

Since antibiotic treatment and *C. difficile* infection impact directly on the gut microbiota and are only indirectly related to the ageing process, these observations are unlikely to be informative for the microbiota changes with increasing age. Other criteria that are a more reliable measure for healthy and unhealthy ageing are needed for such an approach. The Dundee group addressed this hypothesis by comparing the faecal microbiota in 35 healthy elderly subjects living in the local community with that of 38 elderly patients who were hospitalized. They used real-time PCR techniques with group and species-specific primer sets. The *Bacteroides-Prevotella* group, *F. prausnitzii* and *Clostridium clostridiiformi* were all detected with lower numbers in stool of hospitalized patients when compared with community-living subjects. *Bifidobacteria* showed no significant differences between the groups. However, since the hospitalized subjects also showed a 10-fold lower total bacterial 16S rRNA gene count, the relative abundance of the different bacterial groups did not change with hospitalization (Bartosch et al., 2004). A Dutch study took a similar approach by assessing the faecal microbiota composition in 23 elderly subjects (median age 86 years) living in the same old age centre and receiving the same diet. The subjects were stratified according to the Groningen Frailty Indicator into 13 subjects with low frailty and 10 subjects with high frailty score. This time the total number of bacteria as assessed by hybridization with specific probes did not differ between both groups. Statistically significant differences were seen for the *Lactobacillus/Enterococcus* group (10-fold decrease in the high frailty group) and for *Enterobacteriaceae* (10-fold increase in high frailty group) (van Tongeren et al., 2005). Also the ELDERMET consortium stratified their data according to the health status of their elderly subjects into 83 community-dwelling, 20 outpatients, 15 short-term hospitalized subjects and 60 subjects with long-term residential care. The statistical analysis of the microbiota composition indicated a clear separation between community-dwelling subjects and long-stay home residents. The latter showed a higher proportion of *Bacteroidetes* while the former showed a higher proportion of *Firmicutes* and unclassified bacteria. *Lachnospiraceae* were a key species enriched in the community-living subjects (Claesson et al., 2012). Both groups differed also in faecal metabolome analysis. Acetate, butyrate, propionate were more abundant as metabolites in the community dwellers while glucose, glycine and lipids were at higher faecal levels in the long-term residents. The metabolome data were corroborated by a higher gene count for enzymes involved in the production of short-chain fatty acids (SCFA) in the community dwellers (Claesson et al., 2012). The data fit with current knowledge about bacterial metabolism and gut physiology. SCFA are known nutrients for the colonic enterocytes.

Within the ELDERMET study the community dwellers differed from the long-stay residents and rehabilitation subjects also for other parameters. The community dwellers showed a better score in a number of health/frailty tests than the residents including the calf circumference, which is a good measure of muscle mass and an index for sarcopenia. The co-morbidity index was as expected higher in the long stay residents. Inflammation markers (IL-6 and IL-8) correlated with a specific gut microbiota type confirming data from Biagi and colleagues (2010). Notably, the effect of antibiotic treatment was eliminated as confounding factor from this study.

12.4 AGEING, DIET AND MICROBIOTA

Diet correlated very strikingly with the health status in the ELDERMET study: 8% of the long-stay residents consumed a moderate to high-fat/low-fibre diet while 98% of the community dwellers displayed a low to moderate fat/high fibre diet. Interestingly, the diversity index of the faecal microbiota correlated positively with a low fat and high fibre content of the diet. The change in diet is partly the consequence of the food prepared at residence canteens. Due to a greater co-morbidity in residents compared with community dwellers, the diet change is also a consequence of their compromised physical situation (poor dentition decreasing mastication, dysphagia affecting swallowing, loss of salivation complicating lubrication of food, decreased physical activity resulting in reduced gut motility and thus constipation)—all resulting in a trend to offer 'easier' food items. Since food changes are expected to change the metabolism of gut bacteria and thereby also the microbiota composition, we are here confronted with a complicated epidemiological situation. Is the microbiota change observed in the long-stay residents a consequence of the diet change or a consequence of their deteriorating health or even one of the causal factors leading to health decline? An answer could be provided by a prospective study looking into an elderly cohort before and when a deterioration of the health status occurs. If the microbiota changes with decreasing health, but before diet changes occur, gut microbiota composition could be a driver for unhealthy ageing. If microbiota composition changes only secondarily after diet changes, microbiota changes are consequences of unhealthy ageing or even simpler of diet change. The ELDERMET study addressed this question by analysing the diet and microbiota type in residents according to residence time. Within 1 month after transfer to residence, all subjects had changed to the long stay-typical diet, but it took a year for the microbiota to get clearly separated from that of the community dwellers. Therefore microbiota changes do not precede, but follow the changes in health status of elderly subjects. In that study microbiota changes were the consequence of unhealthy ageing.

12.5 NUTRITIONAL INTERVENTIONS: RESISTANT STARCH

A recent study explored the effect of short-term feeding of a high-fat/low-fibre versus a low-fat/high-fibre diet given to 10 healthy adults for 10 days. Wide variation of microbiota composition was observed between the subjects at baseline and a 10-day intervention was not able to impose a diet-induced change in microbiota composition as determined by 16S rDNA sequencing. The authors concluded that changes in microbiota composition (expressed as alternative enterotype states) can only achieved by long-term dietary changes (Wu et al., 2011). Only few studies explored the impact of diet changes on the faecal microbiota using microbiota analysis. One study from UK investigated the effect of feeding diets rich in resistant starch (RS), rich in wheat bran and a low-carbohydrate/high-protein diet, respectively, to 14 obese human volunteers (Walker et al., 2011). 16S rDNA sequencing done with six subjects showed significant diet-induced changes for two species, namely *Eubacterium rectale* and *Ruminococcus bromii,* which accounted for 4% and 2% of all bacterial sequences. The inter-individual difference between the subjects was greater than the diet-induced intra-individual changes. A clearer picture emerged from qPCR analysis conducted with all 14 volunteers. It revealed significant increases of ruminococci in most volunteers after change to the diet rich in resistant starch. The change corresponded to a 10-fold increase in number such that *Ruminococcus* represented 25% of the total bacterial 16S rRNA. The change occurred within 3 days after diet change, but the microbiota returned as quickly to the baseline composition after stopping this diet. A few subjects showed a rise in *E. rectale* during this diet, but only two subjects showed increased counts for bifidobacteria. The other diets had no consistent effects.

Notably, this observation of a specific effect of resistant starch diet on *R. bromii* (and *E. rectale*) confirms reports from two different groups working with subjects from different continents (Abell et al., 2008; Martínez et al., 2010). When 46 healthy adults from Australia got resistant starch as a supplement to their diet at two different concentrations compared with a control diet in a cross-over design, diet-associated DGGE bands were detected in the stool. Half of the bands, which increased by the nutritional intervention were identified as *R. bromii*. A quantitative PCR showed that *R. bromii* increased from about 4.9% to 7.9% after supplementation with RS (Abell et al., 2008). In a US study 10 young adults received diets supplemented with native starch and two forms of RS in a cross-over format: RS2 was granular starch and RS4 was chemically modified starch. Compared with the control starch RS4 showed increases in bifidobacteria (mostly *Bifidobacterium adolescentis*), porphyromonadaceae, but decreases in ruminococcaceae. RS2 showed significant increases in *R. bromii* and *E. rectale*. The RS4-induced increase for *B. adolescentis* was substantial in a subset of the subjects (3–30% of the total bacteria with pyrosequencing) and thus also plainly visible on DGGE analysis (Martínez et al., 2010).

However, the beneficial effects of neither *R. bromii* nor *E. rectale* are established. However, when human stool samples were incubated with various nutrient substrates, the most abundant sequences recovered from starch particles were related to the cultured species *R. bromii, B. adolescentis, B. breve* and *E. rectale* (Leitch et al., 2007). *Eubacterium* belongs to the most abundant known butyrate-producing bacteria in human faeces (Hold et al., 2003). However, only bifidobacteria and lactobacilli have so far been clearly associated with health-promoting effects (Kleerebezem and Vaughan, 2009). What then is the evidence that the prevalence of faecal bifidobacteria could be boosted by nutritional interventions in elderly subjects?

12.6 NUTRITIONAL INTERVENTIONS: PREBIOTICS

A prebiotic has been defined as a non-digestible food ingredient that beneficially affects the host by selectively stimulating the growth and activity of one or a limited number of bacteria in the colon, and thus improves host health (Gibson and Roberfroid, 1995). This is a quite complex definition since it requires for a food ingredient that it should not be hydrolysed and absorbed in the upper part of the intestine, be a selective nutrient for few colonic bacteria, alter the colonic microbiota and induce beneficial health effects for the host. The non-digestible characteristics are associated with some complex carbohydrates and proteins. However, since only anaerobic saccharolytic, but not anaerobic proteolytic activity have been associated with health (anaerobic proteolysis producing in fact harmful compounds), only a handful of complex carbohydrates have qualified as prebiotics like fructooligosaccharides which include both short-chain oligofructose and longer-chain inulin (Hamilton-Miller, 2004). Pioneering work from the MRC Dunn Clinical Nutrition Center at Cambridge/UK showed that these compounds are in vitro selectively fermented by bifidobacteria at the expense of bacteroides, clostridia and coliforms (Wang and Gibson, 1993). In the colonic consortium fructooligosaccharides are metabolized into small chain fatty acids which are used by different host organs (butyrate by the colonic epithelium, propionate and lactate by the liver, acetate by the muscle). Bifidobacteria had immunostimulatory activities when given to elderly subjects as dietary supplement (Gill et al., 2001) to quote only one beneficial effect. Soon later, the Cambridge nutritionists showed that fructooligosaccharides (FOS) increased selectively the faecal counts for bifidobacteria from $10^{8.8}$ to $10^{9.5}$ and $10^{9.2}$ to $10^{10.1}$ cfu g^{-1} faeces, respectively, when oligofructose or inulin was fed to human volunteers (Gibson et al., 1995). German nutritionists achieved with inulin a very similar effect in elderly constipated subjects (Kleessen et al., 1997). Bifidobacteria titres increased in a dose-dependent way from $10^{7.9}$ to $10^{8.8}$ and $10^{9.2}$ cfu g^{-1} faeces when 20 and 40 g inulin per day was fed respectively. Inulin showed a slight beneficial laxative effect. Small chain FOS increased also bifidobacteria from $10^{8.5}$ to $10^{9.2}$ cfu g^{-1} stool and cholesterol excretion from stool in a study with healthy elderly volunteers from France (Bouhnik et al., 2007). However, both values returned to baseline 4 weeks after wash-out. Galactooligosaccharides (GOS) have been extensively used in paediatrics and a study with healthy 70-year-old subjects from UK showed likewise an increase in bifidobacteria from $10^{9.1}$ to 10^{10} cfu g^{-1} stool. GOS had no beneficial effect on cholesterol excretion with the stool, but stimulated natural killer cell activity, phagocytic activity and decreased the production of pro-inflammatory cytokines (interleukin-10 and tumour necrosis factor alpha) compared with placebo (Vulevic et al., 2008). A smaller Bifidobacterium increase was seen in 60-year-old healthy subjects from UK ($10^{8.9}$ to $10^{9.2}$ cfu g^{-1} stool) which was significant only for women (Walton et al., 2012).

Gut microbiota is routinely determined by taking faecal microbiota as a proxy measure. Due to technical difficulties and ethical constraints, biopsies are rarely taken. One exception is the study from Langlands and colleagues (2004) where 60-year-old subjects scheduled for colonoscopy were supplemented for 2 weeks before the intervention with FOS and inulin or no supplement. Biopsy samples from the proximal and distal colon from both groups were cultivated for a panel of bacteria. In both compartments the prebiotic group showed increased bifidobacteria counts compared with the control group ($10^{6.4}$ versus $10^{5.2}$ cfu g^{-1} mucosa). *Lactobacilli* and a specific butyrate-producing group from the *Clostridium* cluster (*Eubacterium*) showed likewise prebiotics-induced titre increases. Total anaerobe counts were unaffected and total aerobes showed a non-significant half-log decrease.

12.7 NUTRITIONAL INTERVENTIONS: PROBIOTICS

In the early 1970s probiotics were described by Sperti as "organisms or substances which contribute to intestinal microbial balance", only to be redefined in the late 1980s by Fuller as "a live food supplement which beneficially affects the host by improving its intestinal microbial balance" (quoted from Gibson and Roberfroid, 1995). The possibilities and problems of probiotics was already highlighted in a study conducted 20 years ago with a *Bifidobacterium* strain which showed natural resistance to streptomycin and rifampicin and could thus be differentiated from the background endogenous bifidobacterial microbiota when given to human volunteers in milk fermented with this strain. One day after oral application, the strain reached a titre of 10^9 cfu g^{-1} stool (Bouhnik et al., 1992). This titre was maintained as long as the oral supplement was given. Two days after stopping the *Bifidobacterium* feeding, the titres gradually decreased and became undetectable a week later. Overall, 30% of the orally applied bifidobacterium survived the gastrointestinal passage, but comparison with an inert control (*Bacillus spores*) suggested that no major amplification of the supplemented *Bifidobacterium* had occurred during in vivo passage. The gut passage was thus a rather passive transit. In healthy elderly subjects from New Zealand, feeding of milk containing various doses of *Bifidobacterium lactis* (known for its immunostimulatory effects; Gill et al., 2001) resulted in a dose-independent increase of faecal bifidobacteria counts from $10^{9.3}$ to $10^{9.8}$ cfu g^{-1} stool. Increases were also seen for faecal lactobacilli and enterococci, while enterobacteria were reduced when bifidobacteria were fed (Ahmed et al., 2007). No marked difference in faecal bifidobacterium concentrations were detected in Finnish elderly nursing home residents fed with a *B. longum*-containing drink compared with a placebo drink. However, when compared with the baseline value, the probiotics-receiving subjects showed a significant increase for *Bifidobacterium bifidum* and *B. breve* (Lahtinen et al., 2009).

The next logical step was combining the rationale of prebiotics and probiotics, by giving a mixture of probiotic bifidobacteria (*B. bifidum* and *B. lactis*) together with an inulin-based prebiotic to 18 healthy 70-year-old women (Bartosch et al., 2005). Total *Bifidobacterium* counts were increased in the symbiotic group ($10^{9.4}$ cfu g^{-1} stool) when compared with the placebo group ($10^{8.3}$ cfu g^{-1}), but not when compared with the symbiotic pre-feeding period. The same observation was made for total lactobacilli counts. The results were confirmed by real-time PCR quantification of rRNA genes for all bifidobacteria. However, significant increases also with respect to the prefeeding period were detected when PCR was done with *B. bifidum*- and *B. lactis*-specific primers. Continuous excretion of the orally applied bifidobacteria was documented for all subjects into the first and for some subjects into the third post-feeding week suggesting limited probiotics persistence in elderly subjects getting synbiotics. Interestingly, supplementation with just inulin induced a significant increase in the endogenous *B. adolescentis* prevalence in the stools of human volunteers (Ramirez-Farias et al., 2009) while a symbiotic combination of inulin with only one bifidobacterium probiotic, namely *B. lactis* Bb-12 in young adults did not induce an increased total bifidobacteria faecal count during the feeding period when compared with the placebo group. Interestingly, total bifidobacterial counts were significantly increased in the post-feeding period, but this could not be attributed to the supplemented probiotic strain. The treatment had only small effects on the faecal clostridia and enterobacteria counts (Palaria et al., 2012).

12.8 OUTLOOK

Whether gut microbiota changes are statistically associated with ageing or are just a biomarker (i.e. a consequence) of or even a driver (i.e. a cause) for the ageing process cannot yet be decided from the available data. The current literature does not even allow assigning a typical and old age-specific composition for the gut microbiota of elderly subjects. Some trends were repetitively observed in old age (decrease of bifidobacteria, increase of enterobacteria), but they were far from universal. Major problems for assigning an old age microbiota profile are the high interindividual variability and the clear impact of geography and diet on gut microbiota composition. Advanced age is probably not a sufficiently clear phenotype. Healthy and unhealthy ageing must certainly be differentiated to get to a more consistent picture. In addition, frailty and diseases come in many forms and each form has most likely its specific impact on the gut microbiota.

Like in the case of resistant starch studies it is important to get a consistent observation from different and independent studies to distil stable signals out of the relative 'noise' of the gut microbiota. Currently, we do not know whether the variability in the gut microbiota composition reflects clear biological rules which we are still unable to read for our limited understanding of the system or whether it represents intrinsic stochastic behaviour. However, sorting out a consistent microbiota picture is only the first step. The next step will be to decipher what changes are potentially detrimental and what re-established prior situations are beneficial. This will not be an easy task since systematic reviews of large epidemiological, nutritional and microbiological data sets will be needed to settle these questions. Finally, from a practical viewpoint knowing what gut microbiota is good and what is bad is not sufficient, we need to know how to get from the bad to the good composition. When limiting the complexity to simple models like gnotobiotic mice colonized with a community of 10 sequenced human gut bacteria, 60% of the microbiota changes following randomized perturbations of simple diets consisting of four defined ingredients can be explained with a statistical model (Faith et al., 2011). The data with the resistant starch dietary intervention are interesting for their consistent effect on specific gut bacteria in three different human populations. Since several microbiota-ageing studies reported decreases of bifidobacteria in old age and since bifidobacteria have an already fairly well-established role as probiotic organisms and since their prevalence can be influenced by specific prebiotic supplements, interventions increasing bifidobacteria and suppressing enterobacteria (another relative constant association with old age) should be conducted in elderly subjects to look for health improvements. Overall, it will be a long way to promote healthy ageing by nutritional interventions which target the gut microbiota. The task will be complex because such trials necessitate the collaboration of doctors, nutritionists, microbiologists and analytical chemists. However, it will be an exciting field for microbial biotechnology approaches and numerous are the people who would profit from such interventions if successful.

REFERENCES

1. Abell, G.C., Cooke, C.M., Bennett, C.N., Conlon, M.A., and McOrist, A.L. (2008) Phylotypes related to Ruminococcus bromii are abundant in the large bowel of humans and increase in response to a diet high in resistant starch. FEMS Microbiol Ecol 66: 505–515.
2. Ahmed, M., Prasad, J., Gill, H., Stevenson, L., and Gopal, P. (2007) Impact of consumption of different levels of Bifidobacterium lactis HN019 on the intestinal microflora of elderly human subjects. J Nutr Health Aging 11: 26–31.
3. Bartosch, S., Fite, A., Macfarlane, G.T., and McMurdo, M.E. (2004) Characterization of bacterial communities in feces from healthy elderly volunteers and hospitalized elderly patients by using real-time PCR and effects of antibiotic treatment on the fecal microbiota. Appl Environ Microbiol 70: 3575–3581.
4. Bartosch, S., Woodmansey, E.J., Paterson, J.C., McMurdo, M.E., and Macfarlane, G.T. (2005) Microbiological effects of consuming a synbiotic containing Bifidobacterium bifidum, Bifidobacterium lactis, and oligofructose in elderly persons, determined by real-time polymerase chain reaction and counting of viable bacteria. Clin Infect Dis 40: 28–37.

5. Biagi, E., Nylund, L., Candela, M., Ostan, R., Bucci, L., Pini, E., et al. (2010) Through ageing, and beyond: gut microbiota and inflammatory status in seniors and centenarians. PLoS ONE 5: e10667.
6. Bouhnik, Y., Pochart, P., Marteau, P., Arlet, G., Goderel, I., and Rambaud, J.C. (1992) Fecal recovery in humans of viable Bifidobacterium sp. ingested in fermented milk. Gastroenterology 102: 875–878.
7. Bouhnik, Y., Achour, L., Paineau, D., Riottot, M., Attar, A., and Bornet, F. (2007) Four-week short chain fructo-oligosaccharides ingestion leads to increasing fecal bifidobacteria and cholesterol excretion in healthy elderly volunteers. Nutr J 6: e42.
8. Claesson, M.J., Cusack, S., O'Sullivan, O., Greene-Diniz, R., de Weerd, H., Flannery, E., et al. (2011) Composition, variability, and temporal stability of the intestinal microbiota of the elderly. Proc Natl Acad Sci USA 108 (Suppl. 1): 4586–4591.
9. Claesson, M.J., Jeffery, I.B., Conde, S., Power, S.E., O'Connor, E.M., Cusack, S., et al. (2012) Gut microbiota composition correlates with diet and health in the elderly. Nature 488: 178–184.
10. Clemente, J.C., Ursell, L.K., Parfrey, L.W., and Knight, R. (2012) The impact of the gut microbiota on human health: an integrative view. Cell 148: 1258–1270.
11. Faith, J.J., McNulty, N.P., Rey, F.E., and Gordon, J.I. (2011) Predicting a human gut microbiota's response to diet in gnotobiotic mice. Science 333: 101–104.
12. Gibson, G.R., and Roberfroid, M.B. (1995) Dietary modulation of the human colonic microbiota: introducing the concept of prebiotics. J Nutr 125: 1401–1412.
13. Gibson, G.R., Beatty, E.R., Wang, X., and Cummings, J.H. (1995) Selective stimulation of bifidobacteria in the human colon by oligofructose and inulin. Gastroenterology 108: 975–982.
14. Gill, H.S., Rutherfurd, K.J., Cross, M.L., and Gopal, P.K. (2001) Enhancement of immunity in the elderly by dietary supplementation with the probiotic Bifidobacterium lactis HN019. Am J Clin Nutr 74: 833–839.
15. Hamilton-Miller, J.M. (2004) Probiotics and prebiotics in the elderly. Postgrad Med J 80: 447–451.
16. Hold, G.L., Schwiertz, A., Aminov, R.I., Blaut, M., and Flint, H.J. (2003) Oligonucleotide probes that detect quantitatively significant groups of butyrate-producing bacteria in human feces. Appl Environ Microbiol 69: 4320–4324.
17. Hopkins, M.J., and Macfarlane, G.T. (2002) Changes in predominant bacterial populations in human faeces with age and with Clostridium difficile infection. J Med Microbiol 51: 448–454.
18. Hopkins, M.J., Sharp, R., and Macfarlane, G.T. (2001) Age and disease related changes in intestinal bacterial populations assessed by cell culture, 16S rRNA abundance, and community cellular fatty acid profiles. Gut 48: 198–205.
19. Kleerebezem, M., and Vaughan, E.E. (2009) Probiotic and gut lactobacilli and bifidobacteria: molecular approaches to study diversity and activity. Annu Rev Microbiol 63: 269–290.
20. Kleessen, B., Sykura, B., Zunft, H.J., and Blaut, M. (1997) Effects of inulin and lactose on fecal microflora, microbial activity, and bowel habit in elderly constipated persons. Am J Clin Nutr 65: 1397–1402.

21. Lahtinen, S.J., Tammela, L., Korpela, J., Parhiala, R., Ahokoski, H., Mykkänen, H., and Salminen, S.J. (2009) Probiotics modulate the Bifidobacterium microbiota of elderly nursing home residents. Age (Omaha) 31: 59–66.

22. Langlands, S.J., Hopkins, M.J., Coleman, N., and Cummings, J.H. (2004) Prebiotic carbohydrates modify the mucosa associated microflora of the human large bowel. Gut 53: 1610–1616.

23. Leitch, E.C., Walker, A.W., Duncan, S.H., Holtrop, G., and Flint, H.J. (2007) Selective colonization of insoluble substrates by human faecal bacteria. Environ Microbiol 9: 667–679.

24. Mariat, D., Firmesse, O., Levenez, F., Guimarães, V., Sokol, H., Doré, J., et al. (2009) The Firmicutes/Bacteroidetes ratio of the human microbiota changes with age. BMC Microbiol 9: e123.

25. Martínez, I., Kim, J., Duffy, P.R., Schlegel, V.L., and Walter, J. (2010) Resistant starches types 2 and 4 have differential effects on the composition of the fecal microbiota in human subjects. PLoS ONE 5: e15046.

26. Metchnikoff, E. (1908) The Prolongation of Life. Optimistic Studies. Putnam's Son. New York and London: The Knickerbocker press [WWW document]. URL http://archive.org/stream/prolongationofli00metcuoft#page/14/mode/2up.

27. Mitsuoka, T. (1992) Intestinal flora and aging. Nutr Rev 50: 438–446.

28. Mueller, S., Saunier, K., Hanisch, C., Norin, E., Alm, L., Midtvedt, T., et al. (2006) Differences in fecal microbiota in different European study populations in relation to age, gender, and country: a cross-sectional study. Appl Environ Microbiol 72: 1027–1033.

29. New York Times (18 January 1908) Book review: the prolongation of life [WWW document]. URL http://query.nytimes.com/mem/archive-free/pdf?res=F40C11FB3C5A17738DDDA10994D9405B888CF1D3.

30. O'Toole, P.W., and Claesson, M.J. (2010) Gut microbiota: changes throughout the lifespan from infancy to elderly. Int Dairy J 20: 281–291.

31. Palaria, A., Johnson-Kanda, I., and O'Sullivan, D.J. (2012) Effect of a synbiotic yogurt on levels of fecal bifidobacteria, clostridia, and enterobacteria. Appl Environ Microbiol 78: 933–940.

32. Ramirez-Farias, C., Slezak, K., Fuller, Z., Duncan, A., Holtrop, G., and Louis, P. (2009) Effect of inulin on the human gut microbiota: stimulation of Bifidobacterium adolescentis and Faecalibacterium prausnitzii. Br J Nutr 101: 541–550.

33. van Tongeren, S.P., Slaets, J.P., Harmsen, H.J., and Welling, G.W. (2005) Fecal microbiota composition and frailty. Appl Environ Microbiol 71: 6438–6442.

34. Vulevic, J., Drakoularakou, A., Yaqoob, P., Tzortzis, G., and Gibson, G.R. (2008) Modulation of the fecal microflora profile and immune function by a novel transgalactooligosaccharide mixture (B-GOS) in healthy elderly volunteers. Am J Clin Nutr 88: 1438–1446.

35. Walker, A.W., Ince, J., Duncan, S.H., Webster, L.M., Holtrop, G., Ze, X., et al. (2011) Dominant and diet-responsive groups of bacteria within the human colonic microbiota. ISME J 5: 220–230.

36. Walton, G.E., van den Heuvel, E.G., Kosters, M.H., Rastall, R.A., Tuohy, K.M., and Gibson, G.R. (2012) A randomised crossover study investigating the effects of

galacto-oligosaccharides on the faecal microbiota in men and women over 50 years of age. Br J Nutr 107: 1466–1475.

37. Wang, X., and Gibson, G.R. (1993) Effects of the in vitro fermentation of oligofructose and inulin by bacteria growing in the human large intestine. J Appl Bacteriol 75: 373–380.

38. Woodmansey, E.J. (2007) Intestinal bacteria and ageing. J Appl Microbiol 102: 1178–1186.

39. Woodmansey, E.J., McMurdo, M.E., Macfarlane, G.T., and Macfarlane, S. (2004) Comparison of compositions and metabolic activities of fecal microbiotas in young adults and in antibiotic-treated and non-antibiotic-treated elderly subjects. Appl Environ Microbiol 70: 6113–6122.

40. Wu, G.D., Chen, J., Hoffmann, C., Bittinger, K., Chen, Y.Y., Keilbaugh, S.A., et al. (2011) Linking long-term dietary patterns with gut microbial enterotypes. Science 334: 105–108.

CHAPTER 13

GUT PHARMACOMICROBIOMICS: THE TIP OF AN ICEBERG OF COMPLEX INTERACTIONS BETWEEN DRUGS AND GUT-ASSOCIATED MICROBES

RAMA SAAD, MARIAM R RIZKALLAH, AND RAMY K AZIZ

13.1 INTRODUCTION

The gut microbiota is the most predominant and most diverse microbial community residing in the human body [1]. It comprises hundreds of microbial species, together constituting about 10 times the number of body cells [2,3], and contributes substantially to human metabolic processes to the extent that up to 36 % of small molecules in human blood are contributed by the gut microbiome [4]. The gut microbiota's impact on drug response and metabolism has been explored since the mid 20th century (reviewed in [5]); however, past studies have mostly focused on assessing the metabolic activity of gut microbial communities on antibiotics and botanicals [6-9]. Meanwhile, the influence of the host genetic makeup on drug response occupied the center stage of personalized medicine research, specifically in the clinical domain, leading to the rise of pharmacogenomic

This chapter was originally published under the Creative Commons Attribution License. Saad R, Rizkallah MR, and Aziz RK. Gut Pharmacomicrobiomics: The Tip of an Iceberg of Complex Interactions Between Drugs and Gut-Associated Microbes. Gut Pathogens 4,16 (2012). doi:10.1186/1757-4749-4-16.

approaches to personalized therapy, while a pivotal player in xenobiotic metabolism, the microbiota, was mostly being overlooked [10,11].

The various metabolic capabilities of the gut microbiota fueled the study of its effects on drug metabolism [11,12]. Several approaches were adopted, including comparisons between metabolic patterns of conventional and germfree mice, biochemical assays of microbial metabolic activities in cultures, and mutagenicity tests [5,6,13]. Population-based approaches, such as investigating the correlation between compositional variations in gut microbiota and response to a particular drug, e.g., digoxin, were followed as well [9].

The evolution of microbial genomics from culture-based (i.e., sequencing genomes of bacterial species after isolating their colonies) to culture-independent strategies (metagenomics—or shotgun sequencing of microbial and viral communities [14,15]) has allowed the identification of the molecular signature of the gut microbiome associated with a certain disease or with altered drug response [16]. To describe this new expansion of pharmacogenomics, we suggested the term pharmacomicrobiomics to denote the effect of microbiome variations on drug disposition and response [17,18]; here, we apply this concept explicitly to the human gut microbiome, the best-studied microbiome for its effect on xenobiotics.

In a broad sense, the term gut pharmacomicrobiomics encompasses the effect of the gut microbiome variations on pharmacokinetic and pharmacodynamic processes [17,19] (See Section "Term disambiguation"). However, to date, the better-documented effects of the human gut metagenome on drugs are those related to metabolism (i.e., effects on pharmacokinetic), either through: (i) the secretion of enzymes that modify the chemical structure of drug molecules, (ii) the secretion of metabolic products that interfere with drug metabolism, (iii) the modification of the levels and activities of liver and intestinal enzymes, or (iv) the modulation of expression of human metabolic genes [16] (Figure 1). Taking into consideration the enormous number of gut-associated microbes, and the extremely large number of diverse genes they encode and pathways they express, understanding the effect of the gut microbiota on human response to drugs is an indispensable step towards providing a comprehensively tailored/personalized therapy that would be more efficient, cost-effective, and with lower adverse drug events [17,20].

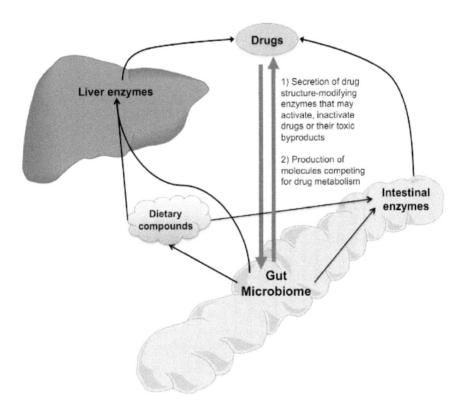

FIGURE 1: Different ways of interactions between the gut microbiome and drugs, sometimes involving dietary compounds or intestinal and liver enzymes. Liver and intestine cartoons were taken from the publicly available clipart of the University of Wisconsin, Madison. URL: http://www.biochem.wisc.edu/medialab/clipart.aspx.

TABLE 1: Role of gut microbiota in the metabolism of dietary compounds and phytochemicals

Chemical (drug or herbal remedy) {CID}	Pharmacological effect	Role of gut microbiota in metabolism	Altered metabolism and subsequent outcome	References
Heterocyclic aromatic amines (HAAs)	Carcinogenic agents	HAAs, originally derived from cooking proteins, are pro-mutagenic compounds known to be carcinogenic to rats and mice reviewed in [30]. Normally upon ingestion of a cooked protein, gut microbiota metabolize these compounds to yield unconjugated mutagen metabolites detectable in urine and stool, and human liver enzymes CYP450 1A1 and 1A2 activate these compounds to the active mutagenic forms. The effect of elevated active mutagens metabolites was reported to be significantly higher in conventional rats than germfree rats. Conventional rats have shown elevated activity of ethoxyresorufin-O-deethylase (EROD), which is a CYP450-dependent enzyme responsible for the biotransformation of HAAs and is increased in the small intestine upon ingestion of fried meat. Thus, the intestinal microbiota is thought to play a central role in HAA metabolism and thereby, in the response to mutagens through enhancing the activity of CYP450 enzymes responsible for the activation of mutagens.	Enhancement of CYP450 activity, deconjugation of HAAs and consequent increased mutagenic activity	[29]
Cycasin {5459896}	Toxic glycoside	Members of the gut microbiota hydrolyze cycasin into the carcinogenic derivative, methylazoxymethanol.	Microbiome-induced hydrolysis leading to direct toxic effect	[7]

TABLE 1: *Cont.*

Chemical (drug or herbal remedy) {CID}	Pharmacological effect	Role of gut microbiota in metabolism	Altered metabolism and subsequent outcome	References
Rutin {5280805}	A quercetin glucoside with angio-protective effects	Several gut anaerobes, e.g., Bacteriodes uniformans, Bacteroides ovatus, and Butrivibrio sp. hydrolyze dietary rutin into its corresponding quercetin aglycone and polyphenols. The release of both the free quercetin aglycone and the phenolic metabolites underlies rutin's mutagenic effect and the further inhibition of platelet aggregation, respectively. The free quercetin aglycone is a mutagen. Furthermore, the administration of rutin has been correlated with the increase of mutagenic activity of other glycosides with mutagenic aglycone component. The increase in glycosidic activity was expected to further increase the release of quercetin; however, the activation of quercetin was decreased in rats fed with rutin in contrast to the free aglycones of other mutagens such as 2-amino-3-methylimidazo [4,5-f] quinoline (IQ), 2-amino-3,4-dimethylimidazo [4,5-f] quinoline (MeIQ), and 2-amino-3,8-dimethylimidazo-[4,5-f] quinoxaline (MeIQx).	Microbiome-induced hydrolysis leading to indirect mutagenic effect	[31]
Aflatoxin B1 {186907}	Carcinogenic myco-toxins	Rats with conventional gut microbiota have shown two-fold increase in aflatoxin concentration in S9 liver fraction. Additionally, an in vivo-modified Ames test showed that rats with conventional gut microbiota have higher number of mutants of the indicator organism, Salmonella Typhimurium TA98, than germfree rats.	Potentiated toxic effects	[31]

TABLE 1: *Cont.*

Chemical (drug or herbal remedy) {CID}	Pharmacological effect	Role of gut microbiota in metabolism	Altered metabolism and subsequent outcome	References
(+)- catechin and (−)-epichatechins {9064, 72276}	Anti-oxidants	The effects of (+)-catechins and (−)-epicatechins on liver and intestinal enzymes have been reported to be different between germfree rats and rats with human gut microbiota. In germfree rats, (+)-catechins and (−)-epicatechins resulted in increase in the levels of liver CYP450 2C11 and (+)- catechins caused elevation in the specific activity of liver Uridine 5'-diphospho-glucuronosyltransferase UGT-chloramphenicol. On the other hand, cytosolic glutathion-S-transferase (GST) levels were higher in rats harboring human gut microbiota upon the administration of (+)-catechins. However, in both germfree and human microbiota inoculated rats, (+)-catechins and (−)-epicatechins increased the specific activity of UGT-4-methyl umbelliferone in the intestine. Furthermore, the specific activity of intestinal UGT-chloramphenicol was higher in rats inoculated with human microbiota.	Indirect potentiating/lowering effect on drug metabolism depending on the type of co-administered drug, the metabolic pathway adapted, and the effect of the resulting metabolite	[32]
2-methoxy esterone	Anti-angiogenic	Members of the gut microbiota are believed to convert 2-methoxy esterone to the active steroid form. This was demonstrated upon incubation of 2-methoxy esterone with isolated rat cecum, where two different reactions were found to take place: oxidoreduction at C17 and demethylation at C2 resulting into the active form.	Oxidoreduction and demethylation resulting in activation of prodrug	[33]
Chlorogenic acid {1794427}	Antioxidant	Gut microbiota metabolize chlorogenic acid to 3-hydroxycinnamic acid and 3-(3-hydroxyphenyl)propionic acid, which are subjects to phase II conjugation followed by excretion in urine. In absence of gut microbiota, chlorogenic acid is metabolized to benzoic acid, which in turn is conjugated with glycine yielding hippuric acid. Gonthier et al. found that the bioavailability of chlorogenic acid relies on its metabolism by gut microbiota [34].	Microbial metabolism resulting in potentiated clinical effect	[34,35]

TABLE 1: *Cont.*

Chemical (drug or herbal remedy) {CID}	Pharmacological effect	Role of gut microbiota in metabolism	Altered metabolism and subsequent outcome	References
Soy-derived phytoestrogens	Xeno-estrogens	Some microbial communities in the gut produce active metabolites from soy-derived phytoestrogens resulting in enhanced efficacy. In addition, the phytoestrogens metabolites produced by gut microbiota are suggested to affect cytochrome P enzymes, which are responsible for estrogen hydroxylation, and therefore result in lower toxic events.	According to the type of microbiota present, toxicity or lower action may result.	[36,37]
Baicalin {64982}	Potential antioxidant, anti-inflammatory and liver tonic	Gut microbiota normally hydrolyze baicalin into its corresponding aglycone baicalein, which is readily absorbable and subject to re-conjugation following absorption. Absence of gut microbiota in germfree rats reportedly resulted in lower levels of baicalin in plasma following oral administration.	Potentiated clinical effect	[38]
Anthocyanins {145858}	Potential anticancer, anti-oxidant and anti-inflammatory	Gut microbes are responsible for the hydrolysis of the glycosidic linkage between the sugar and the aglycone by means of β-glucosidases resulting in the release of the free aglycone active form.	Microbial hydrolysis leading to activation of prodrug	[39]
Genistin {5281377}	Anti-cancer, estrogenic and antiatherosclerotic	Gut microbes hydrolyze the glycosidic linkage between the sugar and the aglycone by means of β-glucosidases resulting in the release of the aglycone active form genistein.	Microbial hydrolysis leading to activation of prodrug	[39]
Naringin {442428}	Anti-oxidant, anti-cancer and blood cholesterol lowering effect	Same as with anthocyanins and genistin, microbial β-glucosidases lead to the release of the free aglycone active form naringenin.	Microbial hydrolysis leading to activation of prodrug	[39]

CID = Chemical ID from the PubChem database (URL: http://pubchem.ncbi.nlm.nih.gov website) [40] is provided in curly braces for all drugs or botanicals.

In this review, we aim at providing an overview of the influence of gut microbiota on drugs, spanning the documented metabolic effects of the microbiota and the different approaches used for their investigation. In addition, we provide an outlook for the future of pharmacomicrobiomics in the context of the Human Microbiome Project (HMP) and for the application of metagenomic approaches as an integral part of pharmacotherapy and personalized medicine.

13.1.1 TERM DISAMBIGUATION

Microbiome and microbiomics

To the best of our knowledge, the term "microbiome" was first suggested in 2000 by the Nobel Laureate, Joshua Lederberg, to describe the sum of microbial genomes associated with the human body, which he described as a part of "the human extended genome" (URL: http://www.project-syndicate.org/commentary/microbiology-s-world-wide-web). Soon after, it was used in the same meaning in literature [21,22]. Currently, however, microbiome is being used to denote two different concepts: (i) the collective microbial genome of a community (i.e., microbial metagenome) or (ii) the sum of all microscopic life forms, viz. microbes, within an environment (i.e., microbiome). Microbiome was initially confined to host-associated metagenomes, but is now being used interchangeably with microbial metagenome (e.g., the Earth Microbiome Project http://www.earthmicrobiome.org/ [23]). The less frequently used term, "microbiomics," describes the study of functional aspects related to the microbiome, including the integration of high-throughput genome-wide data [24].

Pharmacogenomics and pharmacomicrobiomics

Pharmacogenomics [25] is a well-established term that describes the effect of human genome variations on drug disposition and action. The term can certainly be applied not just to the human nuclear and mitochondrial genomes, but also to the human extended genome or the genome of the human supraorganism [18]; yet, to specify the impact of the human-associated microbiome on drugs, we have coined the term pharmacomicrobiomics [17,18], which we consider as a natural expansion of pharmacogenomics, which is likely to spread when more HMP data accrue.

Metabolomics and metabonomics
Those two verbally similar terms have been sometimes used interchangeably to describe the high-throughput study of all genome-encoded metabolites produced by a particular organism or a community; however, Nicholson and coworkers carefully denote the difference between the two terms as they use metabolomics to describe the study of genetically controlled metabolites and fluxes produced by one type of cells or tissues, whereas they define metabonomics as the measurement of metabolites produced by a collection of cells/genomes within a multicellular organism or an ecosystem [26] (the latter once described as the "meta-metabolome" [27]).

13.1.2 ROLE OF GUT MICROBIOTA IN XENOBIOTIC METABOLISM

The influence of the gut microbiota on the metabolism of xenobiotics has been regarded extensively as a response-modifying process, and several mechanisms have been proposed and demonstrated [11]. Gut-associated microbes can alter drug metabolism directly by producing enzymes that degrade or activate the drug molecules, or by competing with drug molecules over the metabolizing enzymes [17,20]. In addition, the gut microbiota may exert its influence by modulating the activity or altering the levels of the host's drug-metabolizing enzymes or by producing enzyme-inducing metabolites that are originally derived from diet [28,29] (Figure 1). Accordingly, the microbiome's response-modifying effect has been widely appreciated in nutrition and toxicology, and the role of gut microbiota in metabolism has initially been investigated in terms of the metabolism of compounds of dietary and botanical origin (Table 1).

TABLE 2: Effect of microbiota on hepatic and intestinal metabolic enzymes [28]

Enzyme	Function	Effect of gut microbiome
Ethoxyresorufin-O-deethylase (EROD)	A CYP450-dependent enzyme responsible for the biotransformation of HAAs	The presence of normal gut microbiota in rats potentiates EROD activity upon ingestion of fried meat
Glutathione S-transferase A 1/2 (GSTA1/2)	Being among the alpha class of GST enzyme family that is preferentially expressed in the colon rather than the liver, it plays a central role in phase II detoxification of xenobiotics. In addition, GSTA1/2 class displays a glutathione peroxidase activity, which underlies its antioxidant and cyto-protective effects.	Measuring GSTA1/2 levels in both germfree rats and microbiota–reassociated rats showed 4- and 5-fold increase in the enzyme level in germfree males and females, respectively.
Glutathione S-transferase A4(GSTA4)	Among the alpha class of GST enzymes that possess high affinity to alk-2-enes	Germfree rats showed 1.5- and 1.9-fold increase in the levels of GSTA4 than microbiota–re-associated rats in males and females, respectively.
Glutathione S-transferase M1 (GSTM1)	GSTM1 is one of the mu class of GSTs which detoxify carcinogens, toxins, drugs and oxidative stress products.	Germfree female rats showed a statistically significant but modest elevation in colonic GSTM1 levels compared to rats with gut microbiota. However, male rats didn't exhibit this elevation. This increase in germfree female rats may be coincidental in spite of the statistical significance.
Epoxide hydroxylase 1 (EPHX1) enzyme	Responsible for the activation and detoxification of xenobiotics as polycyclic aromatic hydrocarbons	Germfree rats showed a substantial increase in the colonic levels of EPHX1 than rats associated with rat gut microbiota.
Epoxide hydroxylase 2 (EPHX2) enzyme	Located in cell cytosol and perixosomes and detoxifies specific peroxides by catalyzing their conversion into dihydrodiols	Germfree rats showed a moderate increase in the colonic levels of EPHX2 than rats associated with rat gut microbiota.
Sulfotransferase 1C2 (SULT1C2) enzyme	Among the SULT1 enzyme subfamily, which conjugates phenolic compounds with sulfo groups obtained from 3'-Phosphoadenosine-5'-phosphosulfate (PAPS)	Germfree female rats showed a statistically significant modest increase (1.6-fold) in colonic levels of SULT1C2.

TABLE 2: *Cont.*

Enzyme	Function	Effect of gut microbiome
Sulfotransferase 1B1 (SULT1B1) enzyme	A member of the SULT1 enzyme subfamily	On the contrary to SULT1C2, germfree male and female rats showed a statistically significant decrease (0.4- and 0.6-fold, respectively) in the enzyme level than gut micro-biota- associated rats.
N-acetyltransferase 1 (NAT1) & N-acetyl-transferase 2 (NAT2) enzyme	Detoxify hydrazine and arylamine drugs	NAT enzyme levels were mod-estly elevated in germfree rats in comparison with rats with conventional gut microbiota.
Glutathione per-oxidase 2 (GPX2) enzyme	A selenium-dependent member of the GPX family of glutathione peroxidase that is present in the epithelium of the gastrointestinal tract	Elevated GPX2 mRNA levels have been correlated with the reintroduction of microbiota in germfree rats.

Additionally, the absence of conventional gut microbiota in germfree mice has been correlated with perturbations in levels of liver and intestinal metabolic enzymes in comparison to their corresponding levels in mice with conventional gut ecosystem [29], and conventional gut microbiotas in human and mice were shown to be associated with a modest elevation in the levels of drug-metabolizing enzymes, such as sulfotransferase1 B1 (SULT1B1) and with reduced levels of other enzymes, such as SULT1C1, NAT1 and NAT2 [28] (Table 2).

13.1.3 IMPACT OF MICROBIOME VARIATIONS ON DRUG RESPONSE AND TOXICITY

Most studies on drug-microbe interactions did not take in consideration the microbiome profile/composition of an individual or a population; however, these variations are the basis of pharmacomicrobiomics, and their study has become possible now that the HMP has been established [3,41], and HMP data have already been made available [1,42].

Several studies associated a particular 16S rRNA microbial signature with specific biomarker metabolites and clinical outcomes. This association has been extended to encompass several conventional drugs such as digoxin and acetaminophen [9,43]. Profiling the signatures of the microbial communities in relation to their metabolic effect on drugs among patients is likely to introduce clinical markers that will dictate treatment regimens tailored in accordance with each patient's resident microbiota [43]. Such regimens, in turn, will modify the current treatment strategies that are based on conventional pathologic and pharmacokinetic parameters to take into account the interindividual perturbations in the gut microbiota and the gut ecosystem. These measures are especially true with the evidence of the sym-xenobiotic metabolism that involves both the host and the associated microbiota to biotransform drugs, including first-line therapies [9,44] (Table 3). As a consequence, microbiome-labile medications may be limited, or their dose readjusted, for certain populations or individuals harboring particular gut microbial community profiles. Several drugs that possess structural similarity to microbial products and are thereby potential candidates of microbial metabolism are yet to be studied.

TABLE 3: Role of gut microbiota in the metabolism of conventional first line therapies and over-the-counter (OTC) drugs

To view Table 3, please view the original version of this article.

13.1.4 A SYSTEMS BIOLOGY VIEW OF THE HOST-MICROBIOTA METABOLOME AND CO-METABOLOME

Previously reported drug-microbe and drug-microbiome interactions have mostly been described as phenotypic observations of drugs being modified by a microbial species, an entire microbial community, or an even more intricate system consisting of a microbial and a human component. However, in many cases the process, biochemical pathway, or specific reaction remains unknown, which renders the analysis of those interactions by reductionist approaches difficult. Instead, exploring the causality of those interactions might require systems approaches such as the metage-nomic analysis of the microbial community followed by the identification of differentially abundant or differentially expressed candidate genes or genomic subsystems [52] involved in those interactions. Yet, metagenom-ic surveys that determine microbial community profiles, gene presence/absence and abundance, or functional classification of sequence fragments are not sufficient to tell a coherent story about the observed phenotypes since a gene's presence does not imply its expression or functionality. Con-sequently, extracting knowledge from those microbiome explorations and translating them into an ultimately tailored therapy requires modeling the human microbiome, variome, and interactions between them via integrat-ing multiple layers of information, including transcriptomic, proteomic, and metabolomic data. Such integration is not always achievable in a sys-tem with this complexity. For instance, a statistically sound correlation between mRNA and protein expression levels in mid-log phase *Saccha-romyces cerevisiae* cells has been hindered by technical limitations [53]. If this was the case with a unicellular organism or with relatively uniform cell lines [54], then further levels of complexity are to be expected in the gut microbiome ecosystem, where communities of unicellular organisms coexist in balance with the human multicellular tissues. Systems biology approaches for such complex communities are inevitable but are still in early development [55,56].

From a holistic perspective, tailoring a pharmacotherapy that accom-modates intraindividual and interindividual variations would take into ac-count the variations in the host's genetic makeup, its associated-microbi-ome, and metabolomic interactions between the host and its associated microbiota (i.e., co-metabolome). With the recognition of the considerable role of the human microbiome and its variations together with the former-ly well-recognized role of the human variome in predicting response to pharmacotherapy, there is a growing demand in both clinical and research domains for proper computational models that are able to comprehensive-ly consider all such aspects of variability [26,53,54]. The best-recognized process in altered drug response, controlled by both human genome and microbiome, is the presystemic metabolism or first-pass effect (reviewed in [57]). Since the metabolism of xenobiotics in humas is performed by host and microbial enzymes, the metabolic process is recognized as combinatorial or "sym-xenobiotic" as recently described [10]. Furthermore, a continuous metabolic interaction, termed metabolome-metabolome interaction, exists between the host and its associated microbiota [10]. Modeling the human/microbiome variations and metabolome-metabolome interactions will provide insights into the metabolism of xenobiotics and thereby allow for accurate predictions for drug response [26].

Nicholson and colleagues [26] attempted to visualize the role of both the host and its associated microbiota in xenobiotic metabolism in the gut by proposing an interesting model, assuming six different cell types in both host and microbiota, every type of which has its own transcriptome and metabolome depending on its role. There is a mutual metabolic exchange between the host and microbiota, and the extracellular compartment contains metabolites generated by both of them. Those metabolites are the result of drug and food metabolism, and might lead to metabolic alterations in both the host and its associated microbiota. This probabilistic model of metabolism was introduced in an attempt to tackle the potential interaction between the different host- and microbiome-related factors that would eventually display a certain outcome for metabolism. The model likens the complex process of drug metabolism to a Japanese Pachinko (pinball machine), where pins represent enzymes and transporters involved in metabolism, holes indicate outlets for metabolites, and pathways are represented by the sequence of pins. According to this model, the final outcome is the increment of the probabilities of collisions between pins and balls [26].

13.1.5 WEB RESOURCES FOR EXPLORING GUT PHARMACOMICROBIOMICS

- **Human variome resources:**
- HVP (Human Variome Project): http://www.humanvariomeproject.org [58]
- HapMap: http://hapmap.ncbi.nlm.nih.gov [59]
- **Human microbiome resources:**
- MetaHIT (Metagenomics of the Human Intestinal Tract): http://www.metahit.eu [42]
- HMP: http://hmpdacc.org [41]

- **Tools or databases for browsing the human microbiome:**
- IMG/HMP: http://www.hmpdacc-resources.org/cgi-bin/imgm_hmp/main. cgi [41]
- myMGDB: http://edwards.sdsu.edu/cgi-bin/mymgdb/show.cgi
- MG-RAST: http://metagenomics.anl.gov [60]
- The SEED Servers: http://www.theseed.org/servers [61]
- **Pharmacogenomics/pharmacomicrobiomics databases:**
- PharmGKB (Pharmacogenomics Knowledge Base): http://www.pharmgkb. org [62]
- PacDB (Pharmacogenetics and Cell Database): http://www.pacdb.org [63]
- CTDB (Comparative Toxigenomics Database): http://ctdbase.org [64]
- The PharmacoMicrobiomics Portal: http://www.pharmacomicrobiomics. org [65]

- **Enzymes/pathways databases:**
- KEGG (Kyoto Encyclopedia of Genes and Genomes): http://www.genome. jp/kegg/ [66]
- Model SEED: http://seed-viewer.theseed.org/seedviewer. cgi?page=ModelView [67]
- BRENDA (BRaunschweig ENzyme Database): http://www.brenda-en-zymes.org [68]

13.1.6 FUTURE ANTICIPATIONS

The current advances in the Human Variome Project [69,70] and the HMP [3,41], together with a battery of publicly available web resources (See Section "Web resources for exploring gut pharmacomicrobiomics") offer a starting point for those interested in drug-microbiome interactions to address several intriguing questions. However, the examples reported previously (e.g., those in Tables 1, 2 and 3) are just the tip of an iceberg of yet-to-be-discovered interactions between the host variome, associated microbiome, their combined metabolome, and chemicals ingested by humans. Ultimately, the study of those interactions in spite of their complexity is driven by the need for devising personalized therapeutic regimens aiming at optimizing drug bioavailability to obtain maximal efficiency and minimal toxicity. Below, we suggest a roadmap of four steps for the development of the nascent field of gut pharmacomicrobiomics and its translation into personalized medicine (Figure 2).

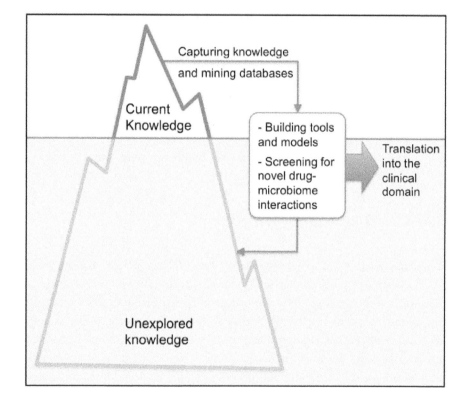

FIGURE 2: A roadmap for the development of the nascent field of gut pharmaco-microbiomics and its translation into the clinical domain.

13.1.7 CAPTURING CURRENT KNOWLEDGE

The first step is to capture and organize the currently available information on drug-microbiome complex interactions by building databases similar to those built for pharmacogenetics, pharmacogenomics, and drug-drug interactions. Concomitant with building databases is developing tools and resources to support discovery by mining those databases and connecting them to microbial genomic databases (e.g., SEED [61], GOLD [71]) metagenomic/microbiome databases, (e.g., MG-RAST [60], myMGDB, HMP [41], METAHIT [42]), and metabolic pathway databases (e.g., KEGG [66], modelSEED [67], BRENDA [68]).

13.1.8 DEVELOPING AND PERFORMING HIGH-THROUGHPUT SCREENS FOR NOVEL DRUG-MICROBIOME INTERACTIONS

In parallel with capturing existing knowledge, there is continuous need for digging deeper into the unknown drug-microbiome interaction space. Addressing this need can be achieved via studies involving high-throughput screens of drugs against human microbiota from different individuals looking at the overall action of these microbiotas on representatives of different drug classes, or, reciprocally, via screening individual resident gut microbes against large libraries of drugs or other chemicals.

13.1.9 DEVELOPING SOFTWARE AND BUILDING MODELS FOR DRUG RESPONSE SIMULATION

The accumulated data in literature pointing out to the response variation mediated by mammalian host variome and microbiome calls for the construction of modeling software that considers all such parameters to provide rational hypotheses or accurate predictions for research [26,55,72]. Developing such modeling software and using it in building models requires encoding data compiled from the literature regarding the host variome, microbiome and co-metabolome, and incorporating these encoded data into a model capable of retrieving an informative index describing the predicted outcome. For instance, Hlavaty and colleagues [73] used a similar approach to construct a predictive model of an apoptotic pharmacogenetic index for infliximab in treatment of Crohn disease. Following data mining, they used SAS® enterprise miner software to analyze all the genetic variants involved with the apoptotic response of infliximab, they managed to develop a new pharmacogenetic index ranging from 0 which denotes diminished response to 3, indicating a powerful response [73].

13.1.10 DATA INTEGRATION AND TRANSLATION INTO THE CLINICAL DOMAIN

The availability of web resources, the generation of more data, and the construction of rigorous models for drug-microbiome interactions will offer a great opportunity to translate this knowledge into diagnostic and clinical measures. In the future, routing clinical practices should include integrating microbiome data and processing them to produce valid assumptions of clinical outcome, based on which the type, dose, and regimen of treatment will be planned for each patient. Accordingly, each case will have its own panel of personalized therapy. For instance, patients harboring gut microbiota known to be associated with elevated levels of metabolic enzymes will be scheduled for higher doses; patients with higher susceptibility to acetaminophen toxicity might either be given a lower dose or an alternative nonsteroidal anti-inflammatory medicine; and patients with a microbiota with higher ability to metabolize digoxin will be scheduled to receive lower dose.

13.2 CONCLUSIONS

Throughout the past five decades, the study of the effect of gut microbiota went through several phases uncovering its ample significance in drug response. With the continuous growth of the HMP and its expansion to cover diverse human populations, it is anticipated that the primary data concerning the common gut microbiome profile and its diversity among humans will be revealed, enabling to pursue further studies on its effect on drug response among populations. However, several steps are yet to be taken in anticipation of the floods of HMP data, including the construction of databases, software, and models that would provide credible predictions of differential clinical outcome and fuel further hypothesis-driven studies whose findings might be integrated into clinical settings.

REFERENCES

1. Human Microbiome Project Consortium: Structure, function and diversity of the healthy human microbiome. Nature 2012, 486:207-214.
2. Savage DC: Microbial ecology of the gastrointestinal tract. Annu Rev Microbiol 1977, 31:107-133.
3. Peterson J, Garges S, Giovanni M, McInnes P, Wang L, Schloss JA, Bonazzi V, McEwen JE, Wetterstrand KA, Deal C, et al.: The NIH Human Microbiome Project. Genome Res 2009, 19:2317-2323.
4. Hood L: Tackling the microbiome. Science 2012, 336:1209.
5. Goldman P, Peppercorn MA, Goldin BR: Metabolism of drugs by microorganisms in the intestine. Am J Clin Nutr 1974, 27:1348-1355.
6. Holt R: The bacterial degradation of chloramphenicol. Lancet 1967, 1:1259-1260.
7. Spatz M, Smith DW, McDaniel EG, Laqueur GL: Role of intestinal microorganisms in determining cycasin toxicity. Proc Soc Exp Biol Med 1967, 124:691-697.
8. Lindenbaum J, Rund DG, Butler VP Jr, Tse-Eng D, Saha JR: Inactivation of digoxin by the gut flora: reversal by antibiotic therapy. N Engl J Med 1981, 305:789-794.
9. Mathan VI, Wiederman J, Dobkin JF, Lindenbaum J: Geographic differences in digoxin inactivation, a metabolic activity of the human anaerobic gut flora. Gut 1989, 30:971-977.
10. Nicholson JK, Holmes E, Wilson ID: Gut microorganisms, mammalian metabolism and personalized health care. Nat Rev Microbiol 2005, 3:431-438.
11. Sousa T, Paterson R, Moore V, Carlsson A, Abrahamsson B, Basit AW: The gastrointestinal microbiota as a site for the biotransformation of drugs. Int J Pharm 2008, 363:1-25.
12. Johnson CH, Patterson AD, Idle JR, Gonzalez FJ: Xenobiotic metabolomics: major impact on the metabolome. Annu Rev Pharmacol Toxicol 2012, 52:37-56.
13. Koch RL, Chrystal EJ, Beaulieu BB Jr, Goldman P: Acetamide–a metabolite of metronidazole formed by the intestinal flora. Biochem Pharmacol 1979, 28:3611-3615.
14. Riesenfeld CS, Schloss PD, Handelsman J: Metagenomics: genomic analysis of microbial communities. Annu Rev Genet 2004, 38:525-552.
15. Edwards RA, Rohwer F: Viral metagenomics. Nat Rev Microbiol 2005, 3:504-510.
16. Haiser HJ, Turnbaugh PJ: Developing a metagenomic view of xenobiotic metabolism. Pharmacol Res 2012.

17. Rizkallah MR, Saad R, Aziz RK: The Human Microbiome Project, personalized medicine and the birth of pharmacomicrobiomics. Curr Pharmacogenomics Person Med 2010, 8:182-193.
18. Aziz RK: Rethinking pharmacogenomics in an ecosystem: drug-microbiome interactions, pharmacomicrobiomics, and personalized medicine for the human supraorganism. Curr Pharmacogenomics Person Med 2012, 10:258-261.
19. Aziz RK, Saad R, Rizkallah MR: PharmacoMicrobiomics or how bugs modulate drugs: an educational initiative to explore the effects of human microbiome on drugs. BMC Bioinforma 2011, 12:A10.
20. Wilson ID: Drugs, bugs, and personalized medicine: pharmacometabonomics enters the ring. Proc Natl Acad Sci USA 2009, 106:14187-14188.
21. Relman DA: New technologies, human-microbe interactions, and the search for previously unrecognized pathogens. J Infect Dis 2002, 186(Suppl 2):S254-S258.
22. Shanahan F: The host-microbe interface within the gut. Best Pract Res Clin Gastroenterol 2002, 16:915-931.
23. Gilbert JA, Meyer F, Antonopoulos D, Balaji P, Brown CT, Desai N, Eisen JA, Evers D, Field D, Feng W, et al.: Meeting report: the terabase metagenomics workshop and the vision of an Earth microbiome project. Stand Genomic Sci 2010, 3:243-248.
24. Egert M, de Graaf AA, Smidt H, de Vos WM, Venema K: Beyond diversity: functional microbiomics of the human colon. Trends Microbiol 2006, 14:86-91.
25. Persidis A: The business of pharmacogenomics. Nat Biotechnol 1998, 16:209-210.
26. Nicholson JK, Wilson ID: Opinion: understanding 'global' systems biology: metabonomics and the continuum of metabolism. Nat Rev Drug Discov 2003, 2:668-676.
27. Ibrahim M, Anishetty S: A meta-metabolome network of carbohydrate metabolism: Interactions between gut microbiota and host. Biochem Biophys Res Commun 2012, 428(2):278-284.
28. Meinl W, Sczesny S, Brigelius-Flohe R, Blaut M, Glatt H: Impact of gut microbiota on intestinal and hepatic levels of phase 2 xenobiotic-metabolizing enzymes in the rat. Drug Metab Dispos 2009, 37:1179-1186.
29. Overvik E, Lindeskog P, Midtvedt T, Gustafsson JA: Mutagen excretion and cytochrome P-450-dependent activity in germfree and conventional rats fed a diet containing fried meat. Food Chem Toxicol 1990, 28:253-261.
30. Sugimura T, Nagao M, Wakabayashi K: Carcinogenicity of food mutagens. Environ Health Perspect 1996, 104(Suppl 3):429-433.
31. Rowland IR: Interactions of the gut microflora and the host in toxicology. Toxicol Pathol 1988, 16:147-153.
32. Lhoste EF, Ouriet V, Bruel S, Flinois JP, Brezillon C, Magdalou J, Cheze C, Nugon-Baudon L: The human colonic microflora influences the alterations of xenobiotic-metabolizing enzymes by catechins in male F344 rats. Food Chem Toxicol 2003, 41:695-702.
33. Axelson M, Sjovall J: Formation of catechol estrogens by intestinal bacterial demethylation of 2-methoxyestrone. Biochim Biophys Acta 1983, 751:162-165.
34. Gonthier MP, Verny MA, Besson C, Remesy C, Scalbert A: Chlorogenic acid bioavailability largely depends on its metabolism by the gut microflora in rats. J Nutr 2003, 133:1853-1859.

35. Gavaghan CL, Nicholson JK, Connor SC, Wilson ID, Wright B, Holmes E: Directly coupled high-performance liquid chromatography and nuclear magnetic resonance spectroscopic with chemometric studies on metabolic variation in Sprague–Dawley rats. Anal Biochem 2001, 291:245-252.

36. Bowey E, Adlercreutz H, Rowland I: Metabolism of isoflavones and lignans by the gut microflora: a study in germ-free and human flora associated rats. Food Chem Toxicol 2003, 41:631-636.

37. Delgado S, Ruas-Madiedo P, Suarez A, Mayo B: Interindividual differences in microbial counts and biochemical-associated variables in the feces of healthy Spanish adults. Dig Dis Sci 2006, 51:737-743.

38. Akao T, Kawabata K, Yanagisawa E, Ishihara K, Mizuhara Y, Wakui Y, Sakashita Y, Kobashi K: Baicalin, the predominant flavone glucuronide of scutellariae radix, is absorbed from the rat gastrointestinal tract as the aglycone and restored to its original form. J Pharm Pharmacol 2000, 52:1563-1568.

39. Selma MV, Espin JC, Tomas-Barberan FA: Interaction between phenolics and gut microbiota: role in human health. J Agric Food Chem 2009, 57:6485-6501.

40. Bolton EE, Wang Y, Thiessen PA, Bryant SH: PubChem: integrated platform of small molecules and biological activities. Annu Rep Comput Chem 2008, 4:217-241.

41. Proctor LM: The Human Microbiome Project in 2011 and beyond. Cell Host Microbe 2011, 10:287-291.

42. Qin J, Li R, Raes J, Arumugam M, Burgdorf KS, Manichanh C, Nielsen T, Pons N, Levenez F, Yamada T, et al.: A human gut microbial gene catalogue established by metagenomic sequencing. Nature 2010, 464:59-65.

43. Clayton TA, Baker D, Lindon JC, Everett JR, Nicholson JK: Pharmacometabonomic identification of a significant host-microbiome metabolic interaction affecting human drug metabolism. Proc Natl Acad Sci USA 2009, 106:14728-14733.

44. Vermes A, Kuijper EJ, Guchelaar HJ, Dankert J: An in vitro study on the active conversion of flucytosine to fluorouracil by microorganisms in the human intestinal microflora. Chemotherapy 2003, 49:17-23.

45. Grundmann O: The gut microbiome and pre-systemic metabolism: current state and evolving research. J Drug Metab Toxicol 2010, 1:105.

46. Steffens LS, Nicholson S, Paul LV, Nord CE, Patrick S, Abratt VR: Bacteroides fragilis RecA protein overexpression causes resistance to metronidazole. Res Microbiol 2010, 161:346-354.

47. Strong HA, Renwick AG, George CF, Liu YF, Hill MJ: The reduction of sulphinpyrazone and sulindac by intestinal bacteria. Xenobiotica 1987, 17:685-696.

48. Strong HA, Warner NJ, Renwick AG, George CF: Sulindac metabolism: the importance of an intact colon. Clin Pharmacol Ther 1985, 38:387-393.

49. Ashida N, Ijichi K, Watanabe Y, Machida H: Metabolism of 5'-ether prodrugs of 1-beta-D-arabinofuranosyl-E-5-(2-bromovinyl)uracil in rats. Biochem Pharmacol 1993, 46:2201-2207.

50. Nakayama H, Kinouchi T, Kataoka K, Akimoto S, Matsuda Y, Ohnishi Y: Intestinal anaerobic bacteria hydrolyse sorivudine, producing the high blood concentration of 5-(E)-(2-bromovinyl)uracil that increases the level and toxicity of 5-fluorouracil. Pharmacogenetics 1997, 7:35-43.

51. Kitamura S, Sugihara K, Kuwasako M, Tatsumi K: The role of mammalian intestinal bacteria in the reductive metabolism of zonisamide. J Pharm Pharmacol 1997, 49:253-256.

52. Overbeek R, Begley T, Butler RM, Choudhuri JV, Chuang HY, Cohoon M, de Crecy-Lagard V, Diaz N, Disz T, Edwards R, et al.: The subsystems approach to genome annotation and its use in the project to annotate 1000 genomes. Nucleic Acids Res 2005, 33:5691-5702.

53. Gygi SP, Rochon Y, Franza BR, Aebersold R: Correlation between protein and mRNA abundance in yeast. Mol Cell Biol 1999, 19:1720-1730.

54. Gry M, Rimini R, Stromberg S, Asplund A, Ponten F, Uhlen M, Nilsson P: Correlations between RNA and protein expression profiles in 23 human cell lines. BMC Genomics 2009, 10:365.

55. Zengler K, Palsson BO: A road map for the development of community systems (CoSy) biology. Nat Rev Microbiol 2012, 10:366-372.

56. Thiele I, Heinken A, Fleming RM: A systems biology approach to studying the role of microbes in human health. Curr Opin Biotechnol 2012.

57. Doherty MM, Pang KS: First-pass effect: significance of the intestine for absorption and metabolism. Drug Chem Toxicol 1997, 20:329-344.

58. Howard HJ, Horaitis O, Cotton RG, Vihinen M, Dalgleish R, Robinson P, Brookes AJ, Axton M, Hoffmann R, Tuffery-Giraud S: The Human Variome Project (HVP) 2009 Forum "Towards Establishing Standards". Hum Mutat 2010, 31:366-367.

59. International HapMap Consortium: The International HapMap Project. Nature 2003, 426:789-796.

60. Meyer F, Paarmann D, D'Souza M, Olson R, Glass EM, Kubal M, Paczian T, Rodriguez A, Stevens R, Wilke A, et al.: The metagenomics RAST server - a public resource for the automatic phylogenetic and functional analysis of metagenomes. BMC Bioinforma 2008, 9:386.

61. Aziz RK, Devoid S, Disz T, Edwards RA, Henry CS, Olsen GJ, Olson R, Overbeek R, Parrello B, Pusch GD, et al.: SEED Servers: high-performance access to the SEED genomes, annotations, and metabolic models. PLoS One 2012, 7:e48053.

62. Owen RP, Altman RB, Klein TE: PharmGKB and the International Warfarin Pharmacogenetics Consortium: the changing role for pharmacogenomic databases and single-drug pharmacogenetics. Hum Mutat 2008, 29:456-460.

63. Gamazon ER, Duan S, Zhang W, Huang RS, Kistner EO, Dolan ME, Cox NJ: PACdb: a database for cell-based pharmacogenomics. Pharmacogenet Genomics 2010, 20:269-273.

64. Davis AP, Murphy CG, Rosenstein MC, Wiegers TC, Mattingly CJ: The Comparative Toxicogenomics Database facilitates identification and understanding of chemical-gene-disease associations: arsenic as a case study. BMC Med Genomics 2008, 1:48.

65. Rizkallah MR SG-E, Saad R, Aziz RK: The pharmacomicrobiomics portal: a database for drug-microbiome interactions. Curr Pharmacogenomics Person Med 2012, 10:195-203.

66. Kanehisa M, Goto S: KEGG: Kyoto encyclopedia of genes and genomes. Nucleic Acids Res 2000, 28:27-30.

67. Henry CS, DeJongh M, Best AA, Frybarger PM, Linsay B, Stevens RL: High-throughput generation, optimization and analysis of genome-scale metabolic models. Nat Biotechnol 2010, 28:977-982.

68. Scheer M, Grote A, Chang A, Schomburg I, Munaretto C, Rother M, Sohngen C, Stelzer M, Thiele J, Schomburg D: BRENDA, the enzyme information system in 2011. Nucleic Acids Res 2011, 39:D670-D676.

69. Ring HZ, Kwok PY, Cotton RG: Human Variome Project: an international collaboration to catalogue human genetic variation. Pharmacogenomics 2006, 7:969-972.

70. Ozdemir V, Rosenblatt DS, Warnich L, Srivastava S, Tadmouri GO, Aziz RK, Reddy PJ, Manamperi A, Dove ES, Joly Y, et al.: Towards an ecology of collective innovation: Human Variome Project (HVP), Rare Disease Consortium for Autosomal Loci (RaDiCAL) and Data-Enabled Life Sciences Alliance (DELSA). Curr Pharmacogenomics Person Med 2011, 9:243-251.

71. Pagani I, Liolios K, Jansson J, Chen IM, Smirnova T, Nosrat B, Markowitz VM, Kyrpides NC: The Genomes OnLine Database (GOLD) v.4: status of genomic and metagenomic projects and their associated metadata. Nucleic Acids Res 2012, 40:571-579.

72. Heinken A, Sahoo S, Fleming RM, Thiele I: Systems-level characterization of a host-microbe metabolic symbiosis in the mammalian gut. Gut Microbes 2013, 4:1-13.

73. Hlavaty T, Ferrante M, Henckaerts L, Pierik M, Rutgeerts P, Vermeire S: Predictive model for the outcome of infliximab therapy in Crohn's disease based on apoptotic pharmacogenetic index and clinical predictors. Inflamm Bowel Dis 2007, 13:372-379.

CHAPTER 14

FAME AND FUTURE OF FECAL TRANSPLANTATIONS: DEVELOPING NEXT-GENERATION THERAPIES WITH SYNTHETIC MICROBIOMES

WILLEM M. DE VOS

Our intestinal tract is colonized since birth by complex communities of microbes that show specific spatiotemporal organizations, differ in composition between individuals, and contribute to health and disease (Zoetendal et al., 2006). Considerable progress has been made in recent years to describe the structure and function of the intestinal microbiota that belong to the major phyla of the *Firmicutes, Actinobacteria, Bacteroidetes, Proteobacteria* and *Verrucomicrobia* (Rajilić-Stojanović et al., 2007). However, the majority of the over 1000 species-like groups of the human intestine have not yet been cultured (Zoetendal et al., 2008). Facilitated by the advances in sequencing technologies, significant attention has been given to culture-independent and high-throughput approaches that generated important baseline information on the intestinal microbiota composition, the description of a reference metagenome of 3.3 Mb, and its structuring into

This chapter was originally published under the Creative Commons Attribution License. de Vos WM. Fame and Future of Faecal Transplantations—Developing Next-Generation Therapies with Synthetic Microbiomes. Microbial Biotechnology *6,4 (2013); pp. 316–325. doi:10.1111/1751-7915.12047.*

clusters, termed enterotypes (Qin and the MetaHit Consortium, 2010; Arumugam and the MetaHit Consortium, 2011; Huttenhower and the Human Microbiome Project Consortium, 2012).

The application of the high-throughput technologies confirmed earlier observations that adults have a unique and stable microbiota (Zoetendal et al., 1998). This has been recently extended by the highly accurate, reproducible and deep analysis of the microbiota of thousands of adults that revealed all of them to have a different composition (J. Salojarvi and W. M. de Vos, unpublished observations using the HITChip, a phylogenetic microarray) (Rajilić-Stojanović et al., 2009). As the systematic analysis of the human microbiota is only recently emerging at this large scale, there are not many studies that addressed the long-term dynamics of the intestinal microbiota. A deeply sampled longitudinal study of two subjects for over a year showed the microbial composition in faecal samples to be rather stable in contrast to that in other body parts, such as skin and oral cavity (Caporaso et al., 2011). Similarly, considerable stability of the of the faecal communities was observed in healthy subjects that were followed for over 10 years and maintained their characteristic personal microbiome (Rajilić-Stojanović et al., 2012). Other longitudinal studies indicated that the microbiota composition is affected by diet, antibiotic use and intestinal transit but possibly also by less well-studied lifestyle factors, such as time zone travelling (Flint et al., 2012; Jalanka-Tuovinen et al., 2011). An inherent determinant of this dynamics could be formed by bacteriophages that are detected in faecal samples and metagenomes (Qin and the MetaHit Consortium, 2010; Minot et al., 2011; Reyes et al., 2012). As typical oscillations have not been observed, it is not yet clear how bacteriophages control the intestinal microbiota but in analogy with other systems, it may be speculated that the intestinal microbiota is in the carrier state with virulent bacteriophages contributing to its stability (de Vos, 1989).

The abundance of accurate approaches to monitor the composition and coding capacity of the intestinal microbiota also greatly advanced the analysis of the differences in intestinal microbiota composition of healthy and diseased subjects. Presently, correlations between specific intestinal microbes or microbial patterns have been determined for several dozens of diseases, varying from severe intestinal inflammations to cancer and obesity, as reviewed recently (de Vos and de Vos, 2012). However, causal relations are scarce and hard to establish, as there are many microbiological, medical and ethical issues to deal with. An exception is the use of faecal transplantations of the intestinal microbiota that is receiving increasing popularity in human interventions since this practice not only provides causal relations but also shows considerable efficacy in treating various diseases, supporting the importance of the intestinal microbiota. Remarkably, there is a large discrepancy between the low-key technology used in this treatment and the sophisticated knowledge of the intestinal microbiome. Hence, this caveat is addressed here with specific attention for next-generation therapies at the interface of medical practice and microbial biotechnology.

14.1 DEVELOPMENT OF FAECAL TRANSPLANTATION: FROM HUMAN TO ANIMALS AND BACK

Long before the discovery of microbes, the concept of transplanting faecal material has been practiced, supporting the often-empirical nature of the medical practice. Records in Chinese medicine documenting the transfer of faecal suspensions date for over 1000 years, as reviewed recently (Zhang et al., 2012). This include the first description by Ge Hong, a medical doctor during the Djong-ji dynasty (fourth century), who could cure patients suffering from food poisoning or severe diarrhoea by making them consume faecal suspensions from healthy donors. Similarly, during the Ming dynasty (16th century) Li Shizen provided detailed descriptions of faecal therapies for the effective treatment of certain abdominal diseases, as noted recently (Zhang et al., 2012). Remarkably, the concept of transferring intestinal samples in veterinary practice was in use around the same time in Europe where the Italian anatomist Fabricius Aquapendente (17th century) described the practice of inoculating rumen fluid presumably into cows that had lost the capacity to ruminate (Borody et al., 2004). This procedure is still practiced today when cud, which is the material that is brought up into the mouth by a cow from its first stomach to be chewed again, is used to inoculate young calves via the oral cavity (Pounden and Hibbs, 1950). In a more extreme situation, this inoculation takes place in adult cows with rumen fluid directly obtained via a fistula from a well-producing cow. This process, also known as transfaunation since both microbes and protozoa are transferred, is an effective therapy in acidosis of cows fed high grain levels that is caused by overgrowth of mainly Streptococcus bovis (Klieve et al., 2003). In the second part of last century, the practice of faecal transplantation was extended to avian species in the so-called Nurmi concept where newly hatched chicks are inoculated by mixtures of chicken faeces (Nurmi and Rantala, 1973). This effectively increased the colonization resistance and protected the chicken from infections, notably from Salmonella spp. Presently, this practice is still in place and freeze-dried preparations of faecal microbiota from pathogen-free chicken are manufactured and commercialized (Stavric, 1992; Nakamura et al., 2002; Revolledo et al., 2009).

Some 50 years ago, human faecal transplantations were again documented in the medical practice by the work of Dr Ben Eiseman (Eiseman et al., 1958). Four enterocolitis patients were treated with faecal enemas (delivery via the colon) and a rapid recovery of all of them was observed. With the knowledge of the present time, these patients probably would have been described as suffering from *Clostridium difficile* infection (CDI). Following this report dozens of reports have appeared showing the success of faecal transplantation in recurrent or chronic CDI and these include over 500 cases as reviewed recently (Gough et al., 2011; Borody et al., 2012). The various avenues used for these and other transplantations, their success in the medical practice and the options for applying microbial biotechnology are discussed below.

14.2 FAECAL TRANSPLANTATION PRACTICE

Transplanting faecal microbiota in its simplest form is the consumption of intestinal microbiota. This is a natural process as it is likely to occur in early life when we are born virtually sterile and are colonized rapidly by specific microbial communities that are only found in the human intestine. So we all start our life with at least one, but most likely multiple, faecal transplantations. This is not an issue to be discussed at the first baby visit, dinner table or before breakfast, as was recently noted (Economist, 2012). Hence, there are a great variety of euphemistic descriptions of the material used, including yellow soup, liquid gold or just Julia Flora, termed after the co-worker who donated the original culture (Schoorel et al., 1980; P. Heidt, pers. comm.). Similarly, the practice itself enjoys over a dozen of terms, the most recent one being "repoopulate" (Petrof et al., 2013). The way the treatment is performed varies considerably and ranges from top to bottom, including simple oral consumption, small intestinal infusion via a nasogastric or naso-duodenal tube, transfer via esophago-gastroduodenoscopy or colonoscopy, or delivery by a colonic retention enema that even can be applied at home. In many cases, the microbial load of the intestinal tract is reduced by a bowel lavage or consumption of laxatives. The delivery mode also explains the wording used for the practice that may vary from faecal duodenal infusion to colonic bowel transplantation. Moreover, often terms as bacteriotherapy or faecal microbiota transplantation are used. However, these do not correctly describe the followed procedure, as the faecal material that is transferred contains more than only microbes as is described below (see also Fig. 1)

14.3 CHARACTERIZATION OF FAECAL MATERIAL FOR TRANSPLANTATION

In contrast to the great interest in the microbial make-up, there are only a few data on the abiotic composition of faecal material. In a thorough study of adults consuming a typical British diet (385 g of carbohydrates, 85 g of protein, 108 g of fat and 22 g of dietary fibre) it was found that on average the faecal discharge was close to 100 g per day and consisted for 75% of water. However, when the dry matter was considered, approximately half (55%) consisted of microorganisms, while the remaining part included fibres such as cellulose, as well as soluble material (24%) (Fig. 1A) (Stephen and Cummins, 1980). The latter also included polymers such as mucus, proteins and fat and expectedly all sorts of small soluble molecules including bile acids that constitute a sink for cholesterol degradation products such as catechol, indols and sulfides that generate the familiar odours, and the characteristic short-chain fatty acids that are produced at a level of up to 100 mM in average faecal samples (Flint et al., 2012). In most faecal transplantations no efforts are made to purify or enrich the microbial fractions and hence the therapeutic preparations contain all or most of these compounds.

Some pre-treatments are done with the faecal samples that are administrated via the upper intestinal tract and include diluting, blending and filtering the faecal microbiota (Vrieze et al., 2012). Protective measures are taken to reduce the exposure to oxygen-rich situations but cannot be prevented. Analysis of the microbiota before or after this treatment did not show major differences (E. G. Zoetendal and W. M. de Vos unpubl. obs.). However, the viability of the preparations has not been tested. This also has not been done for the frozen faecal samples that are used for colonic delivery in CDI patients and also included washing and subsequently storage in cryoprotectants, such as glycerol (Hamilton et al., 2012). This is all of relevance, since it has been reported that the majority of faecal microbes are dead or damaged (Fig. 1B). This is not a surprise as the end-of-the-pipeline fermentations that take place in the colon are not there to preserve viability. The solids contain many toxic components, the most relevant is bile that has powerful antimicrobial properties (Begley et al., 2005). The viability of faecal microbiota has been determined in Dutch subjects consuming a regular diet using advanced flow cytometry with functional fluorescent probes (Ben-Amor et al., 2002). It was observed that about half of the microbes (49%) are dead, one-third are alive (32%), and a smaller fraction is damaged and most likely only can be cultured with specific treatments as described previously (Fig. 1B) (Ben-Amor et al., 2002). This is not likely to happen during the present treatments of faecal transplantation that often require manipulations under less strict anaerobic and protecting conditions than the ones used to preserve viability (Ben-Amor et al., 2002).

In conclusion, it is fair to assume that the vast majority of the transplanted microbes are dead. It cannot be excluded that these, together with other abiotic compounds present in the faecal samples (Fig. 1A), play a role in the success of the faecal transplantations and this is an area that needs further study. Importantly, the viable microbiota that can be recovered from faecal samples shows a non-uniform distribution with less than expected *Bacteroidetes*, some major *Clostridium* groups and *Bifidobacterium* spp. (Ben-Amor et al., 2002). Remarkably, butyrate-producing bacteria such as *Eubacterium hallii* were found to be present in the viable frac-

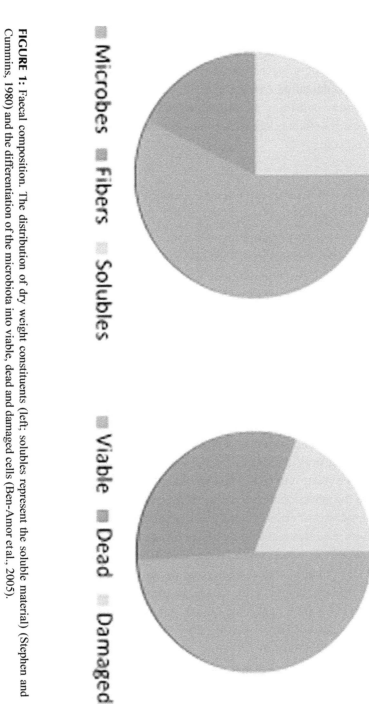

FIGURE 1: Faecal composition. The distribution of dry weight constituents (left; solubles represent the soluble material) (Stephen and Cummins, 1980) and the differentiation of the microbiota into viable, dead and damaged cells (Ben-Amor et al., 2005).

tion. This is of interest as we recently found that *E. hallii*, which converts lactate and acetate into butyrate, was enriched in the ileal microbiota of metabolic syndrome subjects that were cured from their insulin-resistance by faecal transplantation (Vrieze et al., 2012). These differential effects on viability may constitute an important lead for further work that aims to provide cause–effect relations between the transplanted microbiota and the health outcomes.

14.4 PRESENT SUCCESS OF FAECAL TRANSPLANTATION

Following the success of faecal transplantations in the treatment of colitis and recurrent CDI patients in the last 50 years, a variety of other diseases have been targeted. An important one was the first case report in 1989 by Dr Justin D Bennet of Ulcerative Colitis (UC), a severe colitis of the colon (Bennet and Brinkman, 1989). He suffered himself from UC and after describing many unsuccessful treatments he was finally cured by repeated colonic application of large amounts of faecal material from a healthy donor. Since then, many applications in CDI, UC and others have been pioneered, mostly as case studies (Borody and Khoruts, 2011). Presently, successful faecal transplantations have been described for approximately half a dozen of diseases, some of which with large numbers of treated patients (Table 1). There seems not to be a great difference in the success rate when using oral, duodenal and colonic delivery as is evident from the treatment of recurrent CDI. However, in all cases specific precautions are taken in the selection of the donor, varying in stringency from general health to large lists of criteria that have to be met, such as absence of HIV and other viruses, intestinal complaints, or unsafe sex or use of illicit drugs (Vrieze et al., 2013). Apart from CDI and UC, these include irritable bowel syndrome (IBS) that is also characterized by an aberrant microbial composition (Rajilić-Stojanović et al., 2011). In addition, indications exist for the successful treatment of chronic fatigue syndrome (Borody et al., 2012) and multiple sclerosis (Borody et al., 2003) but these are only based on single studies, as has been reviewed recently (Vrieze et al., 2013). An increasing number of studies is also addressing the microbiota composition and function in the donor and the recipient before and after transplantation

(Table 2). This is an important addition to the learning curve and should be standard practice for new interventions as it will contribute to further developing faecal transplantations. Some of the most relevant findings are summarized below.

TABLE 1: Diseases treated by faecal transplantation

Disease	N	Delivery	Reference
C. difficile infection	70	C	Mattila et al. (2012)
C. difficile infection	16	D	van Nood et al. (2013)
Insulin resistance (MetS)	9	D	Vrieze et al. (2012)
Ulcerative colitis	6	C	Borody et al. (2003)
Irritable bowel syndrome	30	C	Andrews et al. (1995)
Chronic fatigue syndrome	60	C	Borody et al. (2012)
Multiple sclerosis	4	C	Borody et al. (2003)
Metabolic acidosis	1	O	Schoorel et al. (1980)
Recolonization after AD	6	O	van der Waaij et al. (1977); Heidt et al. (1983)

The number (N) of described cases is indicated as are the different modes of delivery (D, duodenal; C, colonic or caecal; O, Oral). Studies with the largest number of patients reported are listed. AD, antibiotic decontamination.

14.5 INCREASE IN SOME BUTYRATE PRODUCERS

In the over 500 cases where faecal transplantations have been practiced on recurrent or chronic CDI patients, an average disease resolution of over 95% has been reported (Borody and Campbell, 2012). However, this number may suffer from a publication bias as many studies are small or represent successful case reports. Several recent studies have approached faecal transplantation in CDI in a systematic way with many patients. In a study at Helsinki University, a total of 70 recurrent CDI patients were treated by colonic delivery, resulting in 66 cured patients (94%) (Mattila et al., 2012). In another study in the Amsterdam Medical Centre, a three-arm study was set up where 42 recurrent CDI patients either received vancomycin, vancomycin and a bowel lavage, or all these treatments followed by duodenal infusion of healthy donor faeces (van Nood et al., 2013). After an interim evaluation, the study was stopped by the medical–ethical board since the transplanted patients showed much better recovery than those receiving either of the other treatments—in total 13 of the 16 CDI patients recovered immediately after the faecal transplantation and two of the remaining three after a second infusion. This contrasts markedly with the other treatments that cured either four or three out of 13 with vancomycin, or vancomycin and bowel lavage respectively. Interestingly, the several of these that did not respond to the vancomycin-based treatments received an off-protocol faecal transplantation and 15 of them recovered immediately. Altogether, this resulted in a successful treatment of 30 of the 33 CDI patients (91%). In the latter study the microbiota was studied extensively (van Nood et al., 2013; S. Fuentes and W. M. de Vos, unpubl. obs.). The recurrent CDI patients were all characterized by a consistent and reproducible very low intestinal microbiota diversity that was immediately corrected to donor levels after the faecal transplantation and this stable and healthy situation was followed up for 6 weeks in multiple patients. This analysis extended previous studies in a single (Khoruts et al., 2010) or limited number of subjects with fresh (Shahinas et al., 2012) or frozen faeces (Hamilton et al., 2012) (Table 2). A dramatic increase in *Bacteroidetes,* some *Firmicutes,* including butyrate-producing ones, as well as a reduction in pathobionts belonging to the *Proteobacteria* were observed (van Nood et al., 2013). This all indicated a drastic conversion from a low diversity but highly inflammatory microbiome into that with the characteristics of a healthy microbiota (De Vos and De Vos, 2012). While some individual differences can be observed, the global picture is the same in this and other reported analyses of the microbiota after CDI transplantations (Table 2). This indicates that the nature of the microbiota (fresh or frozen), the delivery mode (duodenal or colonic), or the location, origin or dietary habits of the donors, do not affect the final outcome. It also confirms the earlier observations that the intestinal ecosystem in the CDI patients is so disturbed that the donor microbes rapidly start occupying the available niches resulting in a normally functioning intestinal microbiota (Khoruts et al., 2010).

Most faecal transplantations are performed with stool samples from multiple healthy donors, often family members. Occasionally, transplantations are performed with one or a preferred donor. However, in a recent study a total of 32 recurrent CDI patients were treated with an enema of a mixture of intestinal microbes derived from a single healthy middle-aged donor in 1994, which had been re-cultivated under strict anaerobic conditions for over 10 years (Jorup-Rönström et al., 2012). A simple peptone-yeast medium was used for this subculturing that included egg yolk as a source of cholesterol. Usually such culturing steps decrease the microbial diversity rapidly but the effectiveness of this yet undefined mixture appeared to persist, as 22 out of the 32 patients (69%) could be cured. Remarkably, the mixture was administered as a 30 ml suspension by a 50 cm rectal catheter without prior laxation, although precautions were taken to keep the enema as long as possible. This contrasts with other administration procedures that use usually over 100 g of faecal material that is inserted after bowel lavage. This, the unusual way of delivery, and the nature of the inoculum may be among the factors explaining the lower than elsewhere reported curing rates.

The vast majority of the described studies do not have a control group, most likely as it is not ethical to withheld the best treatment from the patients as the experience with the CDI transplantation indicates (van Nood et al., 2013). Moreover, the selection of a control treatment is far from simple and specifically not in the case of transplantations. However, an elegant solution has been provided in a large study with patients suffering from metabolic syndrome (MetS; Vrieze et al., 2012). Here a control group of nine subjects did not receive faecal transplants from lean donors as the treatment group, but were transplanted with their own faecal samples in a so-called autologous transplantation. Only the treatment group receiving the lean donor transplants showed loss of MetS as evidenced by an increased insulin sensitivity (Table 1). As this study was performed in a blinded way, it represents the first double blind, placebo-controlled faecal transplantation study, adding both credibility and power to the observed results. Moreover, a deep microbiota analysis was also performed in this study and showed less pronounced differences than that after transplantation of the recurrent CDI patients. However, small but reproducible differences could be detected in the cured treatment group, which were absent in the autologous group that received their own microbiota (Vrieze et al., 2013). These included an increase of butyrate-producing bacteria (*Roseburia intestinalis* in the lower and *E. hallii* in the upper intestinal tract) that was accompanied by a reduced number of *Proteobacteria*, including

Escherichia coli (Table 2). This suggests a similar situation, though not so prominent, as observed after the treatment of recurrent CDI patients, viz. a reduction of potential inflammatory Gram-negative bacteria by those that are capable of producing butyrate after faecal transplantation with a healthy donor.

TABLE 2: Lessons learned from transplantations

Patient	Number	Major change	Reference
CDI	1	Increased diversity	Khoruts et al. (2010)
		Increase in *Bacteroidetes*	
CDI	6	Increased diversity—not all successful	Shahinas et al. (2012)
		Increase in *Bacteroidetes* 0026; *Firmicutes*	
		Decrease in *Proteobacteria*	
CDI	3	Increased diversity—like donor in 2/3	Hamilton et al. (2013)
		Increase in *Bacteroidetes* 0026; *Firmicutes*	
		Decrease in *Proteobacteria* 0026; *Actino-bacteria*	
CDI	9	Increased diversity—like donors in 9/9	van Nood et al. (2013)
		Increase in *Bacteroides,* some *Firmicutes*	
		Decrease in Proteobacteria	
MetS	8	Slightly increased diversity	Vrieze et al. (2012)

An unusual study that has received only little attention involves the so-called Julia Flora. This term relates to the faecal microbiota from a healthy donor that was maintained in germ-free mice and could be easily delivered via the oral route (Van der Waaij et al., 1977). This Julia Flora was used to rescue a 3-year-old boy with short bowel syndrome who suffered from metabolic acidosis due to overproduction of d-lactic acid (Schoorel et al., 1980). As described above, acidosis is often encountered in cattle due to *S. bovis* over-growth (Klieve et al., 2003). Here this could be caused by similar mechanism as a higher than normal level of Gram-positive bacteria was observed in the boy's stool. Daily oral administration of the Julia Flora for 5 consecutive days was sufficient to cure the boy and he did not observe any negative effects 9 months after discharge from the hospital (Schoorel et al., 1980).

TABLE 3: Undefined cultures and defined consortia used in microbiota transplantations

Host	Number	Composition	Reference
Germ-free children	2	Two *Bifidobacterium* strains, two spore formers (most likely contaminants of an antibiotic)	Dietrich and Fliedner (1973)
C-section babies	6	Human donor microbiota maintained in germ-free mice	Raibaud et al. (1975)
AD patients	5	Human donor microbiota maintained in germ-free mice	van der Waaij et al. (1977); Heidt et al. (1983)
CDI patients	32	Human donor microbiota subcultured for 10 years	Jorup-Rönström et al. (2012)
CDI mice	20	*S. warneri, E. hirae, L. reuteri, Anaerostipes* sp. nov., *Bacteroidetes* sp. nov., *Enterorhabdus* sp. nov.	Lawley et al. (2012)
CDI patients	6	*E. faecalis, C. innocuum, C. ramosum, B. ovatus, B. vulgatus, B. thetaiotamicron, E. coli* (2), *C. bifermentus, P. productus*	Tvede and Rask-Madsen (1989)
CDI patients	2	***A. intestinalis****, B. ovatus, Bif. adolescentis* (2), ***Bif. longum*** (2), *Bl. producta, C. cocleatum, Col. aerofaciens, D. longicatena* (2), *E. coli, Eub. desmolans,* ***Eub. eligens****, Eub. limosum,* ***Eub. rectale*** (4), *Eub. ventriosum,* ***F. prausnitzii****, Lach. pectinoshiza, L. paracasei, L. casei, Par. distasonis, Raoultella* sp., *R. faecalis, R. intestinalis,* ***Rum. torques*** (2), *Rum. obeum* (2), *S. mitis*	Petrof et al. (2013)

AD, antibiotic decontamination. E., Enterococcus*; C.,* Clostridium*; B.,* Bacteroides*; E.,* Escherichia*; P.,* Propionibacterium*; A.,* Anaerostipes*; Bif.,* Bifidobacterium*; Col.,* Colinsella*; Eub.,* Eubacterium*; F.* Faecalibacterium*; Lach.,* Lachnospira*; Par.,* Parabacteroides*; R.,* Roseburia*; Rum.,* Ruminococcus*; S.,* Streptococcus*; L.,* Lactobacillus*. The species indicated in bold are the main constituents of the mixtures.*

In conclusion, the successes of faecal transplantation range from various levels of colonic inflammation to metabolic diseases. This extends the association of these diseases with the intestinal microbiota by providing a clear causal relation with the faecal components (De Vos and De Vos, 2012). The microbiota analysis confirms and extends this, while providing global insight in how the various taxonomic and functional groups of the recipient are replaced by that of the donor. Moreover, detailed analysis of the microbial changes over time will allow the association of specific bacteria with health status, such as the butyrate-producing *E. hallii* in the case of MetS (Table 2). This type of approaches together with further metagenomic, functional and network analyses will provide a wealth of data that may deliver new leads for defining the minimal microbiome and constructing synthetic microbial communities. This is supported by successes with undefined microbial mixtures, maintained in germ-free mice or subculturing in the laboratory, in curing metabolic acidosis or treating recurrent CDI patients (Schoorel et al., 1980; Jorup-Rönström et al., 2012). Further steps towards the development of synthetic communities are discussed below.

14.6 TOWARDS SYNTHETIC COMMUNITIES

Long before the present interest in our intestinal microbiome and bringing faecal transplantations to the next level, various attempts have been reported on the development of synthetic communities. These are presented here together with the most recently developed mixtures (Table 3).

An unusual set of transplantations that followed intensive treatments with antibiotics to decontaminate the intestinal tract, have described as early as 1973. At this time, isolators were developed to protect patients with immunological deficiencies, such as those treated with acute leukaemia. Some of these studies are detailed here, since it seems that these have escaped the attention of those active in the field of faecal transplantations. In an extensive report describing a complete containment system, it was reported that immune-compromised children and adults could enter a germ-free state after long-term antibiotic treatments (Dietrich and Fliedner, 1973). After the appropriate therapy and cure of the disease in these patients, they had to be colonized in order to enter the ordinary environment. This was performed by a cascade of oral inoculations of single bacterial strains (*Bifidobacteria, Lactobacilli, E. coli* and *Enterococci*), followed by a rectal insertion of a faecal sample from a healthy subject. It was found that each bacterium colonized immediately without symptoms of disease in two of such germ-free children. A single case was described in more detail and included a gnotobiotic child that had been on oral treatment of 500 mg day^{-1} of gentamicin, which was probably contaminated by two aerobic spore-forming bacilli that subsequently colonized. This child received first 10^6 and subsequently 10^{10} cells of different strains of Bifidobacteria, delivered with a milk diet. These inoculated strains grew out to up to approximately 10^8–10^{10} bifidobacterial cells per gram faecal material, outcompeting the spore formers by a factor of 10–1000. After 4 months the faecal transplantation was performed and the child left the isolator (Dietrich and Fliedner, 1973).

Around the same time, faecal transplantations were used to conventionalize caesarean-section (C-section) delivered children, suspected of congenital combined immunodeficiency (Raibaud et al., 1975). Ten days after their delivery, these were fed a suspension of intestinal content of germ-free mice that had been colonized by a diluted human faecal sample. This is the first description of the oral transplantation by a humanized microbiota derived from mice. A similar approach was followed a few years later when a humanized and non-pathogenic microbiota was obtained from a healthy donor, named J.F. (Van der Waaij et al., 1977). The generated microbiota was termed first J.F. flora, and later named Julia Flora (see above and Table 2) and also Human Donor Flora (HDF). Remarkably, during the maintenance in mice, *E. coli* was lost as a major component of the microbiota and mainly consisted of anaerobic bacteria (Heidt et al., 1983). We now know from various studies that the human microbiota in germ-free animals may change rapidly in structure and function (El Aidy et al., 2012). This J.F. flora was used as an oral inoculum to repeatedly (up to five times) recolonize a series of five immunocompromised and hence isolator-kept patients that had been receiving antibiotics in a treatment known as antibiotic decontamination (AD). While virtually sterile before transplantation, the colonic counts rapidly increased after the colonization. However, it was noted that the colonization resistance of the transplanted patients was not as good as that of a normal healthy subject (Van der Waaij et al., 1977). Whether this is due to the composition of the Julia Flora or the impact of the compromised hosts cannot be said but it appeared that the quality of the J.F. flora (then termed Julia Flora) was sufficiently high to cure metabolic acidosis in a young boy (Schoorel et al., 1980; see above).

A series of early but very important experiments with synthetic communities were reported around the same time by Tvede and Rask-Madsen (1989). From 20 intestinal single strain isolates, they selected 10 strains, several of which showed inhibitory activity against *C. difficile* isolated from the six patients with chronic CDI. These patients were treated successfully with faecal samples from healthy relatives or the strain mixture that were all rectally installed. One patient was treated with a faecal enema only, one with a faecal enemas that were unsuccessful and subsequently with the strain mixture, and the remaining four only with the strain mixture that was rectally installed (Table 3). Faecal samples of the patients before these treatments did not contain detectable *Bacteroides* spp. in line with later observations described above (Table 2). This is the first description of a synthetic mixture of intestinal bacteria that shows success in curing five CDI patients from their recurrent CDI. It also showed that the developed mixture was superior to faecal transplantation in the one case tested. The mixture consisted of three Bacteroides spp. that all were inhibited by the patients' C. difficile. However, one *E. coli* strain as well as the *Clostridium bifermentans* and *Peptostreptococcus productus* strains showed antagonistic activity against *C. difficile*. In this context it is relevant to note that recently a two-component modified antimicrobial peptide, thuricin CD, was detected in an intestinal *Bacillus thuringiensis*, which showed strong inhibitory activity against *C. difficile* in vitro and in a distal colon model (Rea et al., 2010; 2011). A long-term follow-up of the patients treated with the synthetic mixture was described and included analysis of the faecal samples by anaerobic culturing (Tvede and Rask-Madsen, 1989). It was observed that mainly the *Bacteroides* spp. colonized and it was suggested that colonization by these bacteria may provide a natural defence against *C. difficile* although synergistics effect of the inhibiting species could not be excluded. These hallmark findings attracted quite some attention but also were criticized as is usually the case when novel approaches are reported. The suggestions that oral therapies with probiotic bacteria or yeasts could be a better approach were adequately rebutted (Seal et al., 1989; Tvede and Rask-Madsen, 1990). The question whether 10 strains are too many or too few has not yet been answered, even not with the molecular approaches available now.

As may be expected from the abundance of the recurrent of chronic CDI, most recent studies in developing synthetic communities have been focusing on this disease. An elegant mouse study was recently reported and included a CDI model that was tested with the best synthetic communities selected via some combinatorial approach. Best results were obtained with a mixture of six species that included some new mouse isolates (Lawley et al., 2012). How the mouse isolates will perform in the human intestinal tract is not known. Similarly, it remains to be seen what regulatory hurdles have to be overcome before human trials can be done with this mixture of mouse strains. However, this study clearly demonstrates the success of an avenue that can be followed to develop, maintain and test synthetic communities for treating CDI patients. This extends the other recent study where a human intestinal microbiota was maintained for over 10 years in the laboratory (Jorup-Rönström et al., 2012; see above). A recent human pilot study re-addressed the issue of using synthetic microbial communities for curing CDI (Petrof et al., 2013). A total of 33 strains of a variety of bacterial groups were isolated from the stool of a healthy donor, combined and cultured, and subsequently used to treat two patients with recurrent CDI who had failed to respond to antibiotic treatments (Table 3). Following delivery by colonoscopy, it was found that the patients were cured while analysis of the resulting intestinal microbiota indicated establishment of some of the new strains. This proof-of-principle study confirms the earlier results of Tvede and Rask-Madsen (1989).

14.7 FUTURE OF FAECAL TRANSPLANTATIONS

Experimental observations ranging from traditional Chinese medicine to those of modern evidence-based medicine, have provided clear evidence that faecal transplantation may work in a series of diseases, recurrent or chronic CDI being the best investigated one (Kelly, 2013; van Nood et al., 2013). The early results initiated in the late seventies and early eighties of large century, with undefined mixtures as well as defined consortia as pioneered by Tvede and Rask-Madsen (1989), indicate strongly that synthetic communities are a feasible approach. This is confirmed by the recent but still anecdotal studies in mice and man (Table 3). There is a clear need to further develop the concept of synthetic microbial communities to treat CDI and possibly other diseases.

The question on how many strains or species are needed, raised over a dozen years ago is still actual. This brings forward the concept of the minimal microbiome that can be defined as the smallest set of microbes and/or microbial functions needed to develop a stable community. Large data sets of microbial communities, their metagenomes and function are being collected worldwide. These can be mined for the networks of microbes and their functions that may provide leads on how such minimal microbiome would look like. Similarly, the analysis of the interactions between intestinal microbes and the host are being studied at a systems level (Martins dos Santos et al., 2010). This will allow the identification of microbial components that can be used to predict the minimal microbiomes. Moreover, there is a great variety of new avenues have been developed that can be followed to isolate and culture new microbial strains, varying from germ-mice to functionalized solid surfaces (Ingham et al., 2007; 2012; Goodman et al., 2011). Hence, there are plentiful possibilities to develop these minimal microbiomes into products based on synthetic microbial communities.

The advantages of synthetic microbial communities are clear as the composition of the synthetic mixtures can be controlled, tested extensively for the absence of undesired pathogens and viruses, and can be reproducibly manufactured. Moreover, the viability can be controlled and optimized. A large number of industrial fermentations rely on this principle and include the aseptic production of freeze-dried or frozen combinations of viable strains such as in the production of multiple strain starter cultures or probiotics (de Vos, 2011). Implementation of these synthetic microbial communities in next-generation therapies would greatly benefit the patients, further advance our understanding of the intestinal microbiome, and intensify the relation between medical practice and microbial biotechnology.

REFERENCES

1. Andrews, P., Borody, T.J., Shortis, N.P., and Thompson, S. (1995) Bacteriotherapy for chronic constipation – long term follow up. Gastroenterology 108: A563.
2. Arumugam, M., and the MetaHit Consortium (2011) Enterotypes of the human gut microbiome. Nature 473: 174–180.
3. Begley, M., Gahan, C.G., and Hill, C. (2005) The interaction between bacteria and bile. FEMS Microbiol Rev 29: 625–651.
4. Ben-Amor, K.A., Breeuwer, P., Verbaarschot, P., Rombouts, E.M., Akkermans, A.D.L., de Vos, W.M., and Abee, T. (2002) Multiparametric flow cytometry and cell sorting for the assessment of viable, injured, and dead bifidobacterium cells during bile salt stress. Appl Environ Microbiol 68: 5209–5216.
5. Ben-Amor, K.A., Heilig, H.G.H., Smidt, H., Vaughan, E.E., Abee, T., and de Vos, W.M. (2005) Genetic diversity of viable, injured, and dead fecal bacteria assessed by fluorescence-activated cell sorting and 16S rRNA gene analysis. Appl Environ Microbiol 71: 4679–4689.
6. Bennet, J.D., and Brinkman, M. (1989) Treatment of ulcerative colitis by implantation of normal colonic flora. Lancet 21: 164.
7. Borody, T.J., and Campbell, J. (2012) Fecal microbiota transplantation: techniques, applications, and issues. Gastroenterol Clin North Am 41: 781–803.
8. Borody, T.J., and Khoruts, A. (2011) Fecal microbiota trans-plantation and emerging applications. Nat Rev Gastroenterol Hepatol 9: 88–96.
9. Borody, T.J., Warren, E.F., Leis, S., and Ashman, O. (2003) Treatment of ulcerative colitis using fecal bacteriotherapy. J Clin Gastroeneterol 37: 42–47.
10. Borody, T.J., Warren, E.F., Leis, S.M., Surace, R., Ashman, O., and Siarakas, S. (2004) Bacteriotherapy using fecal flora: toying with human motions. J Clin Gastroenterol 38: 475–483.
11. Borody, T.J., Leis, S., Campbell, J., Torres, M., and Nowak, A. (2011) Fecal Microbiota Transplantation (FMT) in multiple sclerosis (MS). Am J Gastroenterol 106: S352.
12. Borody, T.J., Nowak, A., Torres, M., Campbell, J., Finlayyson, D., and Leis, S.M. (2012) Bacteriotherapy in Chronic Fatigue Syndrome (CFS): a retrospective review. Am J Gastroenterol 107: S591.
13. Caporaso, J.G., Lauber, C.L., Costello, E.K., Berg-Lyons, D., Gonzalez, A., et al. (2011) Moving pictures of the human microbiome. Genome Biol 12: R50.
14. Dietrich, M., and Fliedner, T.M. (1973) Gnotobiotic care of patients with immunologic deficiency diseases. Transplant Proc 5: 1271–1277.
15. Economist (2012) Microbes maketh man. The Economist, 18 August 2012.
16. Eiseman, B., Silen, W., Bascom, G.S., and Kauvar, A.J. (1958) Fecal enema as an adjunct in the enterocolitis. Surgery 44: 854–859.
17. El Aidy, S., Derrien, M., Merrifield, C.A., Levenez, F., Doré, J., Boekschoten, M.V., et al. (2012) Gut bacteria–host metabolic interplay during conventionalisation of the mouse germfree colon. ISME J. doi: 10.1038/ismej.2012.142
18. Flint, H.J., Scott, K.P., Louis, P., and Duncan, S.H. (2012) The role of the gut microbiota in nutrition and health. Nat Rev Gastroenterol Hepatol 9: 577–589.

19. Goodman, A.L., Kallstrom, G., Faith, J.J., Reyes, A., Moore, A., Dantas, G., and Gordon, J.I. (2011) Extensive personal human gut microbiota culture collections characterized and manipulated in gnotobiotic mice. Proc Natl Acad Sci USA 108: 6252–6257.

20. Gough, E., Shaikh, H., and Manges, A.R. (2011) Systematic review of intestinal microbiota transplantation (fecal bacteriotherapy) for recurrent Clostridium difficile infection. Clin Infect Dis 53: 994–1002.

21. Hamilton, M.J., Weingarden, A.R., Sadowsky, M.J., and Khoruts, A. (2012) Standardized frozen preparation for transplantation of fecal microbiota for recurrent Clostridium difficile infection. Am J Gastroenterol 107: 761–767.

22. Hamilton, M.J., Weingarden, A.R., Unno, T., Khoruts, A., and Sadowsky, M.J. (2013) High-throughput DNA sequence analysis reveals stable engraftment of gut microbiota following transplantation of previously frozen fecal bacteria. Gut Microbes 4: 125–135.

23. Heidt, P.J., van der Waaij, D., Vossen, J.M., and Hendriks, W.D.H. (1983) The use of a human donor flora for recontamination following antibiotic decontamination. Prog Food Nutr Sci 7: 53–63.

24. Huttenhower, C., and the Human Microbiome Project Consortium (2012) Structure, function and diversity of the healthy human microbiome. Nature 486: 207–214.

25. Ingham, C.J., Sprenkels, A., Bomer, J., Molenaar, D., van den Berg, A., van Hylckama Vlieg, J.E., and de Vos, W.M. (2007) The micro-Petri dish, a million-well growth chip for the culture and high-throughput screening of microorganisms. Proc Natl Acad Sci USA 104: 18217–18222.

26. Ingham, C.J., ter Maat, J., and de Vos, W.M. (2012) Where bio meets nano: the many uses for nanoporous aluminum oxide in biotechnology. Biotechnol Adv 30: 1089–1099.

27. Jalanka-Tuovinen, J., Salonen, A., Nikkilä, J., Immonen, O., Kekkonen, R., Lahti, L., et al. (2011) Intestinal microbiota in healthy adults: temporal analysis reveals individual and common core and relation to digestive symptoms. PLoS ONE 6: e23035.

28. Jorup-Rönström, C., Håkanson, A., Sandell, S., Edvinsson, O., Midtvedt, T., Persson, A.K., and Norin, E. (2012) Fecal transplant against relapsing Clostridium difficile-associated diarrhea in 32 patients. Scand J Gastroenterol 47: 548–552.

29. Kelly, C.P. (2013) Fecal microbiota transplantation – an old therapy comes of age. N Engl J Med 368: 474–475.

30. Khoruts, A., Dicksved, J., Jansson, J.K., and Sadowsky, M.J. (2010) Changes in the composition of the human fecal microbiome after bacteriotherapy for recurrent Clostridium difficile-associated diarrhea. J Clin Gastroenterol 44: 354–360.

31. Klieve, A.D., Hennessy, D., Ouwerkerk, D., Forster, R.J., Mackie, R.I., and Attwood, G.T. (2003) Establishing populations of Megasphaera elsdenii YE 34 and Butyrivibrio fibrisolvens YE 44 in the rumen of cattle fed high grain diets. J Appl Microbiol 95: 621–630.

32. Lawley, T.D., Clare, S., Walker, A.W., Stares, M.D., Connor, T.R., Raisen, C., et al. (2012) Targeted restoration of the intestinal microbiota with a simple, defined bac-

teriotherapy resolves relapsing Clostridium difficile disease in mice. PLoS Pathog 8: e1002995.

33. Martins dos Santos, V., Müller, M., and de Vos, W.M. (2010) Systems biology of the gut: the interplay of food, microbiota and host at the mucosal interface. Curr Opin Biotechnol 21: 539–550.

34. Mattila, E., Uusitalo-Seppälä, R., Wuorela, M., Lehtola, L., Nurmi, H., et al. (2012) Fecal transplantation, through colonoscopy, is effective therapy for recurrent Clostridium difficile infection. Gastroenterology 142: 490–496.

35. Minot, S., Sinha, R., Chen, J., Li, H., Keilbaugh, S.A., Wu, G.D., et al. (2011) The human gut virome: inter-individual variation and dynamic response to diet. Genome Res 21: 1616–1625.

36. Nakamura, A., Ota, Y., Mizukami, A., Ito, T., Ngwai, Y.B., and Adachi I, Y. (2002) Evaluation of aviguard, a commercial competitive exclusion product for efficacy and after-effect on the antibody response of chicks to Salmonella. Poult Sci 81: 1653–1660.

37. Nurmi, E., and Rantala, E. (1973) New aspects of Salmonella infection in broiler production. Nature 241: 210–211.

38. Petrof, E.O., Gloor, G.B., Vanner, S.J., Weese, S., Carter, D., Daigneault, M.C., et al. (2013) Stool substitute transplant therapy for the eradication of Clostridium difficile infection: 'RePOOPulating' the gut. Microbiome 1: 3.

39. Pounden, W.D., and Hibbs, J.W. (1950) The development of calves raised without protozoa and certain other characteristic rumen microorganisms. J Dairy Sci 33: 639–644.

40. Qin, J., and the MetaHit Consortium (2010) A human gut microbial gene catalogue established by metagenomic sequencing. Nature 464: 59–65.

41. Raibaud, P., Ducluzeau, R., Ghnassia, J.C., Griscelli, C., Lauvergeon, B., and Moqout, G. (1975) Etablissment d'une flore microbienne dans le tube digest d'enfants axeniques eleves en isolateur. Rev Fr Gynecol 70: 579.

42. Rajilić-Stojanović, M., Smidt, H., and de Vos, W.M. (2007) Diversity of the human gastrointestinal tract microbiota revisited. Environ Microbiol 9: 2125–2136.

43. Rajilić-Stojanović, M., Heilig, H.G., Molenaar, D., Kajander, K., Surakka, A., Smidt, H., and de Vos, W.M. (2009) Development and application of the human intestinal tract chip, a phylogenetic microarray: analysis of universally conserved phylotypes in the abundant microbiota of young and elderly adults. Environ Microbiol 11: 1736–1751.

44. Rajilić-Stojanović, M., Biagi, E., Heilig, H.J.G.H., Kajander, K., Kekkonen, R.A., Tims, S., and de Vos, W.M. (2011) Global and deep molecular analysis of microbiota signatures in fecal samples from patients with irritable bowel syndrome. Gastroenterology 141: 1792–1801.

45. Rajilić-Stojanović, M., Heilig, H.G.H.J., Tims, S., Zoetendal, E.G., and de Vos, W.M. (2012) Long-term monitoring of the human intestinal microbiota composition. Environ Microbiol. doi: 10.1111/1462-2920.12023

46. Rea, M.C., Sit, C.S., Clayton, E., O'Connor, P.M., Whittal, R.M., Zheng, J., et al. (2010) Thuricin CD, a posttranslationally modified bacteriocin with a narrow spec-

trum of activity against Clostridium difficile. Proc Natl Acad Sci USA 107: 9352–9357.

47. Rea, M.C., Dobson, A., O'Sullivan, O., Crispie, F., Fouhy, F., Cotter, P.D., et al. (2011) Effect of broad- and narrow-spectrum antimicrobials on Clostridium difficile and microbial diversity in a model of the distal colon. Proc Natl Acad Sci USA 108 (Suppl. 1): 4639–4644.

48. Revolledo, L., Ferreira, C.S., and Ferreira, A.J. (2009) Prevention of Salmonella Typhimurium colonization and organ invasion by combination treatment in broiler chicks. Poult Sci 88: 734–743.

49. Reyes, A., Semenkovich, N.P., Whiteson, K., Rohwer, F., and Gordon, J.I. (2012) Going viral: next-generation sequencing applied to phage populations in the human gut. Nat Rev Microbiol 10: 607–617.

50. Schoorel, E.P., Giesberts, M.A., and Blom, W. (1980) D-lactic acidosis in a boy with short bowel syndrome. Arch Dis Child 55: 810–812.

51. Seal, D.V., Borriello, S.P., and Piper, M. (1989) Bacteriootherapy for Clostridium difficile diarrhea. Lancet 1: 558.

52. Shahinas, D., Silverman, M., Sittler, T., Chiu, C., Kim, P., Allen-Vercoe, E., et al. (2012) Toward an understanding of changes in diversity associated with fecal microbiome transplantation based on 16S rRNA gene deep sequencing. MBio 3: e00338-12.

53. Stavric, S. (1992) Defined cultures and prospects. Int J Food Microbiol 15: 245–263.

54. Stephen, A.M., and Cummins, J. (1980) The microbial contribution to human fecal mass. J Med Micobiol 13: 45–46.

55. Tvede, M., and Rask-Madsen, J. (1989) Bacteriotherapy for chronic relapsing Clostridium difficile diarrhoea in six patients. Lancet 1: 1156–1160.

56. Tvede, M., and Rask-Madsen, J. (1990) Bacteriotherapy for Clostridium difficile diarrhoea. Lancet 1: 110.

57. Van Nood, E., Vrieze, A., Nieuwdorp, M., Fuentes, S., Zoetendal, E.G., de Vos, W.M., et al. (2013) Duodenal infusion of donor feces for recurrent Clostridium difficile. New Engl J Med 368: 407–415.

58. de Vos, W.M. (1989) On the carrier state of bacteriophages in starter lactococci: an elementary explanation involving a bacteriophage-resistance plasmid. Neth. Milk Dairy J 43: 221–229.

59. de Vos, W.M. (2011) Systems solutions by lactic acid bacteria: from paradigms to practice. Micr Cell Fact 10: S2–S20.

60. de Vos, W.M., and de Vos, E.A.J. (2012) Role of the intestinal microbiome in health and disease: from correlation to causation. Nutr Rev 70: S45–S56.

61. Vrieze, A., Van Nood, E., Holleman, F., Salojärvi, J., Kootte, R.S., Bartelsman, J.F., et al. (2012) Transfer of intestinal microbiota from lean donors increases insulin sensitivity in individuals with metabolic syndrome. Gastroenterology 143: 913–916. e7.

62. Vrieze, A., de Groot, P.F., Kootte, R.S., van Nood, E., and Nieuwdorp, M. (2013) Fecal transplant: a safe and sustainable clinical therapy for restoring intestinal microbial balance in human disease? Best Prac Res Clin Gastroenterol 143: 913–916.

63. van der Waaij, D., Vossen, J.M., Korthals Altes, C., and Hartgrink, C. (1977) Reconventionalization following antibiotic decontamination in man and animals. Am J Clin Nutr 30: 1877–1895.

64. Zhang, F., Luo, W., Shi, Y., Fan, Z., and Ji, G. (2012) Should we standardize the 1,700-year-old fecal microbiota transplantation? Am J Gastroenterol 107: 1755.
65. Zoetendal, E.G., Akkermans, A.D.L., and de Vos, W.M. (1998) Temperature gradient gel electrophoresis analysis of 16S rRNA from human fecal samples reveals stable and host-specific communities of active bacteria. Appl Environ Microbiol 64: 3854–3859.
66. Zoetendal, E.G., Vaughan, E.E., and de Vos, W.M. (2006) A microbial world within us. Mol Microbiol 59: 1639–1650.
67. Zoetendal, E.G., Rajilić-Stojanović, M., and de Vos, W.M. (2008) High throughput diversity and functionality analysis of the gastrointestinal tract microbiota. Gut 57: 1605–1615.

AUTHOR NOTES

CHAPTER 1

Conflicts of Interest
The authors declare no conflicts of interest.

Funding Sources
This study was funded by the National Institutes of Health.

CHAPTER 3

Funding
This work was supported by National Institutes of Health grants P30-ES002109 (pilot project award to SEE and EJA), RO1CA108854 (to SEE), and P01 AI045757, U19 AI046130, U19 AI070352, and P01 AI039671 (to DAH). DAH is also supported by a Jacob Javits Merit award (NS2427) from the National Institute of Neurological Disorders and Stroke and the Penates Foundation and Nancy Taylor Foundation for Chronic Diseases, Inc. The funders had no role in study design, data collection and analysis, decision to publish, or preparation of the manuscript.

Competing Interests
The authors have declared that no competing interests exist.

Acknowledgments
We thank James Versalovic for the gift of ATCC 6475 Lactobacillus reuteri, and special thanks to James G. Fox for encouragement and support.

Author Contributions
Conceived and designed the experiments: TP MK EJA DAH SEE. Performed the experiments: TL TP BJV YMI JRL MK SB SMK AC SEE AP. Analyzed the data: TP CS MK DAH EJA SEE. Contributed reagents/

materials/analysis tools: TP CS EJA. Wrote the paper: TP MK CS DAH EJA SEE.

CHAPTER 4

Funding

This study was supported by a Project Grant (#633240) from the National Health and Medical Research Council of Australia. The funders had no role in study design, data collection and analysis, decision to publish, or preparation of the manuscript.

Competing Interests

I have read the journal's policy and have the following conflicts: JO and LHS are or have been employed by AstraZeneca. This does not alter our adherence to all the PLoS ONE policies on sharing data and materials. The other authors have declared that no competing interests exist.

Acknowledgments

The authors appreciate the assistance of Dr Jane Radford, Shanna Trollip and Jenny Hoffmann with immunohistochemical staining; Dr Helen Ball, Dr Dale Hancock and Luxi Meng with RT-qPCR; and Charlotte Lindgren, Anne-Cristine Carlsson, Lena Amrot Fors and Maria Ericsson with serum assays.

Author Contributions

Conceived and designed the experiments: YYL CRC AJM AD DIC NHH IDC AJH LHS JO. Performed the experiments: YYL CWYH JO LHS. Analyzed the data: YYL CWYH AJH. Contributed reagents/materials/analysis tools: YYL CRC AD JO DIC NHH AJH LHS. Wrote the paper: YYL CWYH CRC AJM AD JO DIC NHH IDC LHS.

CHAPTER 5

Funding

This study was supported by public grants AGL2011-25169 and Consolider Fun-C-Food CSD2007-00063 from the Spanish Ministry of Science and Innovation (MICINN, Spain) The scholarships of AS from CONA-

CYT (México), PGC from CONICET (Argentina) and AM from MICINN are fully acknowledged. The funders had no role in study design, data collection and analysis, decision to publish, or preparation of the manuscript.

Competing Interests

The authors have declared that no competing interests exist.

Author Contributions

Conceived and designed the experiments: YS. Performed the experiments: PGC AS AM. Analyzed the data: PGC AS AM. Wrote the paper: PGC AS YS.

CHAPTER 6

Funding

This work was jointly supported by Korea Yakult Co., Ltd., and the SRC Program (2012-0000644) of the National Research Foundation (NRF) of Korea funded by the Ministry of Education, Science and Technology. The funders had no role in study design, data collection and analysis, decision to publish, or preparation of the manuscript.

Competing Interests

The authors have read the journal,s policy and have the following conflicts. DYP is currently affiliated with Seoul National University. YTA, SHP and CSH are current employees of Korea YaKult Co., Ltd. This work was jointly supported by Korea Yakult Co., Ltd and the SRC Program (2009-0063409) of the NationalResearch Foundation (NRF) of Korea funded by the Ministry of Education, Science and Technology. There are no patents and products in development or marketed product to declare. This does not alter the authors, adherence to all the PLOS ONE policies on sharing data and materials.

Author Contributions

Conceived and designed the experiments: DYP RY MKS MSC. Performed the experiments: DYP SRY. Analyzed the data: DYP RAM. Contributed reagents/materials/analysis tools: YTA SHP CSH MSC. Wrote the paper: DYP RAM MSC.

CHAPTER 7

Acknowledgments
This work was supported by the European Research Council (ERC Starting Grant), the Deutsche Forschungsgemeinschaft and the Robert Bosch Foundation.

CHAPTER 8

Acknowledgments
This work was supported by the agency for the Innovation by Science and Technology in Flanders (IWT Vlaanderen), the Research Council of Ghent University, the Research Foundation Flanders (FWO Vlaanderen), and the Interuniversity Attraction Poles Program of the Belgian Science Policy. Authors wish to thank Amin Bredan for editing the manuscript and Kelly Lemeire and Joke Vanden Berghe for technical assistance.

Supporting Information is available at EMBO Molecular Medicine Online.

The authors declare that there is no conflict of interest.

Funding
Innovation by Science and Technology in Flanders

CHAPTER 9

Author Contributions
BV performed the study design, analysis and interpretation of the data and the writing of the paper. FC and MC performed the DGGE and real time experiments and statistical analysis of the data. MN carried out GC-MS/SPME experiments. PC, MEG and PB coordinated the study. All authors read and approved the manuscript.

CHAPTER 10

Acknowledgments

Thanks to Eibhlís O'Connor, Simone Rampelli, Hugh Harris and Denise Lynch. This review was supported by the (Government of Ireland) Department of Agriculture Fisheries and Food/Health Research Board FHRI award to the ELDERMET project and a Science Foundation Ireland CSET award to the Alimentary Pharmabiotic Centre.

Conflict of Interest

The authors declare no conflict of interest.

CHAPTER 11

Acknowledgments

Pieter Van den Abbeele is a Postdoctoral Fellow from FWO-Vlaanderen (Research Foundation of Flanders, Belgium). Willy Verstraete is coordinator of the Ghent University Multidisciplinary Research Partnership 'Biotechnology for a sustainable economy' (BOF/MRP/005). Finally, Stephen Andersen is thanked for critical revision of this manuscript.

Conflict of Interest

None declared.

CHAPTER 12

Acknowledgments

I thank my colleagues Wolfram Brück for critical reading of the manuscript and Olga Sakwinska for stimulating discussions.

Conflict of Interest

None declared.

CHAPTER 13

Competing Interests

The authors declare that they have no personal or financial competing interests.

Author Contributions

RS reviewed literature, collected data, outlined and drafted the manuscript, and participated in writing the final version. MRR collected data and abstracts, and participated in writing the final version. RKA conceived the article, reviewed literature, and wrote the article in its final format. All authors read and approved the final manuscript.

Acknowledgments

We thank Ms. Radwa Raed Sharaf for critical reading of the draft and help with proofreading the final version.

CHAPTER 14

Acknowledgments

Work by the author was supported by Grant ERC 250172 – Microbes Inside from the European Research Council, Grants 137389 and 141140 from the Academy of Finland and the unrestricted Spinoza Award from the Netherlands Organization for Scientific Research.

Conflict of Interest

None declared.

INDEX